# VALUE
# BY DESIGN

# VALUE BY DESIGN

## Developing Clinical Microsystems to Achieve Organizational Excellence

EUGENE C. NELSON
PAUL B. BATALDEN
MARJORIE M. GODFREY
JOEL S. LAZAR

EDITORS

Foreword by Elliott S. Fisher

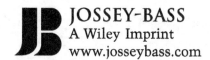

JOSSEY-BASS
A Wiley Imprint
www.josseybass.com

Published by Jossey-Bass
A Wiley Imprint
989 Market Street, San Francisco, CA 94103-1741—www.josseybass.com

Jossey-Bass books and products are available through most bookstores. To contact Jossey-Bass directly call our Customer Care Department within the U.S. at 800-956-7739, outside the U.S. at 317-572-3986, or fax 317-572-4002.

Jossey-Bass also publishes its books in a variety of electronic formats. Some content that appears in print may not be available in electronic books.

**Library of Congress Cataloging-in-Publication Data**

Value by design : developing clinical microsystems to achieve organizational excellence /
Eugene C. Nelson . . . [et al.].
    p. cm.
   Includes bibliographical references and index.
  ISBN 978-0-470-38534-0 (pbk.); 978-0-470-90133-5 (ebk.); 978-0-470-90134-2 (ebk.); 978-0-470-90135-9 (ebk)
 1. Medical care.  2. Medical protocols.  3. Organizational effectiveness.  I. Nelson, Eugene C.
  RA443.V35 2011
  362.1–dc22

                          2010047562

Printed in the United States of America
FIRST EDITION
*PB Printing*     V10009598_041919

# CONTENTS

## Figures

## Tables

*Elliott S. Fisher*

The problems confronting the U.S. health care system are widely recognized: a rising burden of chronic disease;[1] limited capacity to deliver safe, reliable, and effective care (even when the evidence for specific treatments is strong);[2,3] fragmented and poorly coordinated patient care that is frequently impersonal, insensitive to socioeconomic, cultural or ethnic contexts, and poorly aligned with patients' preferences;[4] and rising costs that threaten individual, corporate, and government budgets.[5,6]

As our recognition of the scope of the problems has grown, so has our understanding of the underlying causes of these problems. Although some of the responsibility for poor care rests with our still inadequate health insurance coverage, most policy experts recognize that expanding insurance coverage will do little to address the underlying causes of poor quality and rising costs that afflict even those with excellent insurance. The critical underlying causes include:

- Unclear Aims: failure to be clear about the aims of health care (Is health care a commodity and thus just about making money? Or about better care and better health?);
- Limited Information: inadequate information systems and inadequate information on the risks and benefits of common treatments and the performance of local health systems and providers;
- Disorganized Care: a fragmented and disorganized delivery system that is limited in its capacity to learn or to measurably improve care;
- Flawed Incentives: a payment system that reinforces fragmentation and fosters little or no accountability for the quality and costs of care.

The United States now has an unprecedented opportunity to address these problems. The National Priorities Partnership, a broad multistakeholder coalition including all the major federal health agencies, employers, provider organizations, and consumer groups, has achieved consensus on aims, making explicit the need to improve care, improve health, and reduce costs.[7] The American Reinvestment and Recovery Act (2009) made major policy and funding commitments to improving health information systems, performance measures, and comparative effectiveness research. And the recently passed Affordable Care Act (2010) includes numerous provisions intended to foster delivery system and payment reform. These include: the requirement that the Secretary of Health and Human Services develop a national quality strategy; the creation of a new Center for Medicare and Medicaid Innovation to identify, develop, and test new models of care and payment; authorization and funding to test a broad array of pilot programs (ranging from use of decision-aids to support informed patient choice to the creation of "Health Innovation Zones"); and the creation of a new payment model under Medicare (Accountable Care Organizations) under which physician groups and other providers can take responsibility for defined populations—and be rewarded financially for improving quality and lowering costs. These provisions will set in motion a marked change in the organizational structure, performance measures, and payment methods of the U.S. health care system.

The success of reform, however, will depend upon whether clarity of aims or changes in organization, policy, and payment methods can lead to actual improvements in the health and function of patients, in their experiences of the care, and in the affordability of health care. Policy alone can't change practice: health care professionals must change how they care for patients. The success of reform thus depends upon changes at the front lines of practice—where patients are touched by their clinicians— and in the organizations and systems that support those frontline clinicians.

This book is essential reading for everyone who wants to improve the care that they provide, whether a nurse in the emergency room frustrated by patient flows, a physician in a small office practice trying to improve care for diabetic patients, or a leader of a major health system considering how to become an Accountable Care Organization.

The authors build on decades of work applying scientific principles of improvement to health care and add a key insight drawn from the research of James Brian Quinn:[8] value in health care is produced in small functional units—clinical microsystems— where one or more health professionals work with patients (and their families) to produce a specific health outcome. Microsystems have clinical aims (effective treatment of primary care patients with diabetes), business aims (maintaining income, covering expenses), and shared technology and information. Most importantly, microsystems have inputs, processes, and outputs (including clinical outcomes) that allow their performance to be measured and improved.

Building on this conceptual foundation, the authors describe how health professionals can work with patients, families, and team members within a microsystem to systematically improve performance. The first half of the book focuses on general principles: the theory of microsystems (Chapter 1); engaging patients as partners (Chapter 2); improving reliability (Chapter 3); creating the needed information environment (Chapter 4); and developing plans for how patients traverse a microsystem (Chapter 5). The next four chapters describe specific examples across the care continuum. Finally, Chapter 10 provides a spectacular discussion of how health care leaders can build effective, high-performing delivery systems on the foundation of high functioning clinical microsystems.

Better value is what we badly need in health care. *Value by Design* can help us get there.

## References

1. Thorpe, K. Factors accounting for the rise in health care spending in the United States: The role of rising disease prevalence and treatment intensity. *Public Health*, 2006, *120*(11), 1002–1007.
2. Institute of Medicine, Committee on Quality Health Care in America. *To err is human: Building a safer health system.* Washington, DC: National Academy Press, 2000.

3. McGlynn et al. The quality of health care delivered to adults in the United States. *New England Journal of Medicine*, 2003, *348*(26), 2635–2645.

4. Institute of Medicine Committee on Quality Health Care in America. *Crossing the quality chasm: A new health system for the 21st century.* Washington, DC: National Academy Press, 2001.

5. Orszag, P., & Ellis, P. The challenge of rising health care costs—a view from the Congressional Budget Office. *New England Journal of Medicine*, 2007, *357*(18), 1793–1795.

6. Orszag, P., & Ellis, P. Addressing rising health care costs—a view from the Congressional Budget Office. *New England Journal of Medicine*, 2007, *357*(18), 1885–1887.

7. National Priorities Partnership. *National priorities and goals: Aligning our efforts to transform America's healthcare.* Washington, DC: National Quality Forum; 2008.

8. Quinn, J. *Intelligent enterprise: a knowledge and service based paradigm for industry.* New York: Free Press; 1992.

9. Schaeffer, L. The new architects of health care reform. *Health Affairs (Millwood)*, 2007, *26*(6), 1557–1559.

# IMPROVEMENT AT THE FRONT LINE OF CARE

- Discussion of health care reform has grown ubiquitous in our nation's and states' capitals, in our newspapers, on our television, on the Internet, at the office water cooler, and, of course, within our homes. There is good reason for such discussion and for the deep concerns that prompt it: whether we are employers, politicians, payers, patients, families, or health care professionals, we are also participants in a health care system that too often fails to deliver the quality, safety, and *value* of care we individually and collectively require. But although government policies, community resources, and payer pressures will increasingly shape a health care environment that is more conducive to quality improvement and value creation, the great share of this improvement work must occur at the front line of health care itself in what we call the clinical microsystems, the place where patients, families, and caregivers actually meet. Within these microsystems, clinical needs are most directly linked to clinical resources. Within these microsystems, quality, efficiency, timeliness, service excellence, and innovation can (and must) be built into frontline work processes themselves. The following principles promote quality within clinical microsystems: active attention to quality, safety, and value is no longer an option in health care, but an imperative.
- Quality must be delivered to the right person *by* the right person, at the right place, and at the right time every time.
- Safety must be conceived not merely as a priority in health care design, but as a precondition or prerequisite.
- Value, which can be described as the relationship of quality and safety and outcomes divided by costs over time, requires that we direct our attention to continual removal of unnecessary costs and to using work processes that are (in this era of necessarily limited economic resources) not only effective but also optimally efficient.

Moreover, we must not be content in modern health care to guarantee only clinical quality or only safety or only patient satisfaction or only cost reduction. Instead we must design and manage health systems that are capable of achieving all of these goals all of the time. We will need to do this, finally, in a manner that also increases pride and joy in work of physicians, nurses, and all health professionals who, for the most part, entered this line of work because they wanted to help people and to make a difference.

We have written this book, *Value by Design*, to offer specific guidance on building and improving clinical microsystems. We direct our attention especially to the front line of care because this is where clinical service is actually rendered, success is measured, health care teams learn from experience and modify their work appropriately, patients and families develop their loyalty to the health care system, and patients hopefully recover, maintain, or even generate health. The clinical microsystem is the locus of value creation in health care.

The timing of this book's publication is fortuitous. We believe a *cultural shift* is taking place in the health care quality and safety movement. Until recently, this field was led by a small and tightly linked community of authors and leaders who knew each other well. Only a limited number of high-quality publications were circulated, and new events and developments were communicated quickly and easily among thought leaders in the field and among their colleagues, associates, and acquaintances. This small community was richly connected by shared interests and by collaborative projects and friendship networks that created a generative and enabling context and a fidelity to shared principles, concepts, and methods. The focus of work was on patients, populations, and health professionals.

More recently, however, the culture of the quality movement has shifted. Robust demonstrations of health care improvement are now widely dispersed across multiple sites that are delivering care, conducting research, and educating the next generation of health professionals. Multiple journals and scores of Web sites and blogs now address questions of quality and safety. These provide myriad portals into numerous topics, themes, and programs, both nationally and internationally. Although the primary focus remains on patients, populations, and health professionals, active efforts now align health care delivery with public and community health promotion. Keeping up-to-date in this burgeoning field requires a vigilance that may not be attainable among even well-intended quality practitioners.

We believe the time is therefore right to consolidate, in a single volume, some of what we have learned about *what works* to improve value in health care. We wish to explore durable concepts and methods that have proven useful to clinical microsystems endeavoring to effect meaningful change in diverse real-world settings. We wish to share, as well, a practical framework that has successfully stimulated learning and improvement in microsystem participants and in students who aspire to enter the growing community of quality leaders and practitioners.

## The Dartmouth Institute's Clinical Microsystems Course

In a sense, we (Batalden and Nelson) have been working on this book for more than fifteen years. In 1994 Paul Batalden left the Hospital Corporation of America (HCA) to rejoin forces with Eugene Nelson, who had moved from HCA to Dartmouth in 1992. Dartmouth Medical School's Center for the Clinical Evaluative Sciences (now the Dartmouth Institute for Health Policy and Clinical Practice), under the leadership of Jack Wennberg and Gerry O'Connor, had begun a novel master's degree program to prepare health professionals in health policy, epidemiology, biostatistics, and quality improvement. Dartmouth recruited Batalden to lead the new quality improvement track in the master's degree program and to develop a core curriculum on the fundamentals of modern improvement in health care. The capstone course in this quality track that provides both the content and the structure of our present book was formally named "Continually Improving the Health and Value of Health Care for a Population of Patients: The Design and Improvement of Clinical Microsystems." Offered initially in 1995 and every spring since that time, the *Microsystems Course* (as it is less formally known) remains popular among graduate students, health care administrators, and experienced health care professionals.

The Microsystems Course continues to evolve as new insights are gained and as new applications of modern improvement in health care are tested (and found to work) in the real world. Marjorie Godfrey joined the faculty team in 1999 and has developed numerous useful tools (many of which are featured in this book's action guides) to guide clinical microsystems in the hands-on work of practice self-assessment and change. More recently, Tina Foster and Joel Lazar have joined the core group as well, and have helped further align course principles with the experiential realities of patients, families, and frontline caregivers. The course's theoretical and practical underpinnings come from many sources, with special debt to W. Edwards Deming, James Brian Quinn, Kerr White, Karl Weick, Edgar Schein, Donald Berwick, and Tom Nolan. As time has passed and knowledge has grown, the Dartmouth-based group has authored numerous journal articles on clinical microsystems and a book titled *Quality by Design: A Clinical Microsystems Approach.*

The present book, however, represents our first effort to organize our capstone course material into a single volume for both teaching and value improvement purposes. *Value by Design: Developing Clinical Microsystems to Achieve Organizational Excellence* may be used either as a textbook in health courses like our own, or as a practical guide in the real-world improvement of health care. Because (as we discuss in greater detail in Chapter One) the functions of better patient outcomes, better professional development, and better systems improvement are inextricably linked, we hope and expect our book will serve both purposes simultaneously.

## Organization of the Microsystems Course

The Microsystems Course is based on action-learning methods, skips back and forth from classroom to real-world clinical programs and clinical units, and is outrageously fun to teach. Our own course has thirty to forty students each spring and is made up of an almost equal mix of physicians, nurses, mid-career health professionals, and recently graduated undergraduates. Students organize themselves into teams of three or four; each team is then matched with a particular real-world clinical microsystem that becomes the locus of action-learning throughout the semester. The ten or so clinical microsystems are selected from the surrounding region and are picked to represent different parts of the health care continuum. Our most recent year's sites (2009) included a family practice, a general internal medicine clinic, a pediatric surgery program, an electroconvulsive therapy (ECT) psychiatric treatment center, an ear-nose-and-throat program, a home health agency, a blood bank, an inpatient oncology unit, an infectious disease group, and an ultrasound testing service.

During the course of a ten-week academic term, student teams spend (each week) one half-day in the classroom and one-half to one full day in the field studying their clinical microsystem. The team's study of each particular clinical microsystem is guided by ideas, concepts, and methods covered in class and is specifically based on the *clinical microsystem model.* Student teams complete weekly assignments that contribute to their two final academic products: (1) a twenty-plus page case report assessing the clinical microsystem and making recommendations for improvements, and (2) a poster summarizing the students' assessment of their microsystem and recommendations for improvement. For more detailed information on the Microsystems Course, see the course syllabus, action guides, and three final microsystem case reports written by student teams. These and other resources are available at our Web site, www.clinicalmicrosystem.org.

## The Clinical Microsystem Model

Although specific care processes will of course vary greatly from one clinical microsystem to the next, we have found that a core model is common to the flow of activity in virtually all microsystems. Patients and families enter a system of care with specific health needs; they participate in clinical processes of orientation, assessment, intervention, and reevaluation; and they emerge from that system hopefully with a large or small health benefit, through satisfactory meeting of their needs. Students' and caregivers' rich knowledge of this model permits detailed exploration of care processes and outcomes. This exploration in turn facilitates development and improvement of specific workflows that may improve health outcomes and patient experience, enhance system safety, and reduce associated costs. *This* is value by design! The general clinical microsystem model is shown in Figure P.1. The clinical microsystem model is sometimes referred to as the physiology model (see discussion in Chapters 1 and 2.) The model provides an overarching framework for the spring Microsystems Course, as it does for the present book. The model's strength is its adaptability to any microsystem in any part of the care continuum. We have seen it successfully applied to emergency departments, intensive care units, inpatient medical-surgical units, home health programs, physical rehabilitation programs, nursing home units, outpatient surgical settings, and medical specialty and primary care practices. The model works because, in virtually all caregiving settings, care itself is built from the same *types* of core processes.

- Studying Figure P.1 and the clinical microsystem model, we observe the following: the microsystem's work begins when an individual with a particular health need leaves his everyday environment and *enters* (most often physically but sometimes virtually) a clinical microsystem. This individual can be recognized as one of a population of patients cared for by the microsystem. Attributes of his baseline health status may be depicted with a *value compass* (see discussion in Chapter Four). The value compass

FIGURE P.1  Clinical Microsystem Model.

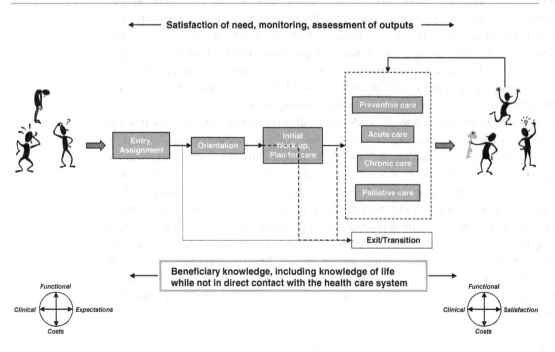

reveals the patient's clinical and functional condition, expectations for goodness of care, and historical costs associated with getting health care and with being ill or injured.

- The individual next receives some *orientation* to the particular microsystem as well as an *initial workup* and *plan of care*, which in turn lead to the delivery of a mix of services (*preventive, acute, chronic, palliative*), based on the patient's health status, preferences, and available resources.

- As time passes, the individual exits the particular clinical microsystem (which can be thought of as *exit/transition* from the microsystem's perspective) and either returns to the everyday social environment or enters another *adjacent* clinical microsystem for the next step in care.

- The goodness of the outcomes of time spent in (or in relationship with) the clinical microsystem can be registered on this individual's *value compass* (measured or unmeasured) at this new point in time. Once again, the individual can be recognized as one member of the population the microsystem has served.

- Two important processes contribute to the linear flow of this model and to the improvement of microsystem performance. The first process is *measurement and monitoring*, which permits assessment of key clinical and performance metrics, primary *outputs* and outcomes, and establishes the degree to which services result in *satisfaction of need* over time. The second process is *knowledge acquisition* about patients, families, and other *beneficiaries* of microsystem service. This *beneficiary knowledge* is specific to immediate needs and to realms of experience external to contact with the microsystem.

## Organization of This Book

We have organized *Value by Design* as we have organized the Microsystems Course itself. Each of the book's ten chapters corresponds to one week in our ten-week course and to detailed exploration of one component of the clinical microsystem model. When we teach the Microsystems Course, the model is shown at the start of every class meeting to orient learners to each new step in their own explorations and to each new step in the clinical care journey of patients, families, and the microsystem itself. At the start of each chapter we provide learning objectives for the unit to indicate what will be covered in the subsequent text. Each chapter concludes with a brief summary, list of key terms, study questions, and discussion topics that serve to broaden and deepen the chapter's (week's) explorations.

Chapters One through Five explore infrastructure elements of the clinical microsystem and show how these elements may be conceptualized, analyzed, designed, and improved to optimize service to patients and families. In Chapter One we define basic terms and explore key concepts that provide a foundation for microsystem design and improvement more generally. Chapter Two highlights the importance of patients as partners, not only in generating caregiving knowledge, but also in creating clinical value. Chapter Three introduces the paired themes of safety and reliability, which are essential to the efficacy and integrity of microsystem care. In Chapter Four we examine the microsystem functions of measuring and monitoring; we observe that these activities entail much more than simple registering of numeric outputs. Indeed, they support and guide our improvement of caregiving activities. Chapter Five directs our attention to the function of patient entry into clinical microsystems: important core processes here include orientation, data acquisition, reliable access, and effective care transitions.

FIGURE P.2   Infrastructual and Experiential Domains of the Clinical Microsystem.

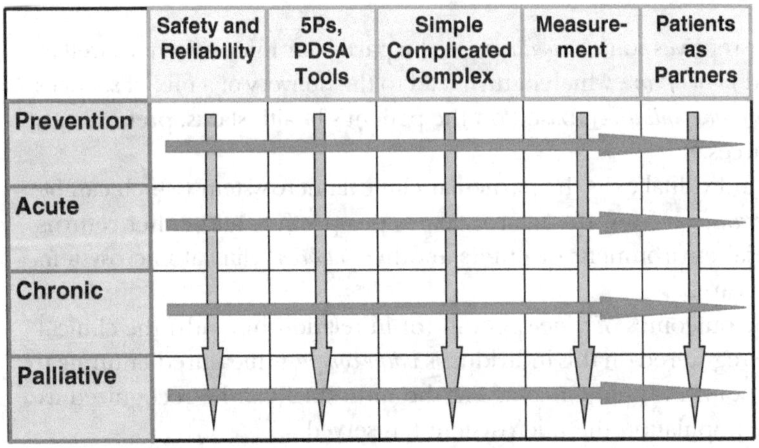

| | Safety and Reliability | 5Ps, PDSA Tools | Simple Complicated Complex | Measure-ment | Patients as Partners |
|---|---|---|---|---|---|
| Prevention | | | | | |
| Acute | | | | | |
| Chronic | | | | | |
| Palliative | | | | | |

In weeks six through nine of the Microsystems Course, and in the corresponding chapters of this book, we maintain the same clear focus on quality improvement and value creation while shifting our perspective. Where our attention previously focused on microsystem processes and infrastructure that support patient care, we now explore more deeply the clinical experiences of patients and families. In Chapters Six through Nine we consider the unique clinical needs, challenges, and opportunities of preventive, acute, chronic, and palliative care.

But we do not view the content of these latter, care-focused chapters as distinct from the infrastructure explorations that preceded them. Quite the contrary, the discussions in Chapters One through Five gain greater relevance as their implications and applications are examined in the context of unique forms of clinical and caregiving experience. As depicted in Figure P.2, we conceptualize the entire microsystem model as something of a grid, with infrastructural domains (such as safety and reliability and measurement and monitoring) represented as vertical columns and clinical experiential domains (preventive, acute, chronic, and palliative care needs) represented as horizontal rows. Throughout the text the reader is invited to give special attention to each of the resulting squares at the intersection of these domain axes. As suggested earlier in this Preface, it is at these points of connection between patients' clinical needs, resources, and care processes that microsystems generate quality, safety, outcomes, and costs that contribute to value.

In Chapter Ten we consider the subject of value creation from one further perspective. After reexamining fundamental principles and discrete practices from earlier chapters, we expand our focus beyond clinical microsystems to meso and macrosystems where quality, safety, and value are achieved on a larger scale. How do we connect the front line to the front office, so that the building blocks of improvement in local contexts support and strengthen one another and stimulate improvement, innovation, and reform across entire health systems?

## Additional Features and Online Resources

We wrote this book with the aim of creating a multifunctional text. *Value by Design* may serve as a course textbook, since its content and structure already reflect the Dartmouth

Institute's Clinical Microsystems Course. Alternatively (or in addition), it may function as a practical guide for real-world improvement in actual clinical microsystems and may function to enhance value in health care settings already familiar to readers. We have made liberal use of case studies, sidebars, and chapter-specific action guides (derived from the Internet-based *Clinical Microsystem Action Guide*) to add texture, tools, depth, and scope. (See www.clinicalmicrosystem.org and select Materials and select Workbooks and select Clinical Microsystem Action Guide).

In using the book as a textbook, educators and learners may take advantage of the model course syllabus for overall planning and management and may then proceed sequentially through each chapter's learning objectives, core material, review questions, and discussion questions. In addition, a set of PowerPoint slides accompanies each chapter and can be accessed at www.clinicalmicrosystem.org. This Web site, developed and administered by one of the editors (Godfrey), has many useful materials and resources, including the Dartmouth Institute Microsystems Course Syllabus, PowerPoint slides, and case studies completed by the Dartmouth Institute Microsystems Course graduate students. Readers should explore the Web site's Resources and Materials sections. Educators will also find a helpful Instructor Guide to offer support in teaching *Value by Design*.

In using the book as a value improvement guide, we recommend that readers familiarize themselves with the content of Chapters One through Five and then selectively explore Chapters Six through Ten and relevant action guides, based on their interests and improvement challenges. Again, this material can be richly enhanced through full use of www.clinicalmicrosystem.org, the free educational Web site where many colleagues from around the world find and contribute resources and knowledge.

One final function of our book and of the Clinical Microsystems Course that informs it is to serve as an invitation. We will have succeeded in our efforts only if we engage educators and students, clinicians, nurses, and other health professionals, leaders and administrators, and, of course, patients and families in the ongoing and essential work of health care improvement. Our health system is deeply in need of improvement, and those of us who work with an awareness of the clinical microsystems are uniquely positioned to perform this necessary work. We invite you to participate, knowing that only by working together can we achieve our common goal of value creation in health care.

We leave you with one further invitation. Our Microsystems Course, like the health care system itself, is an appropriate target for continuous improvement. Fifteen years of design and changes have brought our course to its current state, but there is certainly more work to be done. We expect our readers to experiment with the course material, to modify its content to appropriate educational and clinical contexts, and to engage new learners (new participants in the community of quality improvement and value creation) in ways we have not anticipated. We thus invite all readers of *Value by Design* to share with us their own discoveries. How have the model and materials helped your educational and clinical work? What would be more helpful? Please share your own experiences and insights with us at www.clinicalmicrosystem.org so we can learn together how best to achieve high-value health care, best outcomes for patients and families, and genuine pride in work for health professionals, support staff, and system leaders.

# ACKNOWLEDGMENTS

The principles and practices explored in this text have emerged through nearly two decades of rich conversation and interaction with literally hundreds of individuals and organizations. We are grateful for ongoing engagement with students and system leaders, with health professionals and administrators, and with frontline clinical micro-systems and high performing macrosystems around the world. We have been especially touched and influenced by patients and families who have shared their personal health care journeys, deeply informing our own reflections and insights into health care systems. We wish to acknowledge and thank some of the many collaborators who have contributed materially or intangibly to this collective work and who have asked for so little in return. We ask simultaneously for forgiveness from many others who have made important contributions and yet have been overlooked. It is fitting for teachers to first acknowledge the generative relationships with students, including those involved in the formal education programs of the Dartmouth Institute for Health Policy and Clinical Practice, as well as those we have taught in several parts of the world in short courses during the last fifteen years. These students' curiosity, questions, and critical reflections have made enormous contributions to our thinking about and understanding of clinical microsystems. We wish to thank both past and present leaders of our health system home, Dartmouth-Hitchcock (including Stephen Plume, James Varnum, Nancy Formella, Thomas Colacchio, and Jim Weinstein) for their enduring support and encouragement. These leaders have collectively built our institution into an action-learning lab to test and refine concepts and methods in many clinical programs, including the Spine Center (Bill Abdu, Jim Weinstein), Intensive Care Nursery (Bill Edwards, Caryn McCoy), Children's Hospital at Dartmouth (Paul Merguerian, Sam Casella), Plastic Surgery (Carolyn Kerrigan, Barbara Reisberg), Breast Cancer Program (Dale Collins Vidal), PainFree Program (George Blike, Joe Cravero), Regional Primary Care Center (Cathy Pipas, Diane Andrews, Linda Patchett), and others too numerous to mention.

We also thank leaders of our academic home, the Dartmouth Institute for Health Policy and Clinical Practice at Dartmouth Medical School (including Jack Wennberg, Elliott Fisher, and Gerry O'Connor) for providing a solid platform for our teaching and research on microsystems and high performing health systems.

Our work grows from not only a physical home base, but also an intellectual one. The conceptual underpinnings of this book build directly upon insights from well-known thought leaders in what we consider to be an evolving, worldwide quality and efficiency movement. W. Edwards Deming, James Brian Quinn, Karl Weick, Kerr White, Michael Porter, Paul Bate, Edgar Schein, Donald Berwick, Brent James, and Thomas Nolan are just a few authors and mentors we hold in high esteem whose work has influenced our own thinking, teaching, and writing. Brenda Zimmerman's and Paul Plsek's contributions in the field of complexity science have been essential to our work as well.

We received important assistance early in our study of high performing microsystems in the real world. First, the Institute of Medicine's committee responsible for the groundbreaking *Crossing the Quality Chasm* report also provided support for Julie Johnson and Molla Donaldson to conduct field research on select clinical microsystems. Later, the Robert Wood Johnson Foundation provided generous funding to launch the Clinical Microsystem Research Program. This project generated crucial information we used in our research on microsystems and in our teaching about microsystem performance improvement.

The principles, concepts, and methods upon which microsystem thinking is based have been adapted, advanced, and reinvented by a large number of very progressive health systems (and health system leaders) in the United States. We have learned a great deal from these institutions' efforts to achieve sustainable improvements in performance. Exemplary health systems (and their leaders) include Cincinnati Children's Hospital Medical Center (Jim Anderson, Uma Kotagal, Stephen Muething), Cooley Dickinson Hospital (Craig Melin, Carol Smith), U.S. Department of Defense (Diana Luan), Helen DeVos Children's Hospital at Spectrum Health (Joan Rikli, Amy Atwater), Geisinger Health System (Glenn Steele, Bruce Hamory, Al Bothe, Karen McKinley, Scott Berry), Akron Children's Hospital (John McBride, Elizabeth Bryson, Christine Singh), Maine Medical Center (Rich Peterson, Marjorie Wiggins, Peter Bates, Doug Salvador), North Shore Long Island Jewish Hospital (Fatima Jaffrey, Harry Steinberg), Visiting Nurse Service of New York (Joan Marren), Texas Health Resources (Michael Deegan, Linda Gerbig), and the Veterans Integrated Service Networks 1 (Michael Mayo-Smith, Jim Schlosser, Allan Shirks).

Microsystems are being strategically developed in many other countries as well. We have been grateful for very productive relationships with the Jönköping (Sweden) Academy for the Improvement of Health and Welfare (Johan Thor and Boel Andersson-Gäre) and with the Jönköping County Council Health System, which also leads and hosts the Annual International Clinical Microsystems Network Festival (Göran Henriks, Matts Bojestig, Sven-Olof Karlsson, Agneta Jansmyr, Gerd Ahlström). We have learned a great deal as well from performance improvement leaders in Armenia (Marine Grigoryan, Lusine Hovhannisyan, Karmela Poghosyan), France (Gilles Rault, Karim Laaribi), Northern Ireland (Pedro Delgado), Japan (Shiro Yuasa), Norway (Alf Andreason, Aleidis Skard Brandrud, Hans Asbjørn Holm, Christian von Plessen), Sweden (Michael Bergstrom, Staffan Lindblad, Helena Hvitfeldt), the United Kingdom (Helen Bevan, Laura Hibbs), and Singapore (Peter Chow, Phui Ching Lai).

Several national and regional health profession organizations and programs are making great strides by devising novel ways to deploy microsystem-based improvement across communities of practice. Some of these bright and shining stars are American Board of Internal Medicine (Eric Holmboe, Dan Duffy), Cystic Fibrosis Foundation (Bruce Marshall, Leslie Hazle, Robert Beale, Preston Campbell), Vermont Oxford Network (Jeffrey Horbar, Kathy Leahy), Vermont Program for Healthcare Quality (Cy Jordan), Jeffords Institute at Fletcher Allen Health Care (Randall Messier), Accreditation Council for Graduate Medical Education (David Leach, Ingrid Philibert), American Association of Colleges of Nursing (Joan Stanley), and Indian Health Services through the Institute for Healthcare Improvement (Cindy Hupke). In addition, some extremely talented teachers, advisors, and coaches (including AnnMarie Hess, Kathleen Iannacchino, Lisa Johnson, Neil Korsen, Karen McKinley, Richard Brandenburg, Linda

Patchett, and Victoria Patric) have intelligently and energetically transported microsystem thinking to diverse organizations.

We extend sincere thanks to Paul Gennaro who created our Web site's design and Timothy Good who maintains our Web site, www.clinicalmicrosystem.org, based at Dartmouth Medical School. We are grateful for the graphic work of Coua Early, who has been a frequent collaborator on microsystem diagrams and figures. In addition, our excellent administrative team, Carol Johansen and Joy McAvoy, continue to manage our home base with consummate skill and grace.

We owe a special debt to three terrific people who have opened vital communication channels to the world around us: Andy Pasternack (senior editor, Jossey-Bass, a Wiley imprint), who worked with us on our first microsystem book and who has facilitated our production of this new volume; Steve Berman (executive editor, *Joint Commission Journal on Quality and Patient Safety*), who put in the extra effort required to publish two multipart series on clinical microsystems; and the conscientious and indefatigable Linda Billings, who served as graphic designer and manuscript central for our writing team and who prepared the final version of this entire document in highest quality form. We could not have completed our book without her talent and energy.

Finally, we appreciate the great extent to which our own commitment of time and energy has been sustained by similar commitment from our families. We express our deepest gratitude to Sandy, Alexis, Lucas, and Zachary Nelson; to LaVonne, Maren, and Sonja Batalden; to Tim, Elizabeth, and Jenna Godfrey; and to Barbara, Daniel, and Ben Lazar. Their love and support continue to guide and to inspire us in our work.

**Paul B. Batalden,** MD, is professor of pediatrics and professor of community and family medicine at Dartmouth Medical School. He is the associate director of the Dartmouth-Hitchcock Leadership Preventive Medicine Residency, a combined residency program. He teaches about leadership of improving health care quality, safety, and value at the Dartmouth Institute for Health Policy and Clinical Practice, the Institute for Healthcare Improvement (IHI), and in the Jönköping Academy for the Improvement of Health and Welfare in Sweden. Batalden has helped found, create, or develop many other educational programs, including the IHI Health Professions Educational Collaborative. He is currently researching the multiple knowledge systems that inform the improvement of health and health care.

**Marjorie M. Godfrey,** MS, RN, is co-director of the Dartmouth Institute Microsystem Academy and instructor for the Dartmouth Institute for Health Policy and Clinical Practice at Dartmouth Medical School. Godfrey is a national and international leader of designing and implementing improvement strategies with a focus on adapting clinical microsystem theory. She coaches, consults, and supports health care organizations across the United States and throughout Europe and Asia. She is program advisor and faculty member for many major professional organizations, including the Institute for Healthcare Improvement, the National Cystic Fibrosis Foundation, and the Veterans Administration Health System. Godfrey also collaborates with the American Association of Colleges of Nursing (AACN), developing curriculum to advance nursing faculty knowledge and skills specific to quality, safety, and improvement. She currently is researching the effect of coaching interdisciplinary health care professionals in achieving strategic health care improvement.

**Joel S. Lazar,** MD, MPH, is assistant professor of community and family medicine at Dartmouth Medical School and section chief of Family Medicine at Dartmouth-Hitchcock Medical Center. He serves a diverse clinical population as medical director of Dartmouth-Hitchcock Family Medicine, where he also leads development of practice-based innovation in primary care as director of quality improvement and as a Leadership Steering Committee member of Dartmouth-Hitchcock's Regional Primary Care Center. He served previously as a family physician with the Indian Health Service, and was named chief of staff of Northern Navajo Medical Center in Shiprock, New Mexico, from 1995 to 1996.

**Eugene C. Nelson,** DSc, MPH, is director of Population Health and Measurement for the Dartmouth-Hitchcock Medical Center and professor of community and family medicine at Dartmouth Medical School. He teaches value improvement and population health at the Dartmouth Institute for Health Policy and Clinical Practice. He is a national leader in health care improvement and the development and application of measures of system performance, health outcomes, and population health. He is recipient of the Joint Commission on Accreditation of Healthcare Organizations' Ernest A. Codman award for his work on outcomes measurement in health care. Nelson helped launch the Institute for Healthcare Improvement and served as a founding board member from 1992 to 1998.

**Paul Barach,** MD, MPH, professor of anesthesia and emergency medicine, Centre for Patient Safety, Utrecht University Medical Centre, Utrecht, Netherlands

**Frances C. Brokaw,** MD, MS, assistant professor of medicine and assistant professor of anesthesiology, Dartmouth Medical School; Palliative Medicine Section, General Internal Medicine Section, Dartmouth-Hitchcock Medical Center

**Tina Foster,** MD, MPH, MS, associate professor obstetrics and gynecology and community and family medicine; program director, Dartmouth-Hitchcock Leadership Preventive Medicine Residency Program; associate director, Graduate Medical Education, Dartmouth-Hitchcock Medical Center, Lebanon, New Hampshire

**Julie K. Johnson,** PhD, MSPH, associate professor and deputy director, Centre for Clinical Governance Research, Faculty of Medicine, University of New South Wales, Sydney, NSW 2052 Australia

**Eliza Philippa Shulman,** DO, MPH, clinical instructor, Department of Population Medicine, Harvard Medical School; physician, Harvard Vanguard Medical Associates

**Gautham K. Suresh,** MBBS, MD, DM, MS, associate professor of pediatrics and associate professor of community and family medicine, Dartmouth Medical School; adjunct faculty, the Dartmouth Institute for Health Policy and Clinical Practice; program director, Neonatal-Perinatal Medicine Fellowship Program, Dartmouth-Hitchcock Medical Center

# VALUE
# BY DESIGN

# CHAPTER 1

# INTRODUCING CLINICAL MICROSYSTEMS

Paul B. Batalden

Eugene C. Nelson

Marjorie M. Godfrey

Joel S. Lazar

## LEARNING OBJECTIVES

- Introduce the theory and contexts for microsystems in health care.
- Discuss ways microsystems function in a health care system.
- Summarize important research on microsystems in health care.
- Describe concepts and mechanisms for improving quality and value in clinical practice.

This chapter begins with a *sharp* focus on *clinical microsystems* in health care and then expands its focus to explore contexts for microsystems within the overall health care system. After summarizing some important research on microsystems, the chapter concludes with a discussion on essential elements for making sustainable improvements in the quality and value of health care.

## MICROSYSTEMS IN HEALTH CARE

There was a time when health care was a simpler affair. The doctor-heroes of such classic television programs as *Marcus Welby, M.D.* or *The Cosby Show* modeled practice styles we could recognize in our own personal physicians. Omniscient clinicians delivered care in patients' homes or in a solo office. Unhurried nurses met every clinical need in hospital settings. Health care was embodied in an intimate one-to-one relationship that joined patient with doctor or nurse and that was supported by relatively little medical science. We developed and maintained a romantic view that health care was a professional activity for heroic soloists.[1,2]

**FIGURE 1.1 Many-to-One Diagram.**

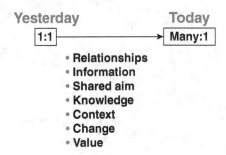

Today, however, that activity, those participants and relationships, and indeed the very goals of health care are much more complex. An interdisciplinary team of clinicians and staff backed up by ancillary services and information technology work in partnership with patient and family members to promote health and to care for health problems. Participants draw upon medical science and biomedical technology that expands at an astonishing (and sometimes overwhelming) rate. Diverse clinical settings with specialized resources, but also unique safety hazards, provide numerous settings in which care may be delivered. Regulators, payers, and *consumers* all have vested interests in quality performance data that are increasingly available for public review. Health care today has grown, for the most part, into a many-to-one relationship as shown in Figure 1.1, where "many" refers to health care professionals and "one" refers to the patient. Health care is now supported by rapidly proliferating biomedical knowledge, expensive technology, and administrative infrastructure.

And yet, if we look again at the sharp end of the health care system, at the place where each patient is in direct contact with health care professionals, we can discern the fundamental building block that remains the foundation of all health care systems. We call this building block the clinical microsystem. *Clinical* reflects the essential priorities of health and care giving. *Micro* reflects the *smallest replicable unit* of health care delivery. *System* reflects that this frontline unit has an aim and is composed of people, processes, technologies, and patterns of information that interact and dynamically transform one another. The clinical microsystem is the place where patients, families, and caregivers meet. It is the locus of value creation in health care.

The theoretical and empirical foundation of clinical microsystem ideas rests upon many decades of pioneering work by such authors as W. Edwards Deming,[3] Kerr White,[4] Avedis Donabedian,[5] and others. But one person in particular, James Brian Quinn, can be regarded as the *father* of clinical microsystem thinking. Professor Quinn, now Emeritus at Dartmouth's Tuck School of Business, conducted research in the early 1990s on the economy's rapidly growing service sector. Quinn wished to understand why some service organizations enjoyed such explosive financial growth and also received accolades from consumers. His research of the world's best of the best service organizations culminated in publication of the seminal work, *Intelligent Enterprise*.[6] Quinn discovered the world's most successful service organizations placed a major focus on what he called the *smallest replicable units* (SRUs) or *minimum replicable units* (MRUs) within their enterprise. These were the places where true value transfer took place, where suppliers interacted directly with the customers, and where service was delivered.

Quinn found the highest performing service organizations had several features in common, including the following:

- The front office was fixated on the ongoing perfection of frontline services within SRUs because value and loyalty are created at the customer-provider interface.
- Quality, efficiency, timeliness, service excellence, and innovation were designed into frontline work processes of SRUs.
- Information flows were engineered into frontline work of SRUs to create supportive, real-time information environments that facilitated swift and correct delivery of services.
- The smallest units of activity within frontline SRUs were measured and tracked over time for monitoring, managing, and improving performance.
- Increasingly rich information environments were created for the frontline SRUs. Data systems were designed to feed information forward and to feed information back so the right information was at the right place at the right time at the right level of aggregation.
- Based on systemic learning, ongoing improvements, and standardization of most effective practices, these *best in the world* service sector leaders could rapidly grow by replicating frontline SRUs through time and across space, reliably extending the delivery of high-value services.

The authors of this text, after reading Quinn's important book, recognized the relevance and prescience of the SRU concept for health care systems. These SRUs, these discrete points of services that unite supplier with customer, are precisely the points that also unite health professionals with patients. The clinical microsystem is the smallest replicable unit of health care. Services are provided or received, and quality, safety, and value are created in microsystems. In this chapter we explore general features of the clinical microsystem, which include its properties, contexts, and empirical supports. In subsequent chapters we examine specific microsystem components that support its optimal function as a self-contained clinical unit and as a building block for larger (macrosystem) health care organizations.

## The Functional Unit in Health Care

Although far-reaching in its practical implications, the notion of a *functional unit* in health care is neither a new nor a radical idea. As long ago as 1935, Dr. Lawrence J. Henderson, who more famously described the Henderson-Hasselbalch acid-base equation taught to chemists, physiologists, and medical students, observed in *The New England Journal of Medicine* that "doctors and patients are part of the same system."[7] More recently, Dr. Staffan Lindblad from the Karolinska Institute in Stockholm, Sweden, has asserted that the clinical microsystem is the *atomic unit* of all health care systems and it is composed of three particles ($P_2I$), a Provider, a Patient, and Information, all of which dynamically interact with one another over brief or extended periods of time.[8] These elements form a system when there is an aim that makes their interdependencies sensible. Figure 1.2 depicts the microsystem as the *atomic unit of health care delivery*.

We have already described the clinical microsystem as the place where patients, families, and caregivers meet. A more formal definition is now useful.

- A *health care clinical microsystem* is the small group of people (including health professionals and care-receiving patients and their families) who work together in a defined setting on a regular basis (or as needed) to create care for discrete subpopulations of patients. As a functioning unit it has clinical and business aims, linked processes,

**FIGURE 1.2   The Simplest Clinical Microsystem.**

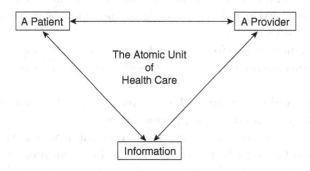

*Source:* Adapted from Staffan Lindblad, MD, September 2007.

a shared information and technology environment, and produces care and services that can be measured as performance outcomes. The clinical microsystem evolves over time and is often embedded in larger systems or organizations. As a living, complex, adaptive system, the microsystem has many functions, which include (1) to do the work associated with core aims, (2) to meet member needs, and (3) to maintain itself over time as a functioning clinical unit.[9]

Zimmerman and colleagues have observed that every complex, adaptive system has structure, processes, patterns, and outcomes.[10] To the extent that we recognize clinical microsystems as living and dynamic entities of this sort, we can also describe and assess them in terms of both structure (or anatomy) and function (or physiology). The anatomy of the clinical microsystem highlights its major structural elements, including its *Purpose, Patients, Professionals, Processes,* and *Patterns,* which together are known as the *5Ps.* To design, implement, and improve frontline clinical services, members of clinical microsystems must first gain self-understanding of their own system's 5Ps. Figure 1.3 depicts structural (anatomical) relationships.

Similarly, caregivers' rich knowledge of the physiology of the microsystem permits detailed exploration of care processes' functional *inputs* and *outputs.* Patients and families enter a system of care with specific health needs; they participate in clinical processes of orientation, assessment, intervention, and reevaluation; and they hopefully emerge from that system satisfied that their health needs have been met. The physiology model is introduced in the Preface as the Clinical Microsystem Model, Figure P.1.

The elements of the anatomy and physiology models offer powerful insights into systematic assessment of clinical microsystem performance, and they enable formulation of sound recommendations for improvement and innovation. Chapter One Action Guide provides the diagram of the anatomy model with detailed description and useful tools for self-assessment of the 5Ps, and the reader is encouraged to use this resource on a frequent basis when engaged in microsystem design and improvement. In addition, the Web site www.clinicalmicrosystem.org offers downloadable tools based on the 5Ps anatomy model, with options to assess and to understand performance of different types of clinical microsystems, including primary care practices, medical homes, specialty medical practices, inpatient care units, neonatal intensive care units, long term care, and supporting microsystems (such as pharmacy, laboratory, and environmental services). The *Assess, Diagnose and Treat* workbook profiles are introduced in Chapter One Action Guide. Two examples of unique clinical microsystems such as primary care

FIGURE 1.3    Anatomy of a Microsystem.

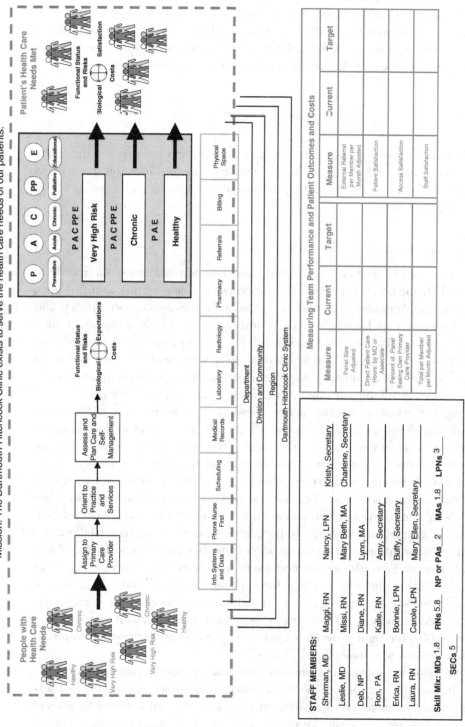

**Building a Clinical Microsystem for Primary Care Patients**

Mission: The Dartmouth-Hitchcock Clinic exists to serve the health care needs of our patients.

and specialty care are outlined; the details and variables of assessing the anatomy of a clinical microsystem then lead to a diagnosis and treatment plan. The Action Guide offers some of the discoveries made through exploring the 5Ps and provides a few examples of what 5Ps might be uncovered by assessing supporting microsystems.

The *physiology model* and *anatomy model* both offer ways to make a systematic assessment of clinical microsystem performance and to formulate informed recommendations for improvement and innovation. More detailed information about using the anatomy and physiology models can be learned at www.clinicalmicrosystem.org.

## A BROADER VIEW OF SYSTEMS AND MICROSYSTEMS

We have introduced the concept of clinical microsystems, and have viewed them first from an up close perspective that highlights local structure and function. Let us now consider systems thinking more broadly and conceptualize clinical microsystems within a larger health care context.

### Systems Dynamics and Embedded Systems

In the second half of the twentieth century, researchers in various disciplines have explored and characterized properties of numerous complex systems, and this work has influenced thinkers and practitioners in academia, commerce, social policy, and medicine. Biologist Karl Ludwig von Bertalanffy was an early investigator of such systems, and developed perspectives and principles of general systems dynamics[11] that have been subsequently adopted and adapted in such diverse fields as sociology,[12] social psychology,[13] quality and productivity improvement,[14] leadership and program development,[15] human factors in high reliability industries,[16] and complexity science.[10,17]

Unifying the common themes across these numerous disciplines, Plsek and Greenhalgh have defined complex adaptive systems as collections of individual agents with "freedom to act in ways that are not always predictable, and whose actions are interconnected so that one agent's actions change the context for other agents."[18] Such systems are notable for their distributed rather than centralized control, for their non-linearity (and non-singularity) of relationship between cause and effect, and for their capacity to learn and to adapt (based on continuous feedback) in a spontaneously self-organizing and reorganizing manner.[10] Importantly, despite their unpredictability at the level of fine detail, complex systems commonly exhibit behavior that is integrated and purposeful. Thus W. Edwards Deming could succinctly assert that "a system is a set of interrelated parts that work together to achieve a common aim."[14] As we shall observe in the present and subsequent chapters, this combination of spontaneity, interconnection, and shared purpose is a key driver of successful work in health care's clinical microsystems. Chapter Eight provides a more extensive discussion of systems thinking in the care of people who have chronic illness.

In addition to this fundamental interconnection of component parts, many systems reveal the further property of multiple *levels* of organization, so that systems and subsystems are actually embedded one inside another. Like Russian matryoshka dolls of increasing size that are nested one inside the next, we can think of systems in nature. For example, cells cohere into organs, then into human beings, families, communities, nations, and finally into all of humanity. Each cell is a system in its own right, and each is intrinsically bound to systems at higher and lower levels. Of course, this nested

FIGURE 1.4   Embedded Provider Units in a Health System.

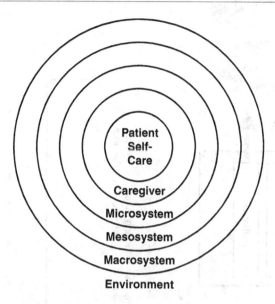

structure adds still further levels of complexity; multilateral relationships and influences exist among components within single levels and also across levels.

In health care this property of embedded systems is especially apparent and important. Figure 1.4 introduces a straightforward *target* design to illustrate the nesting of clinical relationships. At the center of the target, one person links with health-specific information to form a *system* that provides self-care.

Moving out from the target's bull's-eye, we find a patient in relationship with an individual caregiver, then a clinical microsystem, then a mesosystem (of two or more linked clinical and supporting microsystems), then a macrosystem (of interdependent microsystems and mesosystems) that forms a larger organization such as a hospital or integrated health system, then finally a broader environment that can be described in terms of geography, markets, political jurisdictions, regulatory and legal requirements, and biomedical knowledge and technology.

The mesosystem, made up of the linked clinical and supporting microsystems, is part of the embedded systems within the larger organization. Figure 1.5 depicts the relationship of a clinical microsystem with some of the possible supporting microsystems, such as pathology, nutrition, informatics, transportation, and so on, that contribute to the clinical microsystem's processes of care. Every organization will have different supporting microsystems. Figure 1.5 intends to provide an example of supporting microsystems that might exist in one organization.

## The Institute of Medicine's Chain of Effect in Health Care

These ideas about system dynamics have become a major force for change and improvement in health care. In generating its highly influential *Chasm Report*, the Institute of Medicine (IOM) performed its analysis and offered its recommendations based on assumptions of health care *as a system*. The IOM committee responsible for this report identified not individuals but the entire health care system as dysfunctional and unsafe. The entire basic chassis was broken. The report states, "The current care systems cannot

FIGURE 1.5  Supporting Microsystems for a Clinical Microsystem.

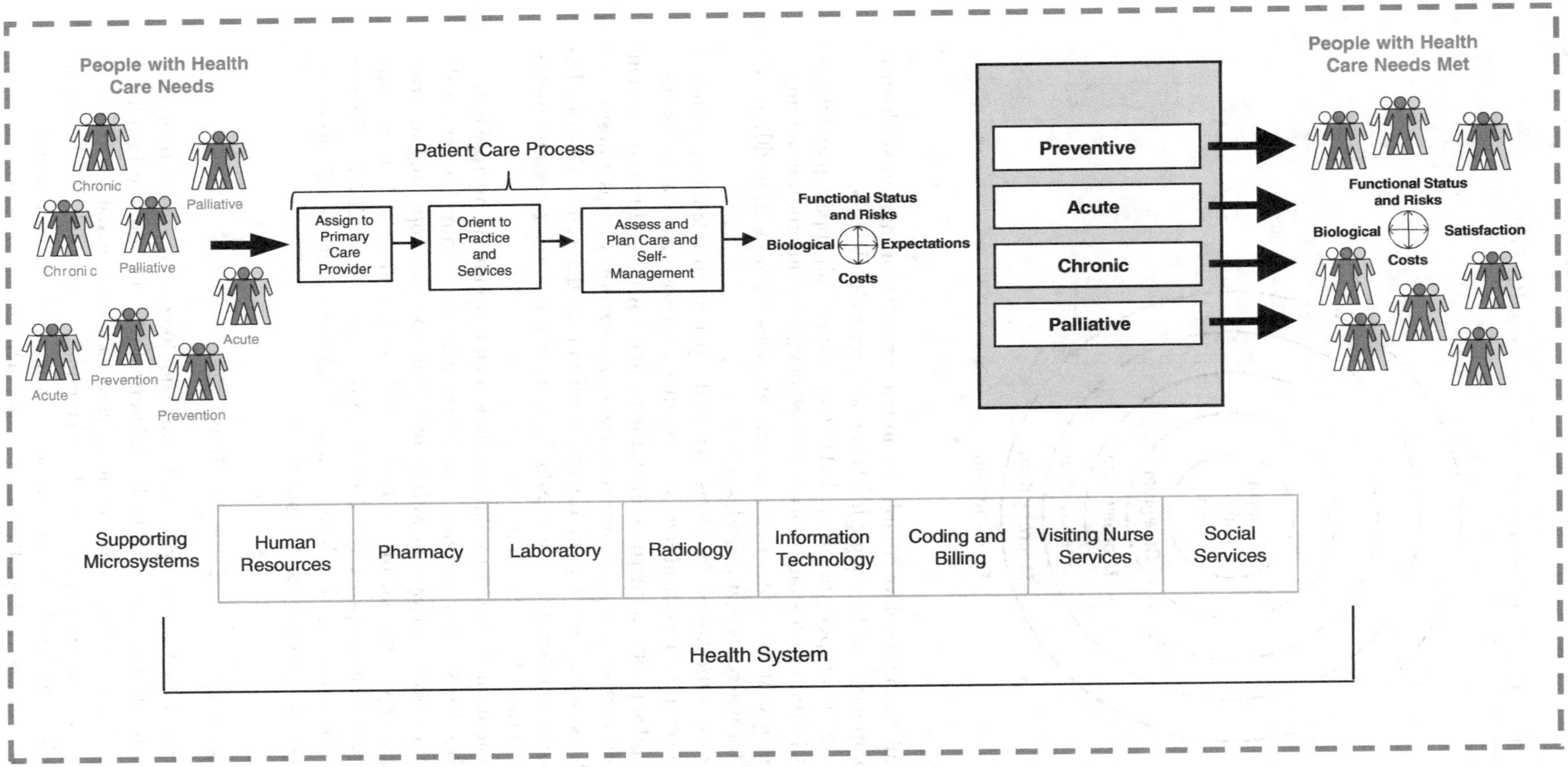

People with Health Care Needs

Chronic
Palliative
Palliative
Acute
Chronic
Prevention
Acute
Prevention

Patient Care Process

Assign to Primary Care Provider → Orient to Practice and Services → Assess and Plan Care and Self-Management

Functional Status and Risks
Biological ⊕ Expectations
Costs

Preventive
Acute
Chronic
Palliative

People with Health Care Needs Met

Functional Status and Risks
Biological ⊕ Satisfaction
Costs

Supporting Microsystems

| Human Resources | Pharmacy | Laboratory | Radiology | Information Technology | Coding and Billing | Visiting Nurse Services | Social Services |

Health System

do the job. Trying harder will not work. Changing systems of care will."[19] The committee asserted that systemic change would require action at all levels of the health care system, and it identified four particular levels that required specific attention:

1. Patient and community
2. Microsystem of care delivery
3. Macrosystem
4. Environmental context

The IOM committee referred to this hierarchy of system levels as the chain of effect in health care improvement.[20] Quality aims of the system were defined broadly and included six related dimensions: health care must be *s*afe, *t*imely, *e*ffective, *e*fficient, *e*quitable, and *p*atient-centered. These system attributes, remembered easily by the mnemonic STEEEP, are themselves interconnected, and imply general and specific targets and interventions for health care improvement and redesign.

## Horizontal and Vertical Levels of the Health Care System

How do we begin to apply general systems thinking to the urgent challenges of health care redesign, improvement, and innovation? Before we turn our attention to the clinical microsystem approach in particular, we will be wise to consider the specific embedding of frontline clinical microsystems in higher nested levels of the meso and macrosystem. Let us imagine, for example, that leaders at all levels of a health care system (for example, a hospital, a multispecialty group practice, or an integrated delivery system) wish to visualize the whole of their system, so that everyone, at all levels, can gain a big-picture view that locates their own work within the larger organization. Figure 1.6 provides such a panoramic view.

The Jönköping County Council health system in Sweden uses a version of this figure to understand both horizontal and vertical dimensions of its organizational structure.

First, analyze the lateral flow of the diagram. At the system's *top* are patients and families interacting with clinical microsystems (the health system's building blocks) and progressing horizontally (from left to right) and through related microsystems on their health care journey. Consider the subjects on this journey: a young mother and father in their first pregnancy who are seeking prenatal, perinatal, and postnatal care, and then effective transition to a primary care clinician in the community; or an octogenarian who fell and broke her hip and will move through hospital admissions, rehabilitation, discharge, and then outpatient services.

Individuals enter each microsystem with specific needs and hope to transition to subsequent settings with the best possible outcomes.

Second, analyze the vertical flow of this same diagram. Here we find, for example, a frontline clinical microsystem such as the local inpatient birthing pavilion, in relationship to a set of inpatient and outpatient clinical and support units. These units in turn form a perinatal and obstetrical institute to care for Jönköping County's maternity population, in relationship to population-specific health care programs with similar aims. These programs are further linked to a nationally organized infrastructure for care of major health conditions or diseases, such as trauma, cardiovascular disease, cancer, and mental illness.

From this high-level and multitiered perspective, all participants can recognize where they fit in the larger system and how their own work contributes to local (micro

FIGURE 1.6    Panoramic View of a Health System.

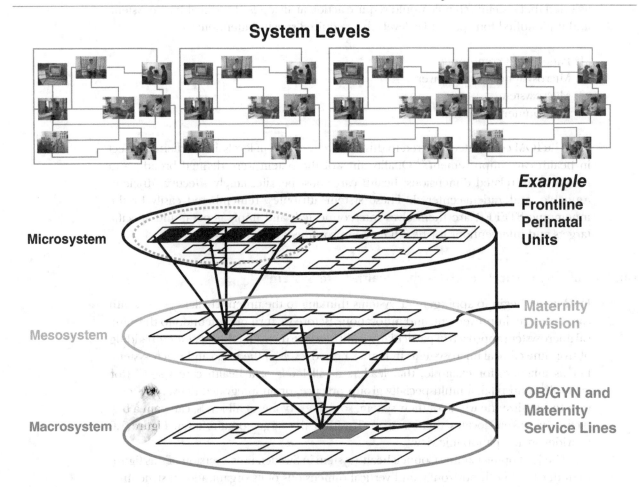

*Source:* Adapted by G. Henriks to include macro, meso, and micro levels, from Langley, G., Moen, R., Nolan, K., Nolan, T., Norman, C., & Provost, L. *The improvement guide: A practical approach to enhancing organizational performance, Second Edition.* San Francisco: Jossey-Bass, An Imprint of John Wiley & Sons, Inc., 2009.

and meso) and global (macro) system aims. Apparent in this analysis is the potential for tension that calls for harmonizing the horizontal and vertical dimensions of care. We observe that health care is experienced by the patient and family in a *horizontal* fashion, with seamless or coordinated or disjointed or defective linkages within and between frontline microsystems. But health care systems themselves are traditionally organized in a *vertical* manner, with attention to organizational structure, chains of command, and *silos* of performance, that is, compartmentalized operation of each department, without real consideration of the whole system or of what needs to happen "upstream" or "downstream" in the flow of care. Leaders at all levels of health care systems must ensure that our traditional emphasis on vertical structures does not distract from efforts to optimize horizontal flow and functioning.

Of course, the *tension* of horizontal and vertical priorities can be positive, so long as reflective leaders are conscious of the dynamic and do not sacrifice quality. Careful consideration of the *architecture* depicted in Figure 1.6 (and of microsystem anatomy and physiology as previously discussed) empowers health care leaders to identify specific areas requiring functional assessment and redesign, so the quality of system performance is improved in all STEEEP dimensions. Some common areas needing attention include leadership development, effective communication, design of coherent meso-systems, patient and family engagement, clarity about mission, vision, values and goals, and relevant measurement within and across all levels of the system.

## Microsystems and Their External Context

Another critical perspective for improvement of clinical microsystems is a map of sur-rounding (external) contexts that provides the view of each microsystem from the inside out. To be successful, every microsystem must interact effectively with other clini-cal and supporting microsystems. Indeed, microsystems depend on each other in the following ways:

- To provide each microsystem with patients to care for
- To receive patients who are discharged after care is complete
- To assist with the provision of need-based specialty and social services
- To provide ancillary services, such as diagnostic tests and assessments
- To administer supporting services, such as informatics, transportation, and nutrition
- To exchange essential information (feed forward and feedback) that facilitates each next step in the patient's journey through microsystems

Figure 1.7 shows the external context map drawn by Godfrey (one of this chapter's authors) for a general practice in one of England's communities. The mapping reveals this particular general practice can engage in a rich mix of health and social resources to provide comprehensive care to individual patients.

Use of an external mapping tool helps microsystem members break traditional patterns of thinking regarding scarcity of resources available to patients and practitio-ners. Indeed, when external relationships are formally mapped in this manner, an abundance of resources is often identified, and insights are gained into common inter-actions, possible improvement or redesign priorities, and functional necessities for cooperative work in the care of patients. Chapter One Action Guide presents more information on the external context of microsystems.

# RESEARCH ON MICROSYSTEMS IN HEALTH CARE

We have considered the benefits of system analysis in general and microsystem assess-ment and intervention in particular. Let us now examine scholarly work that explores the value of this organizing framework in real-world settings. Although research on clinical microsystems is relatively new, a number of important studies and summaries have been published in the last decade. In general, research and evaluation literature on microsystems can be divided into two broad categories: studies that focus on the performance of individual microsystems in specific clinical settings; and studies that address microsystems as elements in the design, improvement, and performance of larger (meso and macro) systems of care.

## Microsystem Research

One of the first published research accounts to use microsystems as an organizing framework was commissioned by the IOM and published in 2000 as a technical report

**FIGURE 1.7** External Mapping of a Clinic in the United Kingdom.

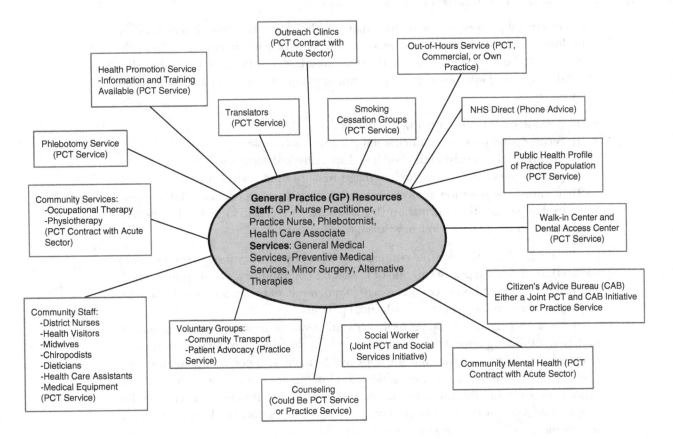

## Examples of Resources Available to General Practice Microsystems

These are examples of some of the resources that may be available to practices. Some are arranged by practices themselves; others are set up as primary care trust (PCT) services to practice populations.

for the Committee on Quality of Health Care in America.[21] In this qualitative assessment, the investigators identified forty-three high performing clinical microsystems, conducted interviews with their leaders, and identified eight core characteristics associated with their superior performance. These characteristics included: constancy of purpose, investment in improvement, alignment of role and training for efficiency and staff satisfaction, interdependence of care team to meet patient needs, integration of information and technology into work flow, continuous measurement of outcomes, supportive larger organization, and connection to community.

A Dartmouth-based team built on this first microsystem study and, with support from the Robert Wood Johnson Foundation, assessed twenty of the best performing clinical microsystems that could be identified in North America.[22] A mixed method study design was employed to sample microsystems from across the care continuum (ambulatory, inpatient, home health, nursing home, and hospice care). Investigators screened more than one hundred fifty potential sites, conducted preliminary interviews at more than fifty sites, and ultimately selected twenty microsystems that appeared to be the best performers. The selection of sites was based on a combination of five complementary methods for identifying *best of the best* clinical sites: literature review,

FIGURE 1.8  The Success Characteristics of
High Performing Clinical Microsystems.

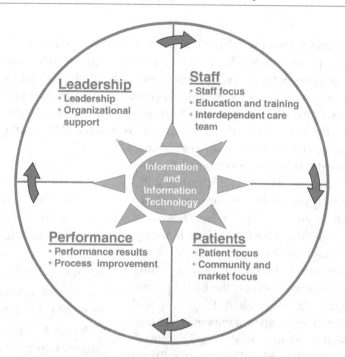

identification of sites that had won quality awards, interviews with national experts to identify exemplary microsystems, prior research, demonstration projects conducted by the IOM and the IHI respectively, and interviews with leaders of some of the leading health care systems in the United States and Canada (asking them to identify *best of the best* microsystems within their large health care systems.) The investigators then conducted multi-day site visits to the twenty top performing sites. Extensive qualitative information was collected based upon individual and group semi-structured interviews with microsystem members and with other staff and leaders in the larger organization. In-depth interviews were supplemented with direct observation of care delivery and with quantitative medical record review of quality metrics and financial data on efficiency and costs.

The research team analyzed all of this information and concluded that these twenty top performing microsystems shared a set of characteristics that combined to produce sustained, superior results. These ten success factors are depicted as dimensions of a microsystem performance wheel, illustrated in Figure 1.8. The success wheel features the following five interrelated components with an information hub at its center:

1. *microsystem leadership actions* (usually through physician and nurse and/or administrative co-leadership) that motivated and guided staff and that gained support from the larger organization
2. focus on the needs of *staff,* who were learning and growing, appreciated by their leaders, and aware of their interdependence
3. primary emphasis on the needs of *patients* and families and on the priorities of local communities and markets
4. full attention to *outcomes and performance results* desired by patients and families and to analysis, improvement, and standardization of effective care *processes*

5. a rich *information environment* and intelligent use of information technology, with recognition of communication's essential role in linking all microsystem participants and activities

The Microsystem Assessment Tool (MAT) is a qualitative tool developed from the research-based microsystem performance wheel. This assessment scheme offers the opportunity for members of microsystems to reflect upon and assess their perceptions of the microsystem before beginning a microsystem development journey. Microsystem members may then reassess six to twelve months later to review their progress. Chapter One Action Guide provides the MAT model, the MAT definitions, and the MAT scoring tool. Although the Dartmouth study focused on top performing clinical systems and identified factors that contributed to superior care, a case study published in 2003 by Weick and Sutcliffe focused on a low performing clinical system in the tragic Bristol Royal Infirmary (BRI) case. In an article aptly titled *Hospitals as Cultures of Entrapment: A Re-analysis of the Bristol Royal Infirmary*, the authors described conditions that contributed to a clinical unit's generation of consistently poor outcomes over a long time span.[23] In this now well-known instance, the BRI, a pediatric cardiac surgery program in the United Kingdom, had consistently higher mortality rates compared to peer programs, and it also failed to achieve the longitudinal decrease in mortality similar programs had experienced. "Why did the Bristol Royal Infirmary continue to perform pediatric cardiac surgeries for almost fourteen years (1981–1995) in the face of poor performance?" asked Weick and Sutcliffe.[23] The authors offered this remarkable conclusion, shown in the sidebar.

Although Weick and Sutcliffe found some clinical microsystems can develop cultures that are resistant to change and can even avoid information that may facilitate such change, Luan[24] explored the shared mental models that can lead to self-sealing entrapment in some clinical microsystems or that can conversely break these negative cycles. Luan examined shared mental models in neonatal intensive care units (NICUs) that were members of the Vermont Oxford Network (VON). She hypothesized NICU staffs shared beliefs regarding either the preventability or inevitability of hospital-acquired infections (HAIs) could predict the actual rate of those infections. Her research was based on the observations of a leading neonatologist, William H. Edwards, that staff in NICUs with the lowest rates of infection believed HAIs were 100 percent preventable by good care processes, whereas staff in high infection rate NICUs believed infections were inevitable. In effect, some staff felt infants were *entitled* to become infected, but then could be cured and saved by rapid diagnosis and treatment.[25]

Luan[24] identified several low and high infection rate NICUs, conducted in-depth interviews with staff, observed care routines and clinical processes, and analyzed mental models with respect to the preventability or inevitability of infection. Her results confirmed the hypothesis: staff expectations of inevitability were self-fulfilling. In NICU microsystems that attributed infection to reversible errors in process of care, HAIs were virtually eliminated over time. In microsystems that believed infections were inevitable, processes were not selectively improved to prevent them, and infection rates ranged from 32 to 54 percent of neonates.

> Culture enables sustained collective action by providing people with a similarity of approach, outlook, and priorities. Yet these same shared values, norms, and assumptions can also be a source of danger if they blind the collective to vital issues or factors important to performance that lie outside the bounds of organizational perception. Cultural blind spots can lead an organization down the wrong path, sometimes with dire consequences. This was the case at the Bristol Royal Infirmary.[23]

In a fourth research project, Homa analyzed the sustainability of clinical microsystem improvements over time.[26] In her careful review of clinical performance at a regional Spine Center, Homa demonstrated clinical staff were able to appropriately increase mental health referrals from 29 percent to 59 percent (for spine patients with emotional difficulties) using microsystem assessment and intervention methodologies. During two subsequent years, however, as attention shifted to other priorities, referral rates dropped back down and actually settled in a zone that was lower than the pre-intervention phase.

Based on extensive interviews with staff and on direct observations of care patterns, Homa concluded that diminished attention to previously successful microsystem processes (such as performance monitoring, corrective response to worsened outcomes, and believing standardized protocols would improve local mental health outcomes) all contributed to the failure of *sustainable* improvement efforts. This study makes clear that long term improvement in clinical microsystems requires attention to not only quality *innovation* (as the Spine Center accomplished in its early phase) but also quality *maintenance*.

Taken together, these intriguing research results suggest the following:

- Microsystems can create either open or self-sealing cultures with respect to better or worse performance.
- Shared mental models are a powerful and often hidden source of both desired and undesired results.
- Initiation of quality improvements does not assure maintenance of them, unless continuous monitoring, reflecting, learning, and responding are built into local microsystem routines.

## Microsystem in Macrosystem Research

As suggested earlier in this chapter, systems are commonly embedded within and mutually influential across multiple levels of organization from micro to macro. The relationships across these levels can also be studied empirically, providing further insight into the function and value of clinical microsystems. Thus, for example, Golton and Wilcock have examined and extensively described the United Kingdom National Health Service's (NHS) early adoption of a microsystem approach in large health systems. In 2003 the NHS Clinical Microsystem (CMS) Awareness and Development program was launched "to investigate the utility and application of the microsystem framework for improvement."[27] The pilot program began in both inpatient acute care hospital and primary care settings spread throughout England. Program leaders deployed coaches to work with microsystems to assess and to improve their performance and to fortify preexisting quality initiatives that were part of Great Britain's major campaign to modernize health care delivery. Action-learning methods (including the 5Ps approach[9]) were used to engage frontline microsystem members in self-assessment, and the Dartmouth Microsystem Improvement Curriculum (DMIC) was adapted to fit the NHS's culture and conditions. The evaluation research report, published in 2005, offers the conclusion in the sidebar.

The initiative has shown that the CMS [Clinical Microsystem] framework is an effective way to promote service improvement and the cohort of pilot sites has used it to good effect. . . . It is relatively easy to adapt microsystems working to complement local improvement initiatives that are already underway. . . . Finally, it is important to emphasize how this initiative has contributed to our understanding of how learning in the work place can produce real benefits for service users . . . it offers some insight into approaches to learning that are close to those we serve and that can be better tailored to meet the needs of learners and the needs of those who depend on them in their care settings.[27]

Works published in 2007 from two leading regional health systems in the United States, Intermountain Health Care in Utah and Geisinger Health System in Pennsylvania, provide different examples of microsystem principles, concepts, and methods in action. These programs have bridged the gap between microsystem and macrosystem by creating innovative mesosystems to serve discrete patient populations.

James and Lazar describe the strategic development of health care delivery programs for patient subpopulations in Utah's highly regarded Intermountain Health care system.[9] This program employs *clinical process models* (CPMs) that design technical quality and evidence-based care into the flow of care for specific patient groups. The CPMs, based on ideas of Deming,[28] Juran,[29] and clinical microsystems,[9] bring together frontline generalists and tertiary and quaternary specialists to continually define the state of the art of evidenced-based care and to embed the provision of this care into regular work routines of health professionals in primary, specialty, and inpatient care settings. A strong information system supports provision of evidence-based care through active decision support tools and constant monitoring of care processes and outcomes, including performance in clinical, cost, and satisfaction domains. Feedback reports on performance are distributed to all relevant frontline clinicians as well as other clinical microsystem members and constantly emphasize the need to find ways to improve performance.

CPMs include modules for health care professionals and also self-management programs for patients and families, who are thus empowered to provide intelligent self-care and to partner effectively with care teams that serve them. The entire CPM infrastructure has been developed by senior leaders to: (1) link frontline microsystems into well-designed mesosystems (that are supported by effective leaders at all levels of the system and a rich information environment) to optimize care within and between microsystems; (2) to provide ongoing means to execute quality planning, quality control, and quality improvement throughout the care continuum and across a large geographic area; and (3) confer upon IHC a competitive advantage, through attention to higher quality care using lower cost methods whenever possible.

Using similar concepts and methods to those employed in Utah, senior leaders in the Geisinger Health System (which offers care in approximately half the state of Pennsylvania and to a third of its population), have refined a novel system, *ProvenCare (SM)*, to provide superior care to diverse clinical populations. *The ProvenCare (SM)* approach focuses on specific patient subpopulations undergoing care episodes, such as open heart surgery, labor and delivery, back surgery, and total joint replacement.[30] Clinical leaders and staffs from contributing microsystems are brought together into functional mesosystems that identify implementable best practices and embed these into structured flows of care. The model is supported by an active information environment that uses state-of-the-art electronic health records (EHRs) and specially designed performance feedback reports that cascade to all levels of the system. Of special note is the use of risk-based pricing and service guarantees, which enable the Geisinger system to explicitly compete in the market on quality and price. Senior leaders of the *ProvenCare (SM)* program link strategy with execution and accountability by engaging microsystem leaders and staff, measuring the quality and costs of performance at all levels of the system, and creating incentives to reward quality and productivity.

## Emerging Microsystem Research in Sweden and the Future

*Bridging the Gaps* is a unique collaborative effort between the County Council of Jönköping (CCJ), Sweden, and four academic schools: Jönköping University, Linnaeus University, Uppsala Clinical Research Center, and Helix Vinn Excellence Center. This national initiative is supported by the Vinnvård research program in Sweden. The gaps to be bridged include those between knowledge and practice, between professionals themselves within multiprofessional organizations, and between different levels and groups within the larger health care system. The vision is multifaceted in the following ways:

- Interactive research will inspire development of new arenas for knowledge exchange and will stimulate new methods for the design of continuous learning, innovation, and improvement.
- Collaborative research will include interactions among frontline microsystems and will generate outstanding examples in practice and research.
- The results of the research (described as new insights, methods, approaches, good examples, and illustrative knowledge) will be integrated into undergraduate AND GRADUATE education, into continuing development activities for health care professionals, and into management training for health care administrative leaders.

Figures 1.9 and 1.10 illustrate the aims, structures, and processes of one of the collaborative efforts sponsored by the County Council of Jönköping that led to increased value for the child and the family.

**FIGURE 1.9  Jönköping County's Child HealthCare Collaboration.**

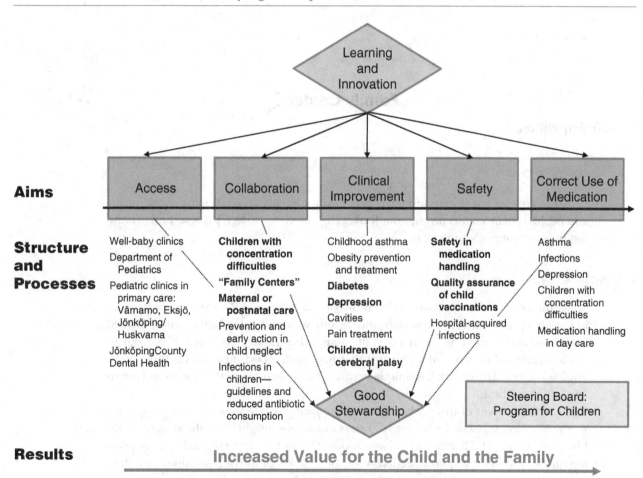

*Source:* Adapted from Henriks and Bardon by Andersson-Gäre.

**FIGURE 1.10** Panoramic View of Jönköping County's Maternity and Newborn Mesosystem.

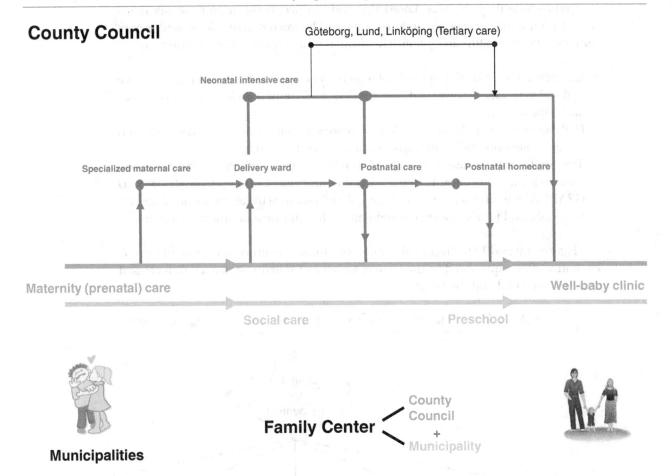

Much research is being conducted by doctoral students in collaboration with faculty and health system leaders throughout Jönköping, Sweden. Table 1.1 lists several promising projects currently underway.

## Organizing for Quality

Some final empirical insights are offered by Bate, Mandel, and Robert in their fascinating study of seven leading hospitals and health systems in the Netherlands, United Kingdom, and United States. Bate et. al. studied health systems that had set out to organize around quality and safety and that had made good progress on their never ending journey. The research is unique because it focuses on both the macro and micro levels of these health care systems.

The final report of this work, *Organizing for quality: The improvement journeys of major hospitals in Europe and the United States,*[31] offers numerous insights into the structure and function of successful health care organizations. The authors first conclude that improving quality and safety requires aligned action at all levels of the organization, including top, bottom, and middle. Second, effective deployment of quality actions generates integration and coordination across the different levels of the organization. Third,

Table 1.1    Bridging the Gaps: Jönköping, Sweden, Research Studies

| Title of Research | Researcher and School |
|---|---|
| *Patient Centered E-Health: An Extended Perspective on Information Systems in Clinical Microsystems?* | Eva Lindholm<br>County Council Jönköping-Qulturum<br>International Business School<br>Jönköping University |
| *Microsystem Theory—A Paradigmatic Change in Health Care?* | Joel Hedegaard<br>School of Education and Communication<br>Jönköping University |
| *The Physician, Learning, and Interprofessional Collaboration— Essential Conditions for Creating Better Patient Results* | Karin Thörne<br>County Council Jönköping-Futurum<br>Health University of Linköping |
| *The Art and Science of Coaching Interdisciplinary Health Care Teams to Achieve Strategic Health Care Improvement* | Marjorie M. Godfrey<br>School of Health Sciences<br>Jönköping University |
| *One Lens Missing? The Clinical Microsystem in a Pedagogical Theory Framework* | Ann-Charlott Norman<br>Växjö University and School of Health Sciences, Jönköping University |
| *Interprofessional Experiences of Quality Improvement Work* | Annette Nygardh<br>School of Health Sciences<br>Jönköping University |
| *Who and What Is in Focus? A Study of Documentation in Electronic Patient Records and Quality Registers* | Eva Gustaffson<br>School of Health Sciences<br>Jönköping University |
| *TechnoOrganizing—Make the Microsystem Work with Efficient Information Provision* | Klas Gäre<br>Jönköping International Business School<br>Linda Askenäs<br>School of Mathematics and Systems Engineering<br>Linné University |
| *Can Complex Adaptive Systems Contribute to the Understanding of Microsystem Thinking?* | Annika Nordin<br>Martin Reiler<br>Jönköping International Business School<br>Jönköping University |
| *Collaboration in health and welfare. Service user participation and teamwork in interprofessional microsystems.* | Susanne Kvarnström<br>School of Health Sciences<br>Jönköping University |

different organizations may take different routes to attain the same goal of safe, high-quality care that is appreciated by patients and families and that enriches the lives of employees. Fourth, local (microsystem-based) communities of practice exert an important and powerful influence on both the quality of patient care and the quality of caregivers' own work experience. In a very real sense, the local communities of practice that thrive in small clinical microsystems provide an antidote to feelings of alienation from being a small part of a larger bureaucratic organization. Fifth, the organization's *mesosystems* can, under some circumstances, positively and proactively align the goals, aspirations, and insights of people in both clinical and administrative service sectors.

Figure 1.11 demonstrates the pivotal integrating and buffering role mesosystems can play in the luminal space between microsystem and macrosystem levels of a health

FIGURE 1.11   Mesosystems as a Connector Entity.

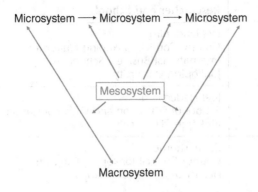

*Source:* Adapted from Bate, P., Mendel, P, & Robert, G. Organizing for quality: The improvement journeys of major hospitals in Europe and the United States. Abingdon, UK: Radcliffe Publishing, 2008.

care organization. Bate finds mesosystems emerging in these high performing organizations that promote alignment and positive interactions within and between linked microsystems (through which patients move horizontally) and that connect direct care delivery work at the front line (microsystems) with strategic and executive work in the front office (macrosytems). Finally, the authors offer a very helpful assessment tool to stimulate organizational response to six universal challenges. The assessment provides discussion opportunities to explore current gaps within and future direction of local quality improvement efforts.

## THREE CONCEPTUAL IMPERATIVES IN THE WORK OF VALUE IMPROVEMENT

We have considered clinical microsystems as *structural* and *functional entities* and have reviewed the small but growing body of *descriptive research* that explores their pivotal role in real-world settings. Before analyzing specific components of clinical microsystems in richer and more practical detail, we introduce three *conceptual imperatives* that may guide microsystem members in the continuous improvement of their work. These imperatives offer some scaffolding upon which more precise manifestations of value can be built in the chapters that follow.

### Imperative Number 1: Engage Everyone in Value Improvement

Implicit in the traditional training of health care professionals, of nursing and support staff, and even of quality administrators, is an artificial distinction between the activities of clinical care and of continuous value improvement. Improvement is deemed as extra (rather than essential) work. It is delegated to special *quality improvement (QI) teams*. It is monitored in contexts that feel foreign or even threatening to clinicians.

Increasingly, however, members of highly effective clinical microsystems recognize that everyone in health care really has two jobs: to do the work and to improve the value of that work. These two functions are inextricably linked in professional activity, and indeed are yoked to a third essential responsibility: all microsystem members "must endeavor *to learn* continually, so that both clinical care and its system-based improve-

FIGURE 1.12   Annotated Sustainable Improvement Triangle.

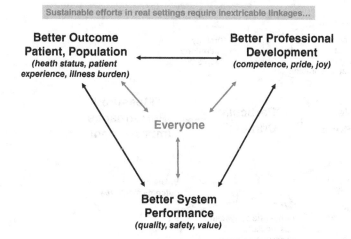

ment are performed with ever-increasing effectiveness and creativity."[32] As depicted in the sustainable improvement triangle of Figure 1.12, the activities of patient care, system performance, and professional development are interdependent and mutually supportive.

In this context, Batalden and Davidoff offer an especially inclusive description of quality improvement, which they define in the sidebar.

Observe in Figure 1.12 that the sustainable improvement triangle has *everyone* at its center. The work of value improvement must be understood not as an extra or a parceled-off function, but as an essential component of everyone's job, every day, in all parts of the system. Observe as well, in this same figure, that arrows emanating from this central term are bidirectional: not only does everyone participate, so too does everyone benefit. Health care professionals, patients and families, researchers, payers, planners, and educators all are rewarded by the mutually achieved outcomes of this important work. Rewards include the following:

The combined and unceasing efforts of everyone—health care professionals, patients and their families, researchers, payers, planners, educators—to make the changes that will lead to better patient outcomes (*health* in physical, psychological, and social domains), better system performance (*care* that is safe, timely, efficient, equitable, and so forth), and better professional development (*learning* new knowledge, skills, and values).[33]

- Better performance measured in terms of improving system quality, safety, and value (or cost)
- Better patient outcomes measured in terms of health status, patient experiences, and actual reductions in the burden of illness
- Better professional development for professionals and staff measured in terms of job satisfaction, competence, pride, joy, and mastery of their work

Because achieving sustainable improvements requires recognition that *every system is perfectly designed to get the results it gets* and because health systems throw off multiple and interdependent results rather than single and isolated outcomes (such as life or death or profits or losses or motivated or demoralized staff), members of clinical microsystems must collectively build new forms of knowledge and skill to support their work.

**FIGURE 1.13    Improvement Equation Annotated:**
**Linking Evidence to Improvement.**

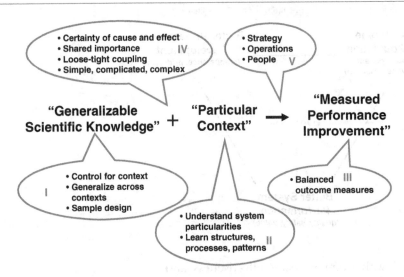

The richly annotated improvement triangle of Figure 1.12, and also the Improvement Equation (Figure 1.13), suggest several knowledge and skill domains that require microsystem mastery. These domains include knowledge of evidence-based practice, appreciation of change management and complexity, deep understanding of local context, capacity to execute change and improvement, and ability to generate and analyze balanced measures of outcomes and costs.

### Imperative Number 2: Work the Improvement Equation

We have learned in the past two decades that development of evidence-based guidelines does not guarantee reliable implementation in real-world clinical settings. McGlynn, for example, reported in an extensive literature review that Americans receive only half of the evidence-based and guideline-specified care for which they are appropriate candidates.[34] Although data from randomized controlled trials and other scientific forms of knowledge are necessary components of real-world clinical quality, these components alone are far from sufficient. Broader forms of knowledge are required.

Pawson and Tilley have developed a framework for program evaluation that is based on a brief equation:[35]

*mechanism + context = outcome*

Batalden and Davidoff have customized and specified this equation for health care:[33]

*generalizable scientific knowledge + particular context → measured performance improvement*

In this seemingly simple formula, the textual elements *and* the syntactic connectors (that is, the + and → signs) embed specific operational tasks and depend upon specific cognitive skills. These tasks and skills are elaborated on in Figure 1.13.

Let us briefly consider the methodologies and special forms of knowledge unique to each *Improvement Equation domain*. Generalizable scientific knowledge derives from decontextualized research and accrues over time. Research designs emphasize controlling for the effects of specific contexts to the greatest degree possible; generalizability is valued, which means specificity of application may be diminished. Particular context knowledge recovers this diminished specificity and focuses upon assessment of local culture and the unique patients, professionals, processes, and patterns (see again the 5Ps) of this clinical setting. In contrast to randomized clinical trials, which eliminate consideration of local context by controlling for it in statistical models, this second knowledge domain focuses sharply on the particular setting and all that contributes to its identity.

Effective integration of both these domains is depicted in the Improvement Equation's + symbol, which suggests methodologies of adaptation and redesign. This *bridging* domain emphasizes reflective planning of specific care algorithms to match locally available resources; it includes management of conflict and negotiation in the context of unique practice histories.

Equally important as a bridging function is activity represented by the Improvement Equation's → symbol, which suggests knowledge necessary for actual execution of change. How is vision communicated, how are stressful transitions managed, how are positive achievements honored and sustained? *Measured performance improvement* permits recognition and analysis of these achievements themselves and is a final knowledge domain necessary for sustainable value creation. Statistical process control charting, graphical data, and other techniques permit monitoring of quality performance and facilitate refinement of improvement efforts over time.

The Improvement Equation's practical relevance becomes apparent in specific clinical contexts. In Chapter Six we elaborate upon the Equation's significance in greater detail and explore (as an extended example) the Equation's value in the design and implementation of preventive care services. The reader is invited to consider other applications as well.

### Imperative Number 3: Frame Problems and Practice Solutions as Simple, Complicated, or Complex

Glouberman and Zimmerman[36] have observed that organizational *problems* of all sorts, including most challenges in health care, may be categorized generally as simple, complicated, or complex. These categories have practical consequences in clinical microsystems. The conceptual framework is discussed in great detail in Chapter Eight, where it is applied specifically to the design and improvement of chronic illness care. Anticipating that discussion, we invite the reader to consider iconic examples in these three activity domains.

As Glouberman and Zimmerman,[36] and later Zimmerman, Lindberg, and Plsek,[10] have described, *baking cookies* is a classically simple problem, and *following a recipe* is a correspondingly simple solution. All ingredients are known and stable. Special expertise is not required, but cooking experience increases success rate. The aim of the recipe is to produce standardized products and the best recipes produce good results every time. Complicated problems and solutions offer similar degrees of certainty, although greater technical knowledge is required to achieve a desired end. *Sending a rocket to the moon*, for example, requires great expertise, but discrete elements of the system are knowable in detail; one successful rocket launch greatly increases the likelihood the next will succeed as well.

Both these examples may be contrasted with the truly complex task of *raising a child*. Recall the discussion of complex adaptive systems earlier in this chapter. Components of such systems are simultaneously interdependent and autonomous. Because these components change both within themselves and in relationship to each other, outcomes are inherently less predictable. Expertise may contribute to better results, but is neither necessary nor sufficient to assure success.

FIGURE 1.14    Simple, Complicated, Complex Framework.

| Simple<br>"Yes/No" | Complicated<br>"If, then…" | Complex<br>"? Maybe" |
|---|---|---|
| Known elements | Elements are knowable | Elements partly known, but they can change… |
| Predictable outcome | Largely predictable outcome | Essentially unpredictable |
| Checklist (or other forcing function) | Algorithm-driven structured orders, decision making | Shared aim, relationship |
| Oxygenation status, smoking cessation, culture before antibiotic, antibiotic in four hours | Antibiotic tolerance/intolerance | Co-morbidities, social situation |
| Low provider autonomy | Variable provider autonomy | High provider autonomy |
| Aim: reliability | Aim: reliability | Aim: resiliency |

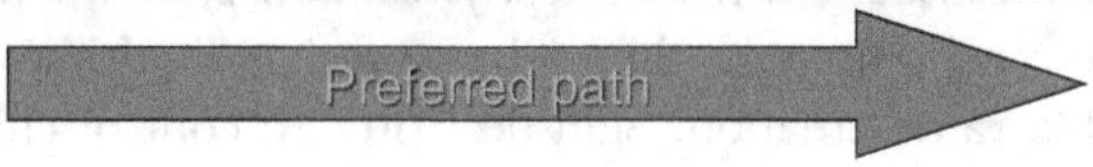

Preferred path

Building on the Glouberman and Zimmerman work, Liu, Homa, Butterly, Kirkland, and Batalden[37] offer practical guidance for people who wish to improve the quality, safety, and reliability of health care systems. This is based on the observation that all clinical microsystems and all health care mesosystems and macrosystems are complex, but not all the activities within these complex systems are themselves complex. It is possible, therefore, to analyze a clinical system, to identify specific challenges that are simple, complicated, or complex, and to improve system performance by matching discrete clinical problems to interventions of comparable simplicity or complexity. Figure 1.14 illustrates the logic of this simple, complicated, complex framework. See Chapter Eight for a more extended discussion.

## CONCLUSION

The road to better value health care has been partially mapped by research on small clinical microsystems and large health care macrosystems. We have focused attention on the sharp microsystem end in particular, for it is here that patients, families, and caregivers meet, and here that services are delivered and safety realized. In these smallest replicable units of the health care system, both quality and costs (and therefore value) are generated. In the upcoming chapters we analyze the actions and the interactions of these microsystem units, and we build from them a working vision of sustainable high-value care.

The ultimate aim of any health care system is to provide high-quality and high-value care for individuals and for populations. Value-based competition, supported by transparent performance measures and value-based payment schemes that reward higher quality, better outcomes, and lower costs, are emerging as a potent force for change in health care. This creates new energy to build knowledge and to redesign care. In order for health systems to respond positively to this new force, they will need to put into place mechanisms to engage all of their employees and staff to provide care and to improve care, by working the improvement equation and by taking effective actions to enhance the reliability and resiliency of care.

## SUMMARY

- Large health care systems (macrosystems) have fundamental building blocks (clinical microsystems), which are the places where patients and families and health caregivers meet.
- Most health care systems are organized vertically, but patients experience care horizontally as they move from their homes and their community into and out of specific clinical microsystems and as they establish, maintain, and terminate caring and curing relationships with individual clinicians and interdisciplinary health care teams.
- The set of clinical microsystems patients move through on their health care journey during an episode of illness, along with ancillary and supporting microsystems that contribute to the patient's care along the way, form a de facto mesosystem that can be analyzed and improved and that can be measured and redesigned to promote better performance.
- Research on specific clinical microsystems and on health systems that adopt a microsystem-smart and enterprise-wide change strategy, reveals the need for alignment and improvement of the health care enterprise at all levels of the system, beginning with leadership and ending with care provided to patients at the sharp end (the clinical microsystem).
- Sustainable improvement requires everyone to focus on better patient or population outcomes, better system performance, and better professional development.
- Real improvements-measured performance is often produced by successful adoption of generalizable scientific knowledge in particular local contexts.
- Although clinical systems are inherently complex they will usually have parts that are simple, parts that are complicated, and parts that are complex. Many problems within systems can be framed as simple, complicated, and complex.

## KEY TERMS

Anatomy model of a microsystem

Clinical microsystem

Clinical process models

Communities of practice

EHR

5Ps

Improvement equation

Macrosystem

Mesosystem

Microsystem

Minimum replicable units or smallest replicable units

$P_2I$

ProvenCare (SM)

Self-sealing cultures

Shared mental models

Sharp end

Simple, complicated, complex framework

STEEEP attributes of quality

Sustainable improvement triangle

Systems thinking

# REVIEW QUESTIONS

1. What are the different *levels* of a health care system? Can you describe a real health care system and point out micro, meso, and macro levels?
2. Think about a person who has a serious injury or illness and describe his or her health care journey. What clinical microsystems might she or he enter as a patient? What ancillary and supporting systems also contribute to care of the patient as his or her journey progresses?
3. What aspects of quality are described by the STEEEP mnemonic?
4. Examine the performance wheel. What are the important dimensions of a high performing clinical microsystem and how might these interact with one another?
5. What are some research findings and implications of the research for health care improvement?
6. What is meant by the term *value* of health care? What can be done to improve the value of care?

# DISCUSSION QUESTIONS

1. How might a clinical microsystem become a culture of entrapment? What are the risks of an entrapment culture, and how might these risks be mitigated?
2. Is it possible to have a system in the absence of a common aim or purpose? What is the aim of a health care system? Do patients and clinicians and health administrators have a shared aim?
3. What is meant by the statement that most health care systems are organized vertically but patients experience care horizontally? How might a health care system be organized to smooth the patient's horizontal flow while improving outcomes and decreasing costs?
4. What are the three corners of the sustainable improvement triangle? How might these be connected and made to interact with each other?

# REFERENCES

1. Morse, G. Health care needs a new kind of hero: An interview with Atul Gawande. *Harvard Business Review*, April 2010, pp. 1–2.
2. Batalden, P., Ogrinc, G., & Batalden, M. (2006). From one to many. *Journal of Interprofessional Care, 20*, 549–551.
3. Deming, W. E. *Out of crisis.* Cambridge: Massachusetts Institute of Technology, Center for Advanced Engineering Study, 1989.
4. White, K. L. *Healing the schism: Epidemiology, medicine, and the public's health.* New York: Springer-Verlag, 1991.
5. Donabedian, A. *The definition of quality and approaches to its assessment.* Ann Arbor, MI: Health Administration Press, 1980.
6. Quinn, J. *Intelligent enterprise: A knowledge and service based paradigm for enterprise.* New York: Free Press, 1992.
7. Henderson, L. Physician and patient as a social system. *The New England Journal of Medicine*, 1935, *212*(18), 819–823.

8. Lindblad, S., *personal communication*. Stockholm, Sweden, 2007.

9. Nelson, E., Batalden, P., & Godfrey, M. *Quality by design*. San Francisco: Jossey-Bass, 2007.

10. Zimmerman, B., Lindberg, C., & Plsek, P. *Edgeware: Insights from complexity science for health care leaders*. Irving, TX: VHA, 1998.

11. von Bertalanffy, K. L. *General system theory: Foundations, development, applications*. New York: George Braziller, 1968.

12. Homans, G. *The human group*. Harcourt, Brace, 1950.

13. Lewin, K. Frontiers in group dynamics. *Human Relations*, 1947, *1*, 5–41.

14. Deming, W. *The new economics for industry, government, education*. (2nd ed.) Cambridge: Massachusetts Institute of Technology, Center for Advanced Engineering Study, 2000, p. 50.

15. Senge, P. *The fifth discipline: The art and practice of the learning organization*. New York: Doubleday/Currency, 1990.

16. Wiener, E., & Nagel, D. C. (Eds.) *Human factors in aviation*. San Diego, CA: Academic Press, 1998.

17. Stacey, R. *Complexity and creativity in organizations*. San Francisco: Berrett-Koehler, 1996.

18. Plsek, P., & Greenhalgh, T. Complexity science: The challenge of complexity in health care. *British Medical Journal*, 2001, *323*(7313), 625–628.

19. Institute of Medicine. *Crossing the quality chasm: A new health system for the 21st century*. Washington, DC: Committee on Quality of Health Care, 2001, p. 4.

20. Berwick, D. (2001). *What hat is on?* Plenary address at the Institute for Health Care Improvement's 12th Annual National Forum, Orlando, FL, December 4, 2001.

21. Donaldson, M., & Mohr, J. *Exploring innovation and quality improvement in health care microsystems: A cross-case analysis*. Washington, DC: Institute of Medicine, 2000.

22. Nelson et al. Microsystems in health care: Part 1. Learning from high-performing front-line clinical units. *Joint Commission Journal on Quality and Patient Safety*, 2002, *28*(9), 472–493.

23. Weick, K. E., & Sutcliffe, K. M. Hospitals as cultures of entrapment: A re-analysis of the Bristol Royal Infirmary. *California Management Review*, 2003, *45*(2), 73–84.

24. Luan, D. M. *The influence of shared mental models of nosocomial bloodstream infections on neonatal intensive care unit infection rates*. Hanover, NH: The Dartmouth Institute of Health Policy and Clinical Practice, Dartmouth Medical School, Dartmouth College, 2009.

25. Edwards, W. H. Preventing nosocomial bloodstream infection in very low birth weight infants. *Seminars in Neonatology*, 2002, 7(4), 325–333.

26. Homa, K. *Evaluating the sustainability of a quality improvement initiative*. Unpublished PhD dissertation, The Dartmouth Institute of Health Policy and Clinical Practice, Dartmouth Medical School, Dartmouth College, 2006.

27. Golton, I., & Wilcock, P. *Clinical microsystems awareness and development programme. Final report*. London: NHS Modernisation Agency, 2005, p. 3.

28. Deming, W. E. *Quality, Productivity and Competitive Position*. MIT Center for Advanced Engineering Studies. Cambridge, MA. 1982.

29. Juran, J., Godfrey, A. B., Hoogstoel, R. E., & Schilling, E. G. *Juran's quality handbook*. (5th ed.) New York: McGraw Hill, 1999.

30. Casale et al. "ProvenCare": A provider-driven pay-for-performance program for acute episodic cardiac surgical care. *Annals of Surgery*, 2007, *246*(4), 613–623.

31. Bate, P., Mendel, P., & Robert, G. *Organizing for quality: The improvement journeys of major hospitals in Europe and the United States*. Abingdon, United Kingdom: Radcliffe Publishing, 2008.

32. Nelson, G., Batalden, P., & Lazar, J. *Practice-based learning and improvement: A clinical improvement action guide*. (2nd ed.) Oak Brook, IL: Joint Commission Resources, 2007, p. 3.

33. Batalden, P., & Davidoff, F. What is "quality improvement" and how can it transform healthcare? *Quality and Safety in Health Care*, 2007, *16*(2–3).

34. McGlynn et al. The quality of health care delivered to adults in the United States. *The New England Journal of Medicine*, 2003, *348*(26), 2635–2645.

35. Pawson, R., & Tilley, N. *Realistic evaluation.* London: Sage, 1997.

36. Glouberman, S., & Zimmerman, B. J. *Complicated and complex systems: What would successful reform of medicare look like?* Ottawa: Commission on the Future of Health Care in Canada, 2002.

37. Liu, S., Homa, K., Butterly, J., Kirkland, K., & Batalden, P. Improving the simple, complicated and complex realities of community-acquired pneumonia. *Quality and Safety in Health Care*, 2009, *18*, 93–98.

The action guides that follow each chapter are designed to offer additional resources, insights, and tools to support and encourage your study of clinical microsystems. Each chapter action guide is designed to complement the chapter content to further advance your skills and abilities to design value into all aspects of care.

## INTRODUCTION TO THE 5PS

Strategic focus on microsystems (the small, functional frontline units that provide most health care to most people) is essential to designing efficient population-based care and services. To begin to increase self-awareness and to assess or diagnose the unique features of any microsystem, use the 5Ps framework. The 5Ps framework can be thought of as a structured and organized method of inquiring into the anatomy of a clinical microsystem. Every complex adaptive system has structure, process, patterns, and outcomes. You can make these features more explicit and analyze them by using the 5Ps framework in your clinical microsystem. The 5Ps framework can help you gain deeper knowledge to inform specific improvement activities rather than make decisions based on intuitive perspectives alone to improve care and services.

## THE CLINICAL MICROSYSTEM PROCESS AND STRUCTURE OF THE 5PS MODEL

The 5Ps framework can be seen within the anatomy of a clinical microsystem as shown in Figure AG1.1. The study of the purpose, patients, professionals, processes, and patterns of any clinical microsystem provides deep insights and perspectives most busy health care professionals do not usually see or understand in their daily work. This knowledge and information comes from both formal analysis and tacit understanding of the clinical microsystem's structure, patients, processes, and its daily patterns of work and interaction.

The 5Ps framework supports understanding of the (1) needs of the major patient subpopulations served by the clinical microsystem, (2) ways the professionals in the microsystem interact with one another, and (3) the ways professionals in the microsystem interact with the processes that unfold to produce critical outcomes.

Deep understanding of the 5Ps framework begins with an interdisciplinary group representing the various clinical microsystem roles exploring the individual "Ps" by answering the following questions.

FIGURE AG1.1   Microsystem Anatomy Model.

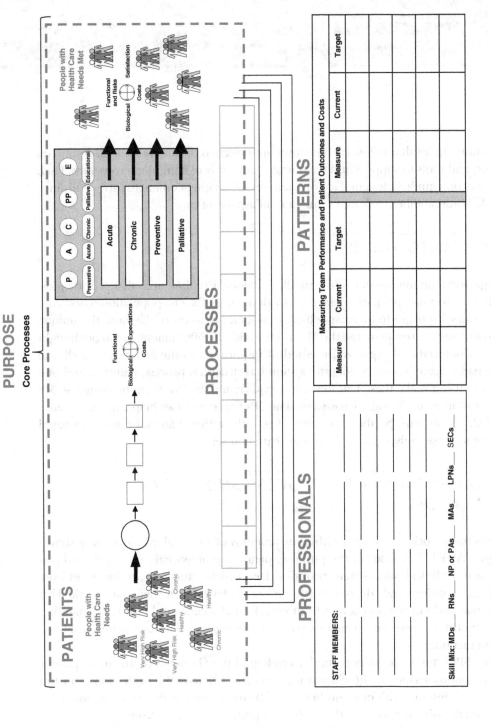

*Know your purpose:* What is our aim? What do we actually intend to make? Fill in this answer: Our system exists to _____. Remember this purpose exists within the context of the population the clinical microsystem seeks to serve.

*Know your patients:* Whom are we caring for? Are there subpopulations we could plan services for differently? What are the most common patient diagnoses and conditions in our care setting? What other microsystems support what we do to meet patients' needs? How satisfied are patients with our clinical microsystem?

*Know your professionals:* Who provides patient care and who are the people supporting the clinical care team? What skills and talents do staff members need to provide the right service and care at the right time? What is the staff morale? What is the role of information technology as a team member?

*Know your processes:* How do we deliver care and services to meet our patients' needs? Who does what in our clinical microsystem? Do our hours of operation match the needs of our patients? What are our core and supporting processes? How does technology support our processes? How do we learn from failures and near misses?

*Know your patterns:* What are the health outcomes of our patients? What are the costs of care? How do we interact within our clinical microsystem? What are the regularly recurring associated or sequential work activities? What does it feel like to work here? How often do we meet to discuss quality and safety in the clinical microsystem? What is leadership like? What traditions and rituals do we have?

When members of the clinical microsystem work together to gain information about their 5Ps, they acquire knowledge and insights that can be used to make long-lasting improvements in the clinical microsystem.

The series of *Assess, Diagnose and Treat* workbooks, otherwise known as the *Greenbooks,* provide the path forward to guide study of the clinical microsystem anatomy and can be found at www.clinicalmicrosystem.org. Each Greenbook offers facts, figures, tools, and questions to consider for each of the 5Ps. The workbook series is intended to offer introductory material and so does not provide an exhaustive list of measures and information. Rather, the data and exploration often stimulate new conversations for those in the clinical microsystem. New perspectives and new insights can lead to new questions and considerations for a rich interdisciplinary conversation.

It is essential in this exploration to attempt to seek measures even if we feel we "just can't get that data here." Measurement and information about patients, professionals, processes, or patterns may not be regularly collected or monitored. Through the use of the many tools and forms in the Greenbooks you can document measures and data through sampling to gain deeper insight into your clinical microsystem. Health care organizations and clinical microsystems historically document and capture financial data and information and have not had the systems or habits to document process information at the clinical microsystem level. Seeking measurement and information about the 5Ps will enhance overall knowledge of the system of care. If the measures shed light on the patterns of population or professional behaviors or helps describe the process of care more deeply, then it is worth pursuing.

It is important to review the Greenbook workbooks and profiles to determine which measures can be easily obtained from your organization before deciding to use the various tools and forms in the Greenbook. The profiles in each Greenbook provide a high-level view and summary of the clinical microsystem 5Ps. Several profiles can be seen in Figures AG1.2, AG1.3, and AG1.4. Increasingly, organizations are collecting many of these previously undocumented measurements and they may be available to the microsystem to help inform action plans and improvements. Examples include

## FIGURE AG1.2   Primary Care Profile.

# Primary Care Practice Profile

**A. Purpose/Aim of Our Clinical Microsystem:** Why does your practice exist?

| Site Name: | Site Contact: | Date: |
|---|---|---|
| Practice Manager: | MD Lead: | Nurse Lead: |

**B. Know Your Patients:** Take a close look into your practice, create a "high-level" picture of the PATIENT POPULATION that you serve. Who are they? What resources do they use? How do the patients view the care they receive?

| Estimated Age Distribution of Patients: | % | List Your Top Ten Diagnoses/Conditions | | Top Referrals (e.g., GI Cardiology) | Patient Satisfaction Scores | | % Excellent |
|---|---|---|---|---|---|---|---|
| Birth–10 years | | 1. | 6. | | Experience via phone | | |
| 11–18 years | | 2. | 7. | | Length of time to get your appointment | | |
| 19–45 years | | 3. | 8. | | Saw who patient wanted to see | | |
| 46–64 years | | 4. | 9. | | Satisfaction with personal manner | | |
| 65–79 years | | 5. | 10. | | Time spent with person today | | |
| 80+ years | | Patients who are frequent users of your practice and their reasons for seeking frequent interactions and visits | Other clinical microsystems you interact with regularly as you provide care for patients (e.g., OR, VNA) | | Patient Population Census: Do these numbers change by season?(Y/N) | # | Y/N |
| % Females | | | | | Patients seen in a day | | |
| Estimated # (unique) Patients in Practice | | | | | Patients seen in last week | | |
| Disease-Specific Health Outcomes | | | | | New patients in last month | | |
| | | | | | Disenrolling patients in last month | | |
| Diabetes HgA1c = | | | | | Encounters per provider per year | | |
| Hypertension B/P = | | | | | **Out of Practice Visits** | | |
| LDL < 100 = | | | | | Condition Sensitive Hospital Rate | | |
| | | | | | Emergency Room Visit Rate | | |

### *Complete "Through the Eyes of Your Patient"

**C. Know Your Professionals:** Use the following template to create a comprehensive picture of your practice. Who does what and when? Is the right person doing the right activity? Are roles being optimized? Are all roles who contribute to the patient experience listed? What hours are you open for business? How many and what is the duration of your appointment types? How many exam rooms do you currently have? What is the morale of your staff?

| Current Staff | FTEs | Comment/ Function | 3 Next Available | | Cycle Time | Days of Operation | Hours |
|---|---|---|---|---|---|---|---|
| Enter names below totals Use separate sheet if needed | | | PE | Follow-up | Range | Monday | |
| | | | | | | Tuesday | |
| MD Total | | | | | | Wednesday | |
| | | | | | | Thursday | |
| | | | | | | Friday | |
| | | | | | | Saturday | |
| NP/PAs Total | | | | | | Sunday | |

Do you offer the following? Check all that apply.

- ☐ Group Visit
- ☐ E-mail
- ☐ Web site
- ☐ RN Clinics
- ☐ Phone Follow-up
- ☐ Phone Care Management
- ☐ Disease Registries
- ☐ Protocols/Guidelines

| Current Staff | FTEs | Comment/ Function | | | |
|---|---|---|---|---|---|
| RNs Total | | | | | |
| LPNs Total | | | | | |
| LNA/MAs Total | | | | | |
| Secretaries Total | | | | | |
| Others: | | | | | |

| Appointment Type | Duration | Comment: |
|---|---|---|
| | | |

| Staff Satisfaction Scores | | % |
|---|---|---|
| How stressful is the practice? | % Not Satisfied | |
| Would you recommend it as a good place to work? | % Strongly Agree | |

Do you use Float Pool? ____ Yes ____ No
Do you use On-Call? ____ Yes ____ No

### *Each staff member should complete the Personal Skills Assessment and "The Activity Survey"

**D. Know Your Processes:** How do things get done in the microsystem? Who does what? What are the step-by-step processes? How long does the care process take? Where are the delays? What are the "between" microsystems handoffs?

1. **Track cycle time for patients from the time they check in until they leave the office using the Patient Cycle Time Tool. List ranges of time per provider on this table**
2. **Complete the Core and Supporting Process Assessment Tool**

**E. Know Your Patterns:** What patterns are present but not acknowledged in your microsystem? What is the leadership and social pattern? How often does the microsystem meet to discuss patient care? Are patients and families involved? What are your results and outcomes?

| | | |
|---|---|---|
| • Does every member of the practice meet regularly as a team? | • Do the members of the practice regularly review and discuss safety and reliability issues? | • What have you successfully changed? |
| • How frequently? | | • What are you most proud of? |
| | | • What is your financial picture? |
| • What is the most significant pattern of variation? | | **\*Complete "Metrics That Matter"** |

FIGURE AG1.3   Specialty Care Profile.

## Specialty Care Practice Profile

**A. Purpose/Aim:** Why does your practice exist?

| | | |
|---|---|---|
| Site Name: | Site Contact: | Date: |
| Practice Manager: | MD Lead: | Nurse Lead: |

**B. Know Your Patients:** Take a close look into your practice, create a "high-level" picture of the PATIENT POPULATION that you serve. Who are they? What resources do they use? How do the patients view the care they receive?

| Estimated Age Distribution of Patients: | % | List Your Top Five Diagnoses | List Your Top Five Procedures | Patient Satisfaction Scores | % Excellent |
|---|---|---|---|---|---|
| Birth–10 years | | 1. | 1. | Experience via phone | |
| 11–18 years | | 2. | 2. | Length of time to get your appointment | |
| 19–45 years | | 3. | 3. | Saw who patient wanted to see | |
| 46–64 years | | 4. | 4. | Satisfaction with personal manner | |
| 65–79 years | | 5. | 5. | Time spent with person today | |
| 80+ years | | | | | |

| % Females | List Your Top Five Referrers | | Patient Population Census: Do these numbers change by season? (Y/N) | # | Y/N |
|---|---|---|---|---|---|
| | Referrer | What are they referring? | | | |
| **Health Outcomes** | | | Patients seen in a day | | |
| | | | Patients seen in last week | | |
| | | | New patients in last month | | |
| | | | Encounters per provider per year | **Out/IN** | |
| | | | Same Day Procedures | | |
| | Emergency Room Visit Rate | | Inpatient Procedures | | |
| | | | In-Clinic Procedures | | |
| | | | Specialty Yield Rate | | |

### *Complete "Through the Eyes of Your Patient"

**C. Know Your Professionals:** Create a comprehensive picture of your practice. Who does what and when? Is the right person doing the right activity? Are roles being optimized? Are all roles who contribute to the patient experience listed? What hours are you open for business? How many and what is the duration of your appointment types? How many exam rooms do you currently have? What is the morale of your staff?

| Current Staff | FTEs | Days/Hours | | | | | | 3 Next Available | | | | Cycle Time | Do you offer any of the following? Check all that apply. |
|---|---|---|---|---|---|---|---|---|---|---|---|---|---|
| | | M | T | W | TH | F | S | New | F/U | OR | Minor | Range | |
| MD Total | | | | | | | | | | | | | Group Visit |
| | | | | | | | | | | | | | E-mail |
| | | | | | | | | | | | | | Web site |
| | | | | | | | | | | | | | RN Clinics |
| NP/PAs Total | | | | | | | | | | | | | Phone Follow-up |
| | | | | | | | | | | | | | Phone Care Management |
| | | | | | | | | | | | | | Registries |
| | | | | | | | | | | | | | Protocols/Guidelines |
| RNs Total | | | | | | | | | | | | | **# Exam Rooms** _____ |
| | | | | | | | | | | | | | **# Minor Rooms** _____ |
| LPNs Total | | | | | | | | | | | | | Supporting diagnostic departments (e.g., respiratory, lab, cardio.) |

| LNA/MAs Total | | | | | | | | | | | | Appt. Type | Duration | Comment |
|---|---|---|---|---|---|---|---|---|---|---|---|---|---|---|
| | | | | | | | | | | | | New Patient | | |
| Others Total | | | | | | | | | | | | Follow-up | | |
| | | | | | | | | | | | | Minor | | |

| | | Staff Satisfaction Scores | | % |
|---|---|---|---|---|
| Secretaries Total | | How stressful is the practice? | % Not Satisfied | |
| Do you use Float Pool? ____ Yes ____ No | | Would you recommend it as a good place to work? | % Strongly Agree | |
| Do you use On-Call? ____ Yes ____ No | | | | |

### *Each staff member should complete the Personal Skills Assessment and "The Activity Survey"

**D. Know Your Processes:** How do things get done in the microsystem? Who does what? What are the step-by-step processes? How long does the care process take? Where are the delays? What are the "between" microsystems handoffs?

1. Track cycle time for patients from the time they check in until they leave the office using the Patient Cycle Time Tool. List ranges of time per provider on this table

2. Complete the Core and Supporting Process Assessment Tool

**E. Know Your Patterns:** What patterns are present but not acknowledged in your microsystem? What is the leadership and social pattern? How often does the microsystem meet to discuss patient care? Are patients and families involved? What are your results and outcomes?

| | | |
|---|---|---|
| • Does every member of the practice meet regularly as a team? | • Do the members of the practice regularly review and discuss safety and reliability issues? | • What have you successfully changed? |
| • How frequently? | | • What are you most proud of? |
| | | • What is your financial picture? |
| • What is the most significant pattern of variation? | | **\*Complete "Metrics That Matter"** |

**FIGURE AG1.4   Inpatient Profile.**

## Inpatient Unit Profile

**A. Purpose/Aim:** Why does your unit exist?

| Site Name: | Site Contact: | Date: |
|---|---|---|
| Administrative Director: | Nurse Director: | Medical Director: |

**B. Know Your Patients:** Take a close look into your unit, create a "high-level" picture of the PATIENT POPULATION that you serve. Who are they? What resources do they use? How do the patients view the care they receive?

| Estimated Age Distribution of Patients: | % |
|---|---|
| 19–50 years | |
| 51–65 years | |
| 66–75 years | |
| 76+ years | |
| % Females | |

| List Your Top Ten Diagnoses/Conditions | |
|---|---|
| 1. | 6. |
| 2. | 7. |
| 3. | 8. |
| 4. | 9. |
| 5. | 10. |

| Patient Satisfaction Scores | % Always |
|---|---|
| Nurses | |
| Doctors | |
| Environment | |
| Pain | |
| Discharge | % Yes |
| Overall | % Excellent |

| Living Situation | % |
|---|---|
| Married | |
| Domestic Partner | |
| Live Alone | |
| Live with Others | |
| Skilled Nursing Facility | |
| Nursing Home | |
| Homeless | |

| Point of Entry | % |
|---|---|
| Admissions | |
| Clinic | |
| ED | |
| Transfer | |
| **Discharge Disposition** | **%** |
| Home | |
| Home with Visiting Nurse | |
| Skilled Nursing Facility | |
| Other Hospital | |
| Rehab Facility | |
| Transfer to ICU | |

| Patient Population Census: Do these numbers change by season? (Y/N) | Y/N |
|---|---|
| Patient Census by Hour | |
| Patient Census by Day | |
| Patient Census by Week | |
| Patient Census by Year | |
| Thirty Day Readmit Rate | |
| Our patients in Other Units | |
| Off Service Patients on Our Unit | |
| Frequency of Inability to Admit Patient | |

| Patient Type | LOS Average | Range |
|---|---|---|
| Medical | | |
| Surgical | | |
| **Mortality Rate** | | |

### *Complete "Through the Eyes of Your Patient"

**C. Know Your Professionals:** Use the following template to create a comprehensive picture of your unit. Who does what and when? Is the right person doing the right activity? Are roles being optimized? Are all roles who contribute to the patient experience listed?

| Current Staff | Day FTEs | Evening FTEs | Night FTEs | Weekend FTEs | Over-Time by Role |
|---|---|---|---|---|---|
| MD Total | | | | | |
| Hospitalists Total | | | | | |
| Unit Leader Total | | | | | |
| CNSs Total | | | | | |
| RNs Total | | | | | |
| LPNs Total | | | | | |
| LNAs Total | | | | | |
| Residents Total | | | | | |
| Technicians Total | | | | | |
| Secretaries Total | | | | | |
| Clinical Resource Coord. | | | | | |
| Social Worker | | | | | |
| Health Service Assts. | | | | | |
| Ancillary Staff | | | | | |

| Admitting Medical Service | % |
|---|---|
| Internal Medicine | |
| Hematology/Oncology | |
| Pulmonary | |
| Family Practice | |
| ICU | |
| Other | |

| Supporting Diagnostic Departments |
|---|
| (e.g., Respiratory, Lab, Cardiology, Pulmonary, Radiology) |

| | | | |
|---|---|---|---|
| Do you use Per Diems? | _____Yes | _____NO | |
| Do you use Travelers? | _____Yes | _____NO | |
| Do you use On-Call Staff? | _____Yes | _____NO | |
| Do you use a Float Pool? | _____Yes | _____NO | |

| Staff Satisfaction Scores | | % |
|---|---|---|
| How stressful is the unit? | % Not Satisfied | |
| Would you recommend it as a good place to work? | % Strongly Agree | |

### *Each staff member should complete the Personal Skills Assessment and "The Activity Survey"

**D. Know Your Processes:** How do things get done in the microsystem? Who does what? What are the step-by-step processes? How long does the care process take? Where are the delays? What are the "between" microsystems handoffs?

**1. Create flow charts of routine processes.**

- a) Overall admission and treatment process
- b) Admit to inpatient unit
- c) Usual inpatient care
- d) Change of shift process
- e) Discharge process
- f) Transfer to another facility process
- g) Medication Administration
- h) Adverse event

**Do you use/initiate any of the following?**
Check all that apply
- ☐ Standing Orders/Critical Pathways
- ☐ Rapid Response Team
- ☐ Bed Management Rounds
- ☐ Multidisciplinary/with Family Rounds
- ☐ Midnight Rounds
- ☐ Preceptor/Charge Role
- ☐ Discharge Goals

**Capacity**   # Rooms _____   # Beds_____

**# Turnovers/Bed/Year _____**

**Linking Microsystems** (e.g., ER, ICU, Skilled Nursing Facility )

**2. Complete the Core and Supporting Process Assessment Tool**

**E. Know Your Patterns:** What patterns are present but not acknowledged in your microsystem? What is the leadership and social pattern? How often does the microsystem meet to discuss patient care? Are patients and families involved? What are your results and outcomes?

- Does every member of the unit meet regularly as a team?
- How frequently?
- What is the most significant pattern of variation?

- Do the members of the unit regularly review and discuss safety and reliability issues?

- What have you successfully changed?
- What are you most proud of?
- What is your financial picture?

### *Complete "Metrics That Matter"

patient satisfaction data at the clinical microsystem level or cycle time measure of an office visit.

Key to all the data and information exploration is obtaining recent data because many aspects of the microsystem and organization change over time.

It is often helpful to print the poster-size 5Ps map found at www.clinicalmicrosystem.org to post the 5Ps data on a wall to create a big-picture view of your clinical microsystem. This poster display also serves as a teaching aid to engage other interdisciplinary members of your microsystem in learning more about your system of care. Some examples of how the 5Ps have informed microsystem improvement efforts are noted in Table AG1.1.

Increasingly, organizations are engaging supporting microsystems to improve their awareness of their purpose, patients or customers, professionals, processes, and patterns. A few examples of supporting microsystems include the following: dietary, respiratory, laboratory, radiology, ultrasound, medical records, environmental services and admissions. The method of assessment is similar to the process used to assess a clinical microsystem, but it has been adapted for the supporting microsystem focus. The goal is to provide services to patients so patients are kept in the 5Ps, and customers are added to reflect the dual beneficiaries of the supporting microsystem. Table AG1.2 provides an example of a few supporting microsystems, such as laboratories, environmental services, and admissions. It also provides examples of some of the "Ps" to be considered.

## EXTERNAL MAPPING TOOL

The external mapping tool (Figure AG1.5) identifies resources outside the clinical microsystem. The tool demonstrates the abundance of resources the microsystem can explore and helps identify relationships (or those that may benefit from additional attention) to attain the best results for patients and families.

Use the blank external mapping tool to increase awareness of current state and potential relationships to build your system to achieve optimal patient or population outcomes. Instructions for using the mapping tool follow.

1. Name the clinical microsystem under study.
2. Identify the subpopulation of patients to focus on and identify resources.
3. List the specific health care needs of the identified subpopulation of patients.
4. Identify the external *contributors* who are in the best position to optimize care for the population. Document the information in each box around the microsystem. Add boxes as you identify additional resources.
5. Based on the patient view, circle the names of the most valued contributors.
6. Circle the most important contributor rectangles.
7. Identify the relationships or *connections* between the clinical microsystem and the contributors.
   a. Illustrate the relationships with a blue line.
   b. Where there is a dominant flow of information between the microsystem and the contributor, indicate this with an arrowhead in the direction of the flow.
   c. When there is an opportunity to improve the connection, make the connecting lines red.
8. Based on this assessment, identify improvement opportunities to enhance patient or population care and outcomes.

Table AG1.1   Assessing Your Practice Discoveries and Actions: The 5Ps

| Know Your Patients | Discoveries | Actions Taken |
|---|---|---|
| 1. Age distribution | About 30% of our patients are greater than 66 years old. | Team designed special group visits to review specific needs of this age group, including physical limitations and dietary considerations. |
| 2. Disease identification | We do not know what percentage of our patients have diabetes. | Team reviewed coding and billing data to determine approximate numbers of patients with diabetes. |
| 3. Health outcomes | Do not know what the range of HbA1c is for our patients with diabetes, or if they are receiving appropriate ADA-recommended care in a timely fashion. | Team conducted a chart audit with 50 charts during a lunch hour. Using a tool designed to track outcomes, each member of the team reviewed 5 charts and noted the finding on the audit tool. |
| 4. Most frequent diagnosis | We had a large number of patients with stable hypertension and diabetes seeing the physician frequently. We also learned that during certain seasons we had huge volumes of pharyngitis and poison ivy. | Designed and tested a new model of care delivery for stable hypertension and diabetes, optimizing the RN role in the practice using agreed-upon guidelines, protocols, and tools. |
| 5. Patient satisfaction | We don't know what patients think unless they complain to us. | Implemented the point-of-service patient survey, which patients completed and left in a box before leaving the practice. |
| **Know Your Professionals** | **Discoveries** | **Actions Taken** |
| 1. Provider FTE | We were making assumptions about provider time in the clinic without really understanding how much time providers are out of the clinic with hospital rounds, nursing home rounds, and so on. | Changed our scheduling process and used RNs to provide care for certain subpopulations. |
| 2. Schedules | Several providers are gone at the same time every week, so one provider is often left and the entire staff works overtime that day. | Evaluated the scheduling template to even out each provider's time to provide consistent coverage in the clinic. |
| 3. Regular meetings | The doctors meet together every other week. The secretaries meet once a month. | Began holding entire practice meeting every other week on Wednesdays to help the practice become a team. |
| 4. Hours of operation | The beginning and the end of the day are always chaotic. We realized we are on the route for patients between home and work, and they want to be seen when we are not open. | Opened one hour earlier and stayed open one hour later each day. The heavy demand was better managed and overtime dropped. |
| 5. Activity surveys | All roles are not being used to their maximum. RNs only room patients and take vital signs, medical assistants do a great deal of secretarial paperwork, and some secretaries are giving out medical advice. | Roles have been redesigned and matched to individual education, training, and licensure. |

Table AG1.1    Assessing Your Practice Discoveries and Actions: The 5Ps (Continued)

| Know Your Processes | Discoveries | Actions Taken |
|---|---|---|
| 1. Cycle time | Patient lengths of visits vary a great deal; there are many delays. | The team identified actions to eliminate and steps to combine; they learned to prepare the charts for the patient visit before the patient arrives. The team now holds daily huddles to inform everyone on the plan of the day and to review relevant issues. |
| 2. Key supporting processes | None of us could agree on how things get done in our practice. | We created a detailed flowchart of our practice to determine how to streamline and to do so in a consistent manner. |
| 3. Indirect patient pulls | The providers are interrupted in their patient care process frequently. The number one reason is to retrieve missing equipment and supplies from the exam room. | Based on the variation of demand for the practice care and services, a critical review of the staff scheduling was conducted to determine if there was matching of available staff to the varied demands by session of the day and day of the week. Through difficult discussion and review of the purpose of the practice, new schedules were negotiated and tested to better meet patient demand. The new staff schedules for all professionals were more evenly matched to the demand of patients resulting in less stress and volume overload than the group had previously experienced. Patients expressed higher satisfaction. |
| Know Your Patterns | Discoveries | Actions Taken |
| 1. Demand on the practice | There are peaks and lows for the practice, depending on day of the week, session of the day, or season of the year. | The team identified actions to eliminate and steps to combine, and learned to prepare charts for the patient visit before the patient arrives. The team now holds daily huddles to inform everyone on the plan of the day and to review relevant issues. |
| 2. Communication | We do not communicate in a timely way, nor do we have a standard forum in which to communicate. | Every other week practice meetings are held to help communication and e-mail use by all staff and to promote timely communication. |
| 3. Cultural | The doctors don't really spend time with nondoctors. | The team meetings and heightened awareness of behaviors have helped improve this. |
| 4. Outcomes | We really have not paid attention to our practice outcomes. | We began tracking and posting results on a data wall to keep us alert to outcomes. |
| 5. Finances | Only the doctors and the practice manager know about the practice money. | Finances are discussed at team meetings and everyone is learning how to make a difference in financial performance. |

*Note:* HbA1c = glycosylated hemoglobin; ADA = American Diabetes Association; URI = upper respiratory infection.

Table AG1.2  Supporting Microsystem 5Ps

| Supporting Microsystem | Purpose | Patients or Customers | Professionals | Process | Patterns |
|---|---|---|---|---|---|
| Laboratory | The laboratory exists to provide all aspects of testing and reporting of necessary diagnostic studies to support delivery of patient care. | Outpatients, inpatients, providers, external organizations with referred diagnostic studies | Laboratory technicians, secretaries, phlebotomists | Obtaining specimens, accessioning specimens, conducting tests, reporting results | Errors in accessioning, delays in reporting, frequency of overall laboratory meetings to discuss safety and processes, communication between laboratory departments |
| Environmental Services | Environmental services exist to create the cleanest environment that supports patient care in all settings of the organization. | Patients, staff, vendors, patient units, families, all visitors to the organization | Environmental technicians, housekeepers | Maintaining organization and microsystem hygiene and appearance; maintaining microsystem-specific activities such as cleaning beds and changing linens to support admission and transfer processes | High-volume bed turnover areas, time from patient discharge to cleaned bed, frequency of standard cleaning of public areas, communication processes for all staff, number of falls related to wet surfaces, frequency of meetings to discuss safety and improvement |
| Admissions | Admissions exist to support the patient and family in their interaction with the organization through admission, transfer, and discharge. | Patients, families, providers, patient units, emergency departments (ED), all inpatient and outpatient diagnostic departments, referring organizations, insurance companies | Admission clerks, registration clerks | Preregistration of patients prior to procedures and admissions, real-time registration of patients in ED and unplanned admissions, coordinating patient placement for admissions and transfers, registration of advance directives | Number of admissions per day per unit, frequency of missing information on admission documentation, percentage of patients with advance directives, communication processes with key contacts in organization facilitating admissions and transfers, frequency of all admission staff meetings to discuss improvement |

**FIGURE AG1.5  External Mapping Tool.**

Exploring the external context of the clinical microsystem for improving the health of a given subpopulation of patients

1. Clinical microsystem name: _____

2. Subpopulation of patients: _____

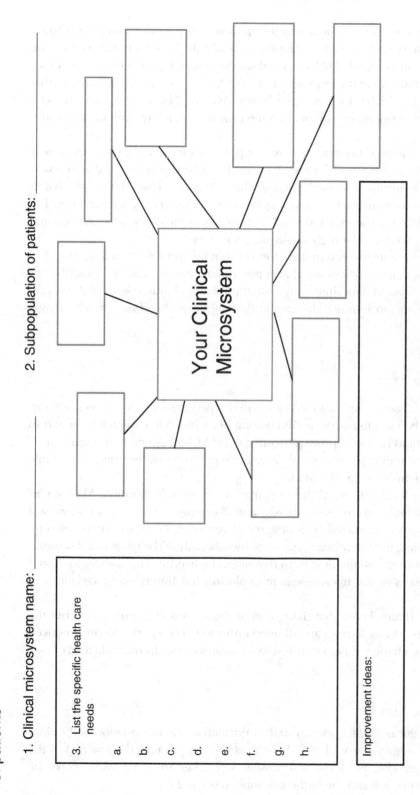

3. List the specific health care needs

a.

b.

c.

d.

e.

f.

g.

h.

Improvement ideas:

Circle the most important contributor rectangles. Illustrate the relationships with a blue line. Add an arrowhead if the direction of the relationship is clear. If the relationship can be significantly improved, use red for the line.

*Source:* © February 10, 2003 Ruth Kennedy, NHS, UK/MM Godfrey, Trustees of Dartmouth College. Revised March 23, 2004.

# MICROSYSTEM ASSESSMENT TOOL (MAT)

The clinical microsystem relies on a systems approach to provide clinical care based on theories from organizational development, leadership, and improvement. The Microsystem Assessment Tool (MAT) is based on the original qualitative research conducted at Dartmouth where the ten *success characteristics* were identified in practices that provide high-quality, high-value care (see Figure AG1.6). The success characteristics reflect what people working in high performing practices say about their work and also how they work.

The MAT can be used to assess the baseline performance of a clinical microsystem before starting the improvement journey. The MAT can be readministered after a year to determine advancement toward success characteristics. This qualitative tool is intended to provoke conversation and inquiry based on success characteristics. For example, one might use the tool and ask, "What does this mean for my microsystem?" "How might we work toward a high performing scenario?"

Many improvements succeed in the short run but fail to be sustained or spread to other areas. Sometimes practices are challenged by barriers that are best described as constraints on the system. Working to improve the specific characteristics of the microsystem will allow you to improve the system that supports the clinical work in your microsystem.

## Description and Use of MAT

The Microsystem Assessment Tool (MAT) was developed from the ten success characteristics and can be used to assess the functioning of an individual microsystem and to help staff understand how to improve performance. MAT is designed to be used quickly and easily by clinical microsystem members to evaluate their own frontline unit. Table AG1.3 provides definitions for the MAT.

Based on the local context of the organization, many will distribute MAT via an electronic survey tool such as *Survey Monkey* and *Zoomerang*. Other organizations will use hard copy surveys tabulated by a designated resource. Once the survey is completed and reported, the interdisciplinary team members should engage in a discussion specific to the findings and the next steps that might be fruitful. The discussion should involve all members of the microsystem in exploring the findings and variations in the results.

It should be remembered that fixing one of the success characteristics is not the ultimate goal. The characteristics are all interconnected. The special blend produced by combining the characteristics often results in improvement in multiple areas.

## Guidelines for Scoring with MAT

There are 12 categories (3 categories are in the Information and Information Technology section). Each category is scored as 0, 1, or 2, where 0 represents the low end of the spectrum, 1 the middle, and 2 the best possible score. For an overall MAT score, the lowest possible score is 0 and the highest possible score is 24.

Table AG1.4 is an example of a worksheet to tally the responses to the MAT.

FIGURE AG1.6  Microsystem Assessment Tool.

## Microsystem Assessment Tool

Instructions: Each of the success characteristics (as, leadership) is followed by a series of three descriptions. For each characteristic, *please* **_check_** the description that **_best describes_** your current microsystem and the care it delivers OR use a microsystem you are MOST familiar with.

| | Characteristic and Definition | | Descriptions | | |
|---|---|---|---|---|---|
| **Leadership** | **1. Leadership:** The role of leaders is to balance setting and reaching collective goals, and to empower individual autonomy and accountability through building knowledge, respectful action, reviewing and reflecting. | ☐ Leaders often tell me how to do my job and leave little room for innovation and autonomy. Overall, they don't foster a positive culture. | ☐ Leaders struggle to find the right balance between reaching performance goals and supporting and empowering the staff. | ☐ Leaders maintain constancy of purpose, establish clear goals and expectations, and foster a respectful positive culture. Leaders take time to build knowledge, review and reflect, and take action about microsystems and the larger organization. | ☐ Can't Rate |
| | **2. Organizational Support:** The larger organization looks for ways to support the work of the microsystem and coordinate the hand-offs between microsystems. | ☐ The larger organization isn't supportive in a way that provides recognition, information, and resources to enhance my work. | ☐ The larger organization is inconsistent and unpredictable in providing the recognition, information, and resources needed to enhance my work. | ☐ The larger organization provides recognition, information, and resources to enhance my work and makes it easier for me to meet the needs of patients. | ☐ Can't Rate |
| **Staff** | **3. Staff Focus:** There is selective hiring of the right kind of people. The orientation process is designed to fully integrate new staff into culture and work roles. Expectations of staff are high regarding performance, continuing education, professional growth, and networking. | ☐ I am not made to feel like a valued member of the microsystem. My orientation was incomplete. My continuing education and professional growth are not being met. | ☐ I feel like I am a valued member of the microsystem, but I don't think the microsystem is doing all that it could to support education and training of staff, workload, and professional growth. | ☐ I am a valued member of the microsystem and what I say matters. This is evident through staffing, education and training, workload, and professional growth. | ☐ Can't Rate |
| | **4. Education and Training:** All clinical microsystems have responsibility for the ongoing education and training of staff and for aligning daily work roles with training competencies. Academic clinical microsystems have the additional responsibility of training students. | ☐ Training is accomplished in disciplinary silos, as nurses train nurses, physicians train residents. The educational efforts are not aligned with the flow of patient care, so that education becomes an "add-on" to what we do. | ☐ We recognize our training could be different to reflect the needs of our microsystem, but we haven't made many changes yet. Some continuing education is available to everyone. | ☐ There is a team approach to training, whether we are training staff, nurses, or students. Education and patient care are integrated into the flow of work in a way that benefits both from the available resources. Continuing education for all staff is recognized as vital to our continued success. | ☐ Can't Rate |
| | **5. Interdependence:** The interaction of staff is characterized by trust, collaboration, willingness to help each other, appreciation of complementary roles, respect, and recognition that all contribute individually to a shared purpose. | ☐ I work independently and I am responsible for my own part of the work. There is a lack of collaboration and a lack of appreciation for the importance of complementary roles. | ☐ The care approach is interdisciplinary, but we are not always able to work together as an effective team. | ☐ Care is provided by an interdisciplinary team characterized by trust, collaboration, appreciation of complementary roles, and recognition that all contribute individually to a shared purpose. | ☐ Can't Rate |
| **Patients** | **6. Patient Focus:** The primary concern is to meet all patient needs – caring, listening, educating, and responding to special requests, innovating to meet patient needs, and smooth service flow. | ☐ Most of us, including our patients, would agree that we do not always provide patient-centered care. We are not always clear about what patients want and need. | ☐ We are actively working to provide patient-centered care and we are making progress toward more effectively and consistently learning about and meeting patient needs. | ☐ We are effective in learning about and meeting patient needs – caring, listening, educating, and responding to special requests, and smooth service flow. | ☐ Can't Rate |

*Source:* © Julie K. Johnson, MSPH, PhD.

## Microsystem Assessment Tool (continued)

| | Characteristic | Definitions | | |
|---|---|---|---|---|
| **Patients** | **7. Community and Market Focus:** The microsystem is a resource for the community; the community is a resource for the microsystem; the microsystem establishes excellent and innovative relationships with the community. | ☐ We focus on the patients who come to our unit. We haven't implemented any outreach programs in our community. Patients and their families often make their own connections to the community resources they need. | ☐ We have tried a few outreach programs and have had some success, but it is not the norm for us to go out into the community or actively connect patients to the community resources that are available to them. | ☐ We are doing everything we can to understand our community. We actively employ resources to help us work with the community. We add to the community and we draw on resources from the community to meet patient needs.<br><br>☐ Can't Rate |
| **Performance** | **8. Performance Results:** Performance focuses on patient outcomes, avoidable costs, streamlining delivery, using data feedback, promoting positive competition, and frank discussions about performance. | ☐ We don't routinely collect data on the process of outcomes of the care we provide. | ☐ We often collect data on outcomes of the care we provide and on some processes of care. | ☐ Outcomes (clinical, satisfaction, financial, technical, safety) are routinely measured, we feed data back to staff, and we make changes based on data.<br><br>☐ Can't Rate |
| | **9. Process Improvement:** An atmosphere for learning and redesign is supported by the continuous monitoring of care, use of benchmarking, frequent tests of change, and a staff that has been empowered to innovate. | ☐ The resources required (in the form of training, financial support, and time) are rarely available to support improvement work. Any improvement activities we do are in addition to our daily work. | ☐ Some resources are available to support improvement work, but we don't use them as often as we could. Change ideas are implemented without much discipline. | ☐ There are ample resources to support continual improvement work. Studying, measuring, and improving care in a scientific way are essential parts of our daily work.<br><br>☐ Can't Rate |
| **Information and Information Technology** | **10. Information and Information Technology:** Information is THE connector of staff to staff, patients, staff to staff, needs with actions to meet needs. Technology facilitates effective communication and multiple formal and informal channels are used to keep everyone informed all the time, listen to everyone's ideas, and ensure that everyone is connected on important topics. *Given the complexity of information and the use of technology in the microsystem, assess your microsystem using A, B and C.* | | | |
| | **A. Integration of Information with Patients** | ☐ Patients have access to some standard information that is available to all patients. | ☐ Patients have access to standard information that is available to all patients. We've started to think about how to improve the information they are given to better meet their needs. | ☐ Patients have a variety of ways to get the information they need and it can be customized to meet their individual learning styles. We routinely ask patients for feedback about how to improve the information we give them.<br><br>☐ Can't Rate |
| | **B. Integration of Information with Providers and Staff** | ☐ I am always tracking down the information I need to do my work. | ☐ Most of the time I have the information I need, but sometimes essential information is missing and I have to track it down. | ☐ The information I need to do my work is available when I need it.<br><br>☐ Can't Rate |
| | **C. Integration of Information with Technology** | ☐ The technology I need to facilitate and enhance my work is either not available to me or it is available but not effective. The technology we currently have does not make my job easier. | ☐ I have access to technology that will enhance my work, but it is not easy to use and seems to be cumbersome and time consuming. | ☐ Technology facilitates a smooth linkage between information and patient care by providing timely, effective access to a rich information environment. The information environment has been designed to support the work of the clinical unit.<br><br>☐ Can't Rate |

Table AG1.3    Microsystem Assessment Tool (MAT) Definitions

| Characteristic | Definition |
|---|---|
| Leadership | The role of leaders is to balance setting and reaching collective goals and to empower individual autonomy and accountability through building knowledge, respectful action, and reviewing and reflecting clinical microsystem performance. |
| Organizational support | If a microsystem is part of a larger health care system, the larger organization looks for ways to support the work of the practice and coordinate the handoffs between the practice and other microsystems. |
| Staff focus | There is selective hiring of the right kind of people. The orientation process is designed to fully integrate new staff into culture and work roles. Expectations of staff are high regarding performance, continuing education, professional growth, and networking. |
| Education and training | All clinical microsystems have responsibility for the ongoing education and training of staff and for aligning daily work roles with training competencies. Academic clinical microsystems have the additional responsibility of training students. |
| Interdependence | The interaction of staff is characterized by trust, collaboration, willingness to help each other, appreciation of complementary roles, respect, and recognition that all contribute individually to a shared purpose. |
| Patient focus | The primary concern is to meet all patient needs by caring, listening, educating, responding to special requests, innovating to meet patient needs, and providing smooth service flow. |
| Community and market focus | The practice is a resource for the community; the community is a resource to the practice; the practice establishes excellent and innovative relationships with the community. |
| Performance results | Performance focuses on patient outcomes, avoidable costs, streamlining delivery, using data feedback, promoting positive competition, and frank discussions about performance. |
| Process improvement | An atmosphere for learning and redesign is supported by the continuous monitoring of care, use of benchmarking, frequent tests of change, and a staff that has been empowered to innovate. |
| Information and information technology | Information connects staff to patients, staff to staff, and needs with actions to meet needs. Technology facilitates effective communication; multiple formal and informal channels are used to keep everyone informed all the time, to listen to everyone's ideas, and to ensure everyone is connected and informed on important topics. |

Table AG1.4   Microsystem Assessment Tool (MAT) Worksheet

| Characteristic | 0 (Lowest) | 1 (Middle) | 2 (Best) | Totals |
|---|---|---|---|---|
| Leadership | | | | |
| Organizational support | | | | |
| Staff focus | | | | |
| Education and training | | | | |
| Interdependence | | | | |
| Patient focus | | | | |
| Community and market focus | | | | |
| Performance results | | | | |
| Process improvement | | | | |
| Integration of information with patients | | | | |
| Integration of information with providers and staff | | | | |
| Integration of information with technology | | | | |
| TOTALS | | | | |

FIGURE AG1.7   Microsystem Assessment Tool (MAT) Scores.

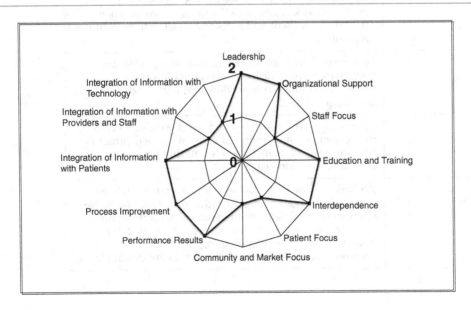

*Source:* Julie K. Johnson, MSPH, PhD.

## Interpretation of Scores

A score of less than 2 for any success characteristic indicates a potential area for improvement. The radar chart in Figure AG1.7 shows one way to display MAT scores.

If your microsystem has a score of 10 or less, you are probably spending a lot of your time each day working around defects in processes of care. (Some observers have estimated up to one-third of a clinician's time and efforts are wasted by dysfunctional workflow processes.) A score of 18 or higher indicates that overall your practice is functioning well. The MAT is not only a diagnostic tool to help identify where your practice can improve, but it can also, if used for follow-up, help track your progress over time.

# PARTNERING WITH PATIENTS TO DESIGN AND IMPROVE CARE

Eugene C. Nelson

Joel S. Lazar

Marjorie M. Godfrey

Paul B. Batalden

## LEARNING OBJECTIVES

- Explore the fundamental aim of health care.
- Describe foundational concepts and models helpful when partnering with patients.
- Discover ways to gain insight about what is important to patients in a specific process and to design patient-centered care.
- Specify tactics to partner with patients to assess health status, to set health goals, to establish plans of care, and to execute care plans by engaging the patient.
- List methods for designing patient-centered care and for promoting patient partnerships.

Chapter One provided a panoramic view of health care and systems of care with a sharp focus on frontline clinical microsystems (the places where patients and interdisciplinary providers meet and interact). This chapter will focus on the patients who hope to derive benefit from the care and services they receive through their one-on-one interactions with health care professionals. This chapter will cover several important subjects, including the aim of health care and the need to partner with patients; conceptual models that contribute to an appreciation of patients as partners in health care; and methods for designing patient-centered care and partnering with patients to achieve desired outcomes.

## THE AIM OF HEALTH CARE AND THE NEED TO PARTNER WITH PATIENTS

If we accept Chapter One's basic premise that health care value is created in complex adaptive systems and that such systems (micro, meso, and macro) are composed of individual agents with "freedom to act in ways that are not always predictable, [but] whose actions are interconnected so that one agent's actions change the context for other agents,"[1] then we are invited to recognize the necessarily active role of trained professionals, of patients, and of patients' families in creating value. Dr. Henderson observed early in the twentieth century that "a physician and a patient make up a social system."[2] Even today we grapple with the rich opportunities inherent in this observation. To assert (as we do) that clinical care must be *patient-centered* does not imply that patients are mere passive recipients of care that is designed and delivered by external sources. Rather, patients and their families are active agents and indeed partners in the creation, preservation, and restoration of their own health; clinical microsystems must endeavor continually to recognize and to engage this active agency.

What are the implications, both conceptual and practical, of engaging patients and families as partners in care? In all cultures and in all recorded time, from earliest societies to the present day, the essential role of healer, shaman, or clinician has been to preserve the health and functioning of individuals within their own communities.[3] Both the World Health Organization (WHO) and the Institute of Medicine (IOM), in their widely accepted definitions of health, emphasize that the fundamental aim of health care is to advance, preserve, or restore individuals' biological, physical, mental, and social functioning, so they can enjoy the best quality of life attainable.[4,5] But neither the responsibility nor the capacity to achieve this aim resides solely with trained health professionals, nor with the sophisticated technologies that have come to support the work of contemporary medicine. As the experience of illness has grown more complex in modern times (see discussion in Chapters Eight and Nine), and as Western societal values have shifted from paternalism toward personal autonomy, the rich collaboration of clinical teams with patients and families has proven to be desirable and essential to delivering effective health care and to achieving optimal health.

Consider, in Table 2.1, the Institute of Medicine's (IOM's) Ten New Rules for providing health care in the twenty-first century, and note how these contrast with implicit assumptions of the recent past and even present day. Of course, these rules are not prescriptive; no regulatory agency or professional society formally enforces them. Rather, they are *de*scriptive of the unspoken beliefs that inform actual health care activities. Effective clinical micro, meso, and macrosystems recognize the impact

Table 2.1 Ten New Rules for the Twenty-First Century Health Care System

| Current Approach | New Rule |
|---|---|
| 1. Care is based primarily on visits. | **Care is based on continuous healing relationships.*** |
| 2. Professional autonomy drives variability. | **Care is customized according to patient needs and values.** |
| 3. Professionals control care. | **The patient is the source of control.** |
| 4. Information is a (*medical*) record. | **Knowledge is shared and information flows freely.** |
| 5. Decision making is based on training and experience. | **Decision making is *shared and* is evidence-based.** |
| 6. *Do no harm* is an individual responsibility. | Safety is a system property. |
| 7. Secrecy is necessary. | Transparency is necessary. |
| 8. The system reacts to needs. | **Needs are anticipated.** |
| 9. Cost reduction is sought. | Waste is continuously decreased. |
| 10. Preference is given to professional roles *and prerogatives more than to teamwork and the system working well for patients.* | Cooperation among clinicians is a priority. |

*Source:* Institute of Medicine. *Crossing the quality chasm: A new health system for the 21st century.* Washington, DC: Committee on Quality of Health Care, 2001, p. 67.

*Bold text added to highlight rules that place a premium on partnering with patients.
**Words and phrases in italics have been added by the authors.

of these unspoken beliefs on the design and implementation of their own work processes and increasingly shift toward behaviors that manifest the more modern and collaborative approach.

Careful reflection upon the IOM's ten simple rules (particularly those in bold type) reveals that a new conception of patient centeredness and clinical partnership will greatly facilitate the work of health care and will support the achievement of both individual and population health goals. Consider first the extent to which those goals depend upon behaviors that only patients and families can enact. The majority of health care costs and diseases and disabilities in our society are associated with shortfalls in personal prevention and with development of preventable injuries and chronic illness.[6] The role of clinical microsystems in this context is not to bestow preventive knowledge upon patients and families, but to activate them through collaborative problem solving toward informed self-care (see Chapters Six and Eight for further discussion).

Consider also the simple math that underscores the necessity of patient and family engagement:

$$(3 \times 20) + (1 \times 60) = 120 \text{ minutes per year the average patient spends with clinician.}$$

$$(60 \times 24 \times 365) - 120 = 525,480 \text{ minutes per year the average patient}$$
$$\text{spends on own away from clinician.}$$

It is unrealistic and also clinically unwise to assume patients will experience their brief time within formal health care settings as the central focus of their lives. We view ourselves as people first (not as patients) and we make our own personal health care decisions within the context of our larger lives. Clinical microsystems must actively seek understanding of this context and must couple their own biomedical knowledge with experiential (personal, familial, cultural, financial) knowledge that only patients possess. Again, partnering with patients can mutually broaden the perspectives of all participants; partnering is essential for sharing pertinent information, negotiating clinical priorities, and enacting agreed-upon health care plans.

Moreover, effective prevention of both acute and chronic illness depends upon individuals' capacity and motivation to engage in regular *self-care*. As the sidebar demonstrates, self-care is essential to the optimization of clinical value, improving health, and reducing costs for both patients and payers.

## HIGH-VALUE CARE AND SELF-CARE STATISTICS

Many Americans are staggering under the burden of illness. More than 130 million people, almost half of all Americans, are living with one or more chronic conditions, and chronic problems account for 70 percent of all deaths.[1] The number of days per year Americans report feeling unhealthy is high and getting higher. Americans report they suffer from poor physical and mental health on more than 40 days per year and this rate is increasing. Ratings of poor health are common among adults and range from 5 percent (for people ages 25 to 34) to 30 percent (for people 75 years and older).[2] Not only are chronic diseases and poor health common today, but the lifestyle-based risk factors that generate illness are increasing as well: 20 percent of Americans smoke,[1,3] fewer than 50 percent exercise regularly,[1,3] more than 15 percent report binge drinking,[3] 74 percent need to improve their diet,[3] and more than 30 percent of adults are obese.[3,4]

### The Value of Partnering with Patients

It is clear the path to best health care value leads to increasing the ability and motivation of people and families to take care of themselves. Partnering with patients to help them adopt healthy lifestyles can decrease health risks, increase the experience of good health and functioning, and prevent illness and injury. Helping patients self-manage using clinically effective and evidence-based methods can keep them out of doctors' offices, emergency rooms, and hospitals, even when patients are faced with acute and chronic problems. If the goal is to achieve the desired outcomes at the lowest real cost to patients and to society, then the highest value health care must take full advantage of self-care.

### References

1. Center for Disease Control and Prevention. *Chronic diseases and health promotion*. Retrieved August, 4, 2010, from www.cdc.gov/nccdphp/overview.htm
2. National Center for Chronic Disease Prevention and Health Promotion. *Health-related quality of life*. Retrieved August, 4, 2010, from http://apps.nccd.cdc.gov/HRQOL
3. Institute of Medicine. *State of the USA health indicators: Letter report*. Washington, DC: National Academy of Sciences, December, 9, 2008.
4. Ogden, C., Carroll, M. D., McDowell, M. A., Flegal, K. M. *Obesity among adults in the United States—no change since 2003–2004*. Hyattsville, MD: National Center for Health Statistics, 2007. NCHS Data Brief No. 1. Retrieved August, 4, 2010, from www.Cdc.Gov/nchs/data/databriefs/db01.Pdf

Several dimensions of partnering with patients honor the IOM's new rules for health care in the twenty-first century. We first examine conceptual models that illuminate various dimensions of patient-centeredness in microsystem design and clinical intervention. We then consider specific methods for gaining knowledge of patients at the front line of care, and we review diverse methods for engaging patients in their own care and in improving health care systems, too. In Chapters Six through Nine, our discussion returns to manifestations of patient partnering in the specific contexts of preventive, acute, chronic, and palliative care.

## CONCEPTUAL FRAMEWORKS FOR PARTNERING WITH PATIENTS

### Core Concepts

The Institute for Patient and Family-Centered Care recognizes the essential value of patient partnership in planning, delivering, and evaluating health care services. This organization identifies the following four core concepts of patient- and family-centered care:[7]

*Dignity and Respect:* Patient and family perspectives are honored and their beliefs, priorities, and cultural backgrounds are routinely elicited and incorporated into planning and implementing care.

*Information Sharing:* Patients and families receive unbiased information in a manner that is both comprehensive and comprehensible. Information exchange is bilateral, reflecting the mutually beneficial knowledge of all participants.

*Participation:* Patients and families are supported and empowered to participate in decision making at the level they choose and to engage actively in self-care to the extent they are able.

*Collaboration:* Patient and family are invited to participate in institutional planning, in program and policy development, in professional education, and in evaluation of services.

We can see that each of these core concepts suggests specific tactics for partnering with patients and families. These tactics range from staff training in cultural competence to implementation of chronic disease self-management support groups to formal appointment of patient representatives on hospital planning committees. Other examples will be considered in greater detail later in this chapter.

### Target Diagram and Clinical Microsystem Model

One advantage of the clinical microsystem model is its own intense focus upon patient priorities and experiences. Recall the target diagram in Chapter One (Figure 1.4) that depicts interdependent systems embedded one inside the next. The center of this target (the bull's-eye or innermost ring) is the patient's own system of self-care, which is practiced by one's self or along with one's family. This innermost self-care system interacts with and is influenced by the clinician-patient system (second ring out) and the clinical microsystem (third ring out). We observe that the effects of professional health care systems (no matter how scientifically grounded and technologically enriched) are necessarily mediated by patient and family self-care systems at the diagram's center.

**FIGURE 2.1**    Clinical Microsystem Physiology Model.

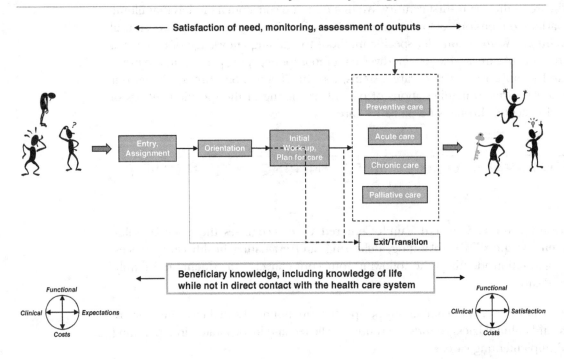

Therefore, these various systems need to be concordant. Symptoms of discord include not only patients who do not (or cannot) adhere to recommended care, but also microsystems that fail to incorporate patient preferences and priorities into those same care recommendations.

Consider also the clinical microsystem physiology model depicted in Figure 2.1. An individual enters a specific clinical microsystem, and then is recognized as *the patient*. As the process of care unfolds, a diagnostic and therapeutic plan is tailored to the unique needs, values, desires, and capabilities of this particular person at this specific point in time. Based on the initial impact of this care, the plan is dynamically modified and recalibrated to match patient needs and capabilities as care objectives continue to evolve. Again, the essential dynamic is partnership itself. Patient input is continually required to identify clinical needs, to negotiate care that addresses these needs, and to evaluate the *rightness* of that care as circumstances change.

## Kano Model of Satisfaction with Services

Patient satisfaction is an important marker of patient centeredness and of clinical value because it captures the capacity of microsystems to anticipate, to meet, and even to surpass patients' expectations. Noriaki Kano's model of customer satisfaction provides another important perspective on the need to partner effectively with patients.[8] Clinical microsystems must acquire deep knowledge of patients' wants, needs, values, and priorities, in order to design and deliver care that honors all of these variables. Again, after considering the available treatment options, caregivers must determine which approach best combines biomedical evidence with the expectations and preferences of this patient at this time. If care is to be assembled and delivered in a manner that produces total patient satisfaction, then microsystems must understand how patients define good service and good outcomes. It is the totality of patients' perceptions and judgments

FIGURE 2.2   Kano Model for Understanding Customer Satisfaction.

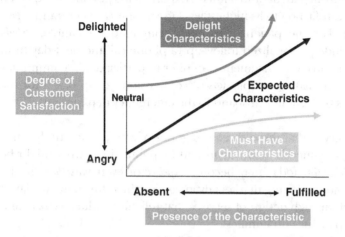

*Source:* Kano, N., Seraku, N., Takahashi, F., & Tsuji, S. Attractive quality and must-be quality. *The Journal of the Japanese Society for Quality Control,* 1984, *14*(2), 39–48.

that, in the end, produces satisfaction, appreciation, respect, and loyalty, all of which redound to the health care system.

Kano provides a sophisticated model that links customer perceptions to overall satisfaction and loyalty.[8] His model is depicted in Figure 2.2 and can be used to elicit the following vital information about patients:

- What are their expectations?
- What are their needs?
- What excites or delights them?
- What angers or disappoints them?

The *Kano framework* suggests there are actually three distinct domains of patient experience that contribute to three separate categories of satisfaction. These interact to produce an overall level of satisfaction, as shown on the vertical axis of Figure 2.2.

- The first category includes *must have* characteristics: features of service so essential they are assumed to be present. They are taken for granted and mainly noticed when missing. The absence of a *must have* characteristic will be perceived as a defect by the patient, and overall level of satisfaction will be low. For example, a middle-age man who presents to his local emergency department with chest pain will assume the presence of such *must have* features as competency (a qualified clinician), technical resources (proper equipment availability), and cleanliness (a "germ free" well-kept exam room).
- The second category includes *expected* characteristics: features of service that are generally anticipated and desired. The more of these features that are present, the higher the level of satisfaction. Continuing the emergency room example above, *expected* characteristics include such features as timeliness (the faster, the better) and pain relief (the more comfort, the better).
- The third category includes *delight* characteristics: features of service neither expected nor anticipated that are perceived by patients who experience them as innovative and

positive. Such features anticipate patients' special and unexpressed needs and generate gratitude and loyalty from patients and families. Experiencing just one unexpected *delight* can raise overall satisfaction to its highest level (assuming *must haves* and *expecteds* are fully realized). For the patient with chest pain in our example, *delight* characteristics may include personalized follow-up (a phone call the next day from emergency department staff), enhancements (an offer to participate in community-based heart healthy programs), or simple acts of compassion (a cup of tea for the worried spouse who has brought her husband to the emergency department).

Kano has further observed that these three categories of satisfaction are dynamic in nature. As experience is gained by individuals and by populations, what might be considered exciting or *delighting* today may become *expected* or even *must have* in the future. In competitive situations, lasting market advantage is gained through avoidance of *must have* breeches and through design of services that reliably produce *expected* and *delightful* experiences for patients and families.

Kano invites us to consider these *expected* and *delight* features not as random acts of kindness, but as planned components of care. Such planning, in turn, requires rich understanding of individual patients and also of discrete populations served by the clinical microsystem. This understanding is gained specifically through partnering with patients, through explicit querying and implicit observing, and through collaborative learning that maintains a clear focus on patients at the center of care.

## Deming Model for Organizing Services as a System of Production

Whereas Kano amplifies our understanding of discrete patient experiences that contribute to overall judgments regarding goodness of care, W. Edwards Deming embeds fundamental knowledge of the patient (or customer or service beneficiary) into an overarching approach to planning, executing, and improving service, based on systems thinking.[9]

*Deming's system model,* modified for health care and depicted in Figure 2.3, is a brilliant adaptation of systems thinking applied to the production and continual improvement of services with a goal of meeting people's needs. Deming's model integrates the customer into the system of production and emphasizes three main clusters of activity:

1. Depicted from left to right across the bottom of Figure 2.3 are sequential steps necessary to produce value that are known as the *value chain* for delivering services. The sequence begins with suppliers and inputs and ends with outputs received by patients and other beneficiaries. For example, a teenage boy with a broken arm enters the emergency department (an input is a patient with need for fracture care) and he exits the emergency department with the fracture being set and a cast on the arm (an output). Another example is a healthy, pregnant twenty-eight-year-old woman who sees her obstetrician for an initial visit (input is a pregnant woman) and eight months later the obstetrician assists the mother in delivering a healthy baby (output is the healthy baby and a still healthy woman).

2. In the upper center and right hand sections of the model are three clustered activities that together garner foundational knowledge about patients, including knowledge about specific patient needs and shared patient and professional vision for ideal service.

FIGURE 2.3    Deming Model: Organizing as a System of Care.

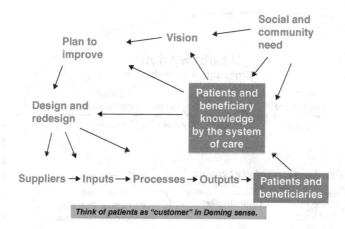

*Source:* Adapted from Deming, W. E. *Out of crisis.* Cambridge: Massachusetts Institute of Technology, Center for Advanced Engineering Study, 1989.

3. To the upper left are represented planning and designing, two activities that focus upon creation of a general plan of service improvement and design (or redesign) of specific activities to realize that improvement.

Of course, because Deming understands health care to be a *system* of production, and because (as we discussed in Chapter One) all elements of complex adaptive systems interact with one another to achieve a common aim, all the parts of Deming's model are linked together and related to one another. But note the critical position of the patient or beneficiary of services. Deming's vision of production is distinctive because he includes the customer, beneficiary, or end user as an integral part of the system of production. Patients or beneficiaries are depicted twice: first, at the end of the value chain because patients are indeed the ultimate recipients of value created within this system; and second, at the diagram's center, where patients serve the key functions of articulating need, forming vision, and contributing to design and improvement of services. We suggest yet another patient role in this system of value production: that of supplier. As suggested above and elaborated on below, patients' self-care activities (which can be supported through microsystem resources) are both a *means* to improved function and a desired *outcome* in the health care process.

## Wagner's Chronic Care Model and Lorig's Self-Management Model

Whereas Kano and Deming offer general service sector models applicable to customer engagement in any service industry, Edward Wagner and Kate Lorig examine patient partnerships directly and articulate specific applications in health care for people with chronic health conditions such as diabetes, arthritis, hypertension, heart failure, and persistent back pain.

In May 1973, Don Etzwiler[10] noted in the *Journal of the American Medical Association* that patients and professionals were partners in the management of diabetes, and that contracts between them could yield clinical benefit. This work and that of several others led Wagner and colleagues to propose a general model of chronic care. The *chronic care*

FIGURE 2.4   Chronic Care Model.

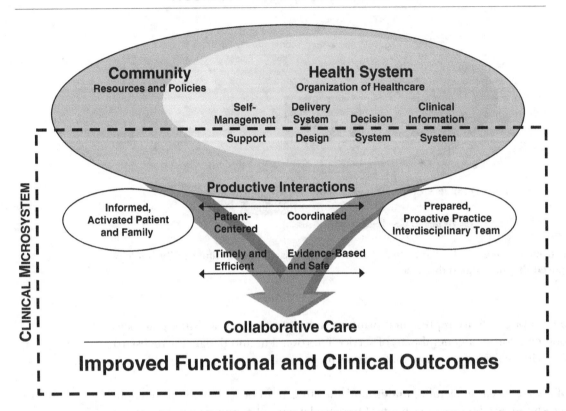

*Source:* Wagner, E. H. Chronic disease management: What will it take to improve care for chronic illness? *Effective Clinical Practice*, August 1998, *1*(1), 22–24.

*model* (also called the *planned care model*, which included additional services such as preventive, acute, and palliative care) is depicted in Figure 2.4;[11,12,13] its key tenets have been rapidly and widely embraced by patients and clinical teams throughout the nation.[14] As introduced in Chapter One, and as further explored in Chapter Eight, the centerpiece of the chronic care model is effective partnership (what Wagner calls *productive interaction*) between an informed, activated patient and family and a prepared, proactive practice team. This interaction builds upon and reinforces key quality characteristics (patient centeredness, timeliness, coordination, efficiency, safety, and evidence-base) and helps generate desired patient outcomes.

Complementing Wagner's emphasis upon the central partnership of patients, families, and clinicians, or practice teams, Kate Lorig and others emphasize the critical role self-care plays in achieving the best possible health outcomes.[15,16] Lorig's *self-management model* promotes patient-professional collaboration as a means of promoting clinically enlightened self-care and family care. The role of professionals in this model is to support patients' and families' acquisition of knowledge, skill, and confidence, so patients and families can become first providers of their own medically appropriate care. Interactive health education methods, combined with more general problem-solving techniques, are employed to foster patient and family self-efficacy, assuring reliability and also adaptability of self-care in patients' daily lives.

If clinical microsystems are to successfully promote patient self-efficacy in this manner, they must design and implement patient or family educational programs with

Table 2.2  Patient Education Program

| Educational Issue | Self-Management Education Content |
|---|---|
| What is taught? | Skills on how to act on problems. |
| How are problems formulated? | Patient identifies problems she or he experiences that may or may not be related to disease. |
| What is the relation of education to the disease? | Education provides skills to address problems associated with chronic conditions. |
| What is the theory underlying the education? | Increased patient confidence in her or his capacity to make life-improving changes (self-efficacy) yields better clinical outcomes. |
| What is the goal? | Increased self-efficacy to improve clinical outcomes. |
| Who is the educator? | A health professional, peer leader, or other patients, often in group settings. |

*Source:* Based on Table 2 in Lorig, K., Bodenheimer, T., Holman, H., & Grumbach, K. Patient self-management of chronic disease in primary care. *Journal of the American Medical Association*, 2002, 288(19), 2469–2475.

specific goals of capability and confidence in mind. Lorig and her associates have demonstrated the efficacy of programs for chronic conditions such as asthma and rheumatoid arthritis in controlled clinical trials. These studies confirm that special forms of patient self-management education can improve health status and decrease costs of care.[15,17] Design features of a rigorous self-management patient education program are listed in Table 2.2.

But although self-management education programs can improve patient health and decrease need for expensive medical care, many individuals lack access to patient-centered training. Programs do not exist in many communities, nor are they consistently offered by patients' principle source of care. Fortunately, however, a growing *medical home* movement within primary care incorporates features championed by both Wagner and Lorig. Medical homes have gained rapid acceptance across the nation, combining patient-centered care coordination with improved clinical microsystem design. In such settings, planned care and self-management support have increasingly become mainstream services.[18,19]

## Amy's Experience in Clinical Microsystems

We have explored the rationale for partnering with patients in the design and implementation of health services, and we have considered several conceptual models that locate such partnership at the very center of care. Before examining specific practical methods to engage patients in the frontline work of clinical microsystems, let us consider a case example that uncovers challenges and opportunities within this special form of partnership.

Shortly after her thirty-fourth birthday, Amy Dressler moved to rural Vermont to teach special education in a small town's elementary school. She had grown up outside New York City, and because she was new to the community had not yet found a primary care physician. Soon after her move, Amy discovered a lump in her breast during a routine self-examination. After consulting with family and exploring resources online and in local newspapers, she called to make an appointment with the Breast Care Program at Dartmouth-Hitchcock Medical Center (DHMC).

Figure 2.5 provides a panoramic view of Amy's health journey during the next seven months of care and treatment. Each rectangular box represents a clinical microsystem she entered and exited in these seven months. Between each rectangular box are the dates of services received. During this intense period, Amy's knowledge grew, including new understanding and skills in the following areas:

- Her diagnosis (breast cancer)
- Her prognosis (unclear in her perception)
- Her treatment options
- What was known and not known based on medical evidence
- How to navigate the complex DHMC health care system
- How to cope with the emotional and physical strain of living with breast cancer
- How to get advice and information from the breast care program coordinator and her team of DHMC professionals
- How to speak up if she experienced unnecessary waits or delays at DHMC
- How to talk with the breast care team staff about both successes and disappointments in her care experience
- How to continue teaching young children while facing a life-threatening condition

Because her medical problem was serious and complex, Amy's care experiences were varied and intense. In her first seven months of care, she had twenty-one visits or overnight stays at DHMC, and she interacted with fourteen different clinical microsystems. When Amy spoke about her care experiences at DHMC, she reported some wonderful *delights* (for example, her relationships with the Breast Care Program Coordinator, with her primary oncologist, and with the Wig Lady who offered exceptional support after initial therapy). On the other hand, Amy also recounted the missing of some *must haves*. Her first meeting with the surgeon was especially disappointing, and on three consecutive occasions she waited almost three hours for Stat lab results that were needed for specification of chemotherapy. The variation in delay in chemotherapy infusion is illustrated in the last two rows with specific time tracking.

As Amy's journey unfolded, she often (but not always) found herself treated as a full partner in her care, as in the following examples:

- She worked closely with her oncologist and the program coordinator on a regular basis to assess her health condition, to consider different treatment options, and to develop or recalibrate a plan of care that fit her preferences (informed decision making).
- She participated in a formal shared decision-making program[20] at DHMC that included thoughtful examination of treatment options and selection of one that best matched her values, preferences, and understanding of therapeutic efficacy.
- She met with the entire medical staff for a frank discussion of some problems and frustrations she experienced as a breast cancer patient.
- She gave a grand rounds presentation to interdisciplinary staff to share one patient's perceptions of care; she did not sugarcoat the disappointments nor did she overplay the delights.
- She interacted with patient peers also undergoing care and with breast cancer survivors to reflect upon her own feelings, experiences, and vision of her future.

FIGURE 2.5 Amy's Breast Cancer Care Journey.

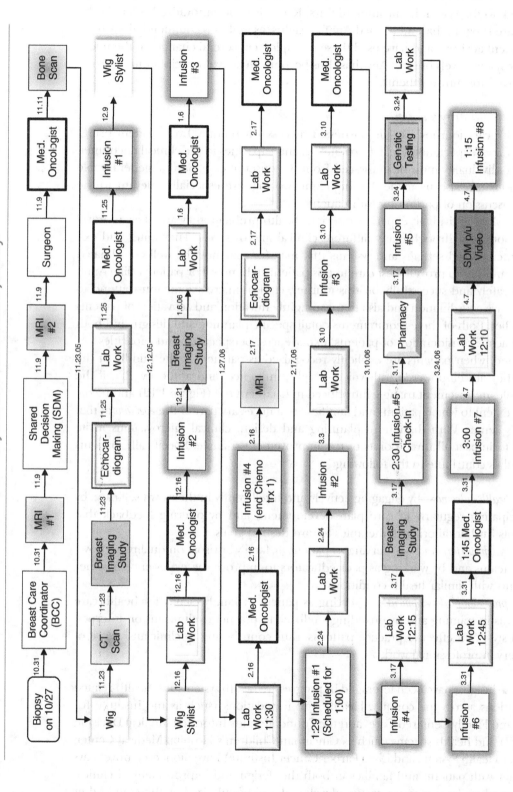

To date, Amy has enjoyed successful remission of her breast cancer. She has benefited greatly from her relationship with DHMC clinicians and staff, and she has also given back to the system in meaningful ways. Receptive and innovative leaders in the Breast Care Program have welcomed Amy's insights, as well as recommendations from other patient advisors, and have used these to implement several changes at the micro and mesosystem levels of care. Amy has thus become an active participant in improvement of care for future patients.

### Reflections on Amy's experience

This health care journey, like all journeys, is necessarily unique. Every patient brings his or her own expectations, beliefs, resources, and capacities to the clinical encounter, and this individuality must be embraced from the onset of care. Several generalizable observations can also be made. We highlight two that are especially relevant to the present discussion of partnering with patients.

First, when individuals experience serious health problem, they are likely to travel on their journeys through many different clinical microsystems. They enter and exit and reenter myriad settings and systems that may (or may not) be well coordinated with one another to provide best care to this patient right now. For patients (like Amy) to travel safely and successfully on this journey, clinical microsystems must attend to effective care coordination and also to meaningful education and activation of patients and families. Both of these requirements entail specific planning and design, and both demand active consideration of patients' experiences, perspectives, and capacities.

Second, when patients are explicitly recognized as partners in the middle of the action, they are empowered with voice, insight, influence, and authority. Recall the sustainable improvement triangle introduced in Chapter One (Figure 1.12) and recognize the extent to which patients and families are a necessary part of the *everyone* at that triangle's center. With thoughtful planning and design, clinical microsystems invite patients to impact all three points of the improvement triangle. Specifically, patients and families contribute to the following:

- *Better health outcomes*—by engaging actively and intelligently in their own self-care, by participating regularly in care plan development, and by offering feedback that permits further tailoring of therapies toward desired goals
- *Better system performance*—by serving as patient or family advisors on quality improvement teams and by working as peer educators to improve the experience of other patients with similar health conditions
- *Better professional development*—by serving as patient or family faculty for health care students in training and by providing feedback to practicing clinicians on interpersonal style and effective practice patterns, thus contributing to clinicians' sense of mastery in professional work

These insights have been leveraged by progressive health systems and health-related organizations across the country. Health care foundations (such as the Institute for Patient and Family-Centered Care[7] and the Foundation for Informed Medical Decision Making[21]) and health systems (such as Cincinnati Children's Hospital Medical Center, Geisinger Health System, and Dana Farber Cancer Institute) have pioneered novel ways to partner with patients and families in both the design and improvement of clinical care. Some specific partnering tactics, developed and popularized by these and other organizations, are reviewed next.

## TACTICS FOR PARTNERING WITH PATIENTS

How then do clinical microsystems partner effectively with patients and families? How specifically are participants empowered to become full partners in the planning, delivering, evaluating, and improving of their own care? We can parse these partnership opportunities into several high-leverage phases central to the process of health care delivery:

1. Assessing the patient's health status
2. Setting health goals with the patient
3. Making decisions about treatment plans
4. Executing the plan of care based on effective self-management

Let us consider specific tactics in each of these high-leverage domains.[22]

### Feed Forward Health Status Assessment

Any plan of individual care must begin with reliable assessment of the patient's *current health status.* This status is necessarily dynamic and shifts over time; assessment must take this personal variation into account. A patient's current health status includes rapidly developing *acute* conditions (such as recent injury or emerging illness) that may be amenable to cure, and underlying *chronic* health conditions (such as diabetes or asthma) that cannot be cured but that may be managed or controlled by ongoing care. In addition, personal behaviors, environment, and physiology expose each of us to health risks that may be mitigated by *prevention* and health promotion activities. Assessment of health status can be complex in these multiple (acute, chronic, and preventive) domains, but powerful (patient-partnering) techniques can greatly facilitate the task. Patient-based *feed forward*[23] reports can enhance clinician-based history and physical examination, and can provide accurate and comprehensive assessment of current health status. Feed forward data and reports refer to moving key information with the patient as patients move from one care setting to the next. Feed forward data systems keep key data about the patient with the patient across time and space.

*Health assessment surveys,* completed by patients before clinician visits, have been used in innovative clinical centers to complement traditional sources of information, to generate more comprehensive and patient-centered health assessments, and to track outcomes over time. Patient-based feed forward systems have been developed for both primary care and specialty care practices, have been deployed in diverse settings, and include the following:

- How's Your Health,[24] initially developed by John Wasson for primary care and more recently adapted to diverse communities and workplaces
- The Group Health Profile,[25] developed by David Grossman and Robert Reid at Group Health of Puget Sound, also initially for primary care and now extended to employee populations
- Spine Condition Survey,[26] developed by James Weinstein at the Dartmouth Spine Center and deployed by Dynamic Clinical Systems, Inc. (DCS),[27] for various patient populations
- Rheumatoid arthritis (RA) patient survey,[28] developed by Staffan Lindblad at the Karolinska Institute and now deployed throughout Sweden for a national RA registry, with future plans to develop pediatric and chronic disease registries

- Autism survey[29] for parents of children with autism, developed by Geisinger Health System to improve and streamline care

Each of these health assessment surveys is completed by the patient or family with a user-friendly, computer-based interface. Pertinent data on current conditions, health behaviors, and functional status are analyzed, summarized, and fed forward to both clinician and patient at the point of care, front-end loading the next steps in the care process. Information is integrated across multiple sources and is used by the clinician and patient partners to set explicit health goals and to formulate explicit plans of care. The survey is then re-administered at regular intervals to measure progress, to adjust treatment plans, and to track outcomes over time.[30] The Karolinska Institute RA Clinic process can be viewed at www.clinicalmicrosystem.org.

## Motivational Interviewing, Patient Contracting, and Goal Setting

Once a full health assessment has been completed, clinician and patient must negotiate relevant and meaningful health goals. Two well-studied techniques, motivational interviewing and patient contracting, can facilitate this goal setting process.

*Motivational interviewing* is a powerful interactive approach that explores and activates a patient's intrinsic motivation and values as a means of stimulating more effective self-care.[31] Patient and clinician together identify health assets and liabilities, with attention to behaviors that contribute to poor health or that confer future health risk. Discrepancies are identified between these risky behaviors and patients' self-articulated health goals; ambivalence is leveraged to focus patient attention on goals of genuine personal concern. Motivational interviewing aims not to convince the patient that one specific behavior change or another is required, but to discover intrinsic motivations that enable self-prioritizing of behaviors that contribute to positive health.

*Patient contracting* has been used for many years to promote patient commitment to a care plan.[10,32,33] The approach is designed to clarify agreement between patient and clinician on a specified health goal and to specify needed resources and mutual responsibilities toward achieving that goal. After negotiating desired behaviors and outcomes, a plan of care is documented in print. Patient and clinician formalize their agreement with a signature, which underscores their shared commitment to the plan. In general a patient contract will indicate the purpose of the health agreement, the actions that will be taken, the methods for keeping track of intended actions, and the plan for reviewing patient and clinician performance. This method reinforces for all parties what will be done, why, by whom, and with what manner of feedback to evaluate success.

## Shared Decision Making and Shared Medical Appointments

When multiple treatment options are available, elicitation of patients' values, preferences, and expectations is especially important. Shared decision making and shared medical appointments can greatly facilitate patients' capacity and confidence to make informed choices.

*Shared decision making* has emerged as not only a powerful clinical aid, but also a field of intense academic study. The Foundation for Informed Medical Decision Making, founded by Drs. Jack Wennberg and Al Mulley, has substantially advanced clinical understanding in this area.[21,34] This work, in turn, has been richly informed by Annette O'Connor's research at the Ottawa Health Decision Center at Ottawa Hospital Research

Institute.[35] When confronted with different (and often difficult) therapeutic options, shared decision-making resources enable patients and families to explore risks and benefits in the context of their own personal preferences.[36,37,38] This process enables individuals to make informed choices guided by medical science, outcomes research, and personal values. It is particularly helpful when clinical stakes are high (as in care of breast cancer, low back pain, or infertility), and when medical evidence provides no strong basis for one therapeutic option over another (as in screening for prostate cancer).

*Shared medical appointments* were initially popularized by Ed Noffsinger[39] and have now gained broad traction in innovative clinical microsystems. These appointments are a form of planned care that allow multiple patients to be seen at the same time. Shared medical appointments combine features of a traditional, private clinician visit with efficiencies and support structure of group visits. In such encounters, patients may receive individual and focused physical examination in conjunction with extended group discussion about specific treatment plans and self-care strategies. Patients are afforded time to discuss their own treatment plans, and are also invited to listen in on discussion of other patients' experiences and therapies. The result is greater breadth of individual learning and greater depth of personal and group support. Shared medical appointments have been adapted to many types of patients and many forms of clinical need.[40] One novel and important application is group facilitation of informed patient choice. For example, DHMC plastic surgeon Dr. Carolyn Kerrigan has used shared medical appointments for several years to support informed decision making in patients with carpal tunnel syndrome and other hand ailments.[41] She observes that these group appointments improve her productivity as a physician and also enhance the quality of her patients' decisions. People can participate in a shared medical appointment after reviewing and agreeing with a written statement on patient confidentiality.

## Health Coaching and Information Prescriptions

We have thus far considered patients' engagement in assessment, goal setting, and decision-making processes. But the ultimate value of these processes will be realized only when patients enact their negotiated plans. Health coaching and information prescriptions are designed to foster actual execution of self-management activities.

*Health coaching* is a high touch approach that has migrated from the field of athletics to the field of health care.[42,43,44] Health coaches work with individual patients to promote knowledge, skills, attitudes, and practices, in the service of actual care plan execution. These coaches (who are most commonly health professionals and specially trained nurses) work with patients over time to foster mastery of knowledge and skills and to develop attitudes and practices that enable effective self-management. The more generalizable outcome of health coaching is not simply management of specific foreseeable events, but broader self-efficacy (a blend of capability and confidence) that will empower patients in novel situations. Self-efficacy has special value in the management of chronic illness, and we discuss this concept further in Chapter Eight.

*Information prescriptions* are a new approach to patient education, inspired by the traditionally written medication prescription.[45,46,47] The idea is disarmingly simple: just as physicians write drug prescriptions to be filled at local pharmacies, so too can health coaches and clinicians write information prescriptions to be filled (or at least stored) in electronic or personal health records. Combining sound patient education principles with mass customization techniques, information prescriptions automate the process

# PLASTIC SURGERY, ACCESS, AND SHARED MEDICAL APPOINTMENTS

Plastic Surgery Section Chief at Dartmouth-Hitchcock Medical Center, Carolyn Kerrigan, MD, organized an interdisciplinary improvement team to improve quality and value for plastic surgery patients. After reviewing their 5Ps (purpose, patients, professionals, processes, and patterns) and available data, the team concluded that access to care needed to be improved.

The Plastic Surgery Microsystem Purpose was "Improving Form and Function for Better Living."

Their mission included the following:

- Provide timely, courteous, and compassionate care of the highest quality.
- Maximize patient satisfaction.
- Use the most current medical evidence to care for patients.
- Initiate and accept change toward improvement.
- Create a harmonious and fulfilling work environment.

The 5Ps revealed new patients had to wait three to six months for an initial appointment, or for a minor procedure, and two to five months for a major procedure. These findings supported the aim to improve access to care. Discussion revealed that many return appointments were scheduled out of habit rather than because patients needed to return. By reducing the number of follow-up appointments, more appointment slots would be available for new patients.

Shared Medical Appointments (SMA) were developed to improve patient ability to be seen when they wanted to be seen and to standardize the process of care for informed decision making and informed consent. The goals of SMA development included the following:

- Promote patient understanding of disease or condition.
- Make better-informed medical decisions and give informed consent to treatment.
- Promote adherence to recommended treatments and therapies.
- Integrate peer support into health care experience.
- Better address psychosocial needs.
- Increase quality of care and outcomes.

The metrics tracked to determine success of SMAs included patient, employee, and physician satisfaction; financial productivity; time to third appointment; and numbers of patients seen.

One patient offered this typically positive feedback after implementation of SMAs.

> Hello. Thank you very much for making my recent visit with you and the staff so welcoming, informative, and worthwhile. I felt very comfortable in the group setting, and think it is an excellent format for providing information and attention to women who have individual needs but shared concerns.

The following improvements were also reported after implementation of SMAs:

- Patients reported an improvement in discussion of "all my questions" from 62 percent to 82 percent.
- Patients' overall rating of information increased from 82 percent to 92 percent.
- Productivity increased from 3 patients seen in 135 minutes in the traditional model to 12 patients seen in 120 minutes in the SMA model.
- Overall staff satisfaction increased from a score of 2.6 to 3.9 on a scale ranging from 1 to 5.

of education and stimulate patients' acquisition of essential knowledge, attitudes, skills, and practices. One prescription might read as noted in the sidebar.

Patients receive a written copy of this instruction in the form of an actual prescription, and are stimulated to successfully execute the treatment plan they have negotiated with their health care team.

> Take a brisk walk with dog twenty minutes, three times per week; may increase to thirty minutes four times per week; goal is improved exercise tolerance, five-pound weight loss, and healthier heart; please phone me at office if experiencing difficulty.

## PATIENTS AS INFORMANTS AND ADVISORS

In this chapter we have recognized collaboration as a core concept of the Institute for Patient and Family-Centered Care, and we have understood this term to signify not only patients' participation in their own care, but also their contribution to the care of others through feedback, institutional planning, and program and policy development. Amy's participation in grand rounds and interdisciplinary staff meetings was one example of such collaboration. Indeed, many powerful methods enable clinical microsystems to gain deeper knowledge of patients' and families' knowledge and experience, and to harness this for more general improvement of care processes.[48] In this section we briefly examine some of these approaches (see Chapter Two Action Guide for more detailed information).

### Using Direct Observations to Improve Care

Improvement begins with observation and reflection.[49] Before improving care we must understand the current state of affairs. Who is doing what, in what way, and under what conditions? What results are obtained, and how do these results vary in predictable or unpredictable ways? Direct observation can be incorporated into the daily work of clinical microsystems (through participant observation), or it can be performed in a special manner by trained professionals in collaboration with selected patients. Thus, for example, to facilitate clinical improvement in real time, Amy was followed in her breast cancer care journey by a Quality Fellow. The Fellow observed, documented, and reported findings to the medical director and to an interdisciplinary team. Many fruitful improvement projects begin with special observations of the current state, through group communication of field notes, and through depiction of these insights in process flow diagrams and even physical maps of the workplace. Refer to Chapter Two Action Guide for worksheets that guide the activity of direct observation.

### Interviews and Surveys

Complementing the process knowledge gained through direct observation is survey information acquired from participants in the care process itself, including patients, families, clinicians, technicians, and support staff. All these microsystem members bring different experiences and perceptions to the greater work; all have a different understanding of what works, what fails, what adds value and what does not, what delights and what disappoints. Participant knowledge can be gathered effectively through interviews, surveys, and occasional focus groups.[50,51,52] In general, open-ended interviews are an appropriate initial technique; these in turn can generate more specific questions that are best explored through follow-up fixed-response surveys. Again, see Chapter Two Action Guide for more information on interviews and surveys.

## Value Stream Mapping

*Value stream mapping*[53] is one especially powerful and versatile method of microsystem self-inquiry that helps prepare for the design of more ideal future states. This robust approach integrates different types of available process information, identifies discrete process elements that add direct value for the end user, and exposes other elements that fail to add (or even diminish) such value. Value stream maps are functional pictures that illuminate various process features such as work flows, decision points, information flows, timing (waits, delays, cycle times), interactions, and specific quality characteristics. Individual steps in the overall flow of activity are assigned their own data points in the overall mapping process.

In health care, the patient and family are often viewed as customers at the end of the *value chain*. In this context, a primary use of clinical value stream mapping is exploration of sequential care process steps with patients and families themselves at the end point. The aim is to understand how each step contributes to overall value (best outcome, lowest cost, least amount of time) from the patients' and families' perspectives. This process knowledge empowers clinical microsystems to redesign care with patient-customer needs clearly in view. Chapter Two Action Guide offers more specific information on value stream mapping techniques.

## Patients and Families as Committee Members and Advisors

Users of any health care system possess deep knowledge and broad experience that can benefit the system. Frontline microsystems and institutional macrosystems have increasingly sought to harness this important resource and to engage patients and family members as formal or informal members of work committees and institutional advisory boards. Clinicians and staff may recommend patients they believe would function effectively in this role. Alternatively, review of satisfaction surveys may reveal individuals who propose consistently constructive ideas.[7]

Who is the *ideal* patient representative or advisor? The Institute for Patient and Family-Centered Care[7] recommends that microsystems and macrosystems seek patients or family members who demonstrate the following characteristics:

- Represent the community served by the health system
- Share insights and information about their experiences in ways that others can learn from
- Show concern for more than one issue or agenda
- Listen well and respect others' perspectives
- Speak comfortably and candidly in a group
- Interact well with many different kinds of people
- Work in partnerships with others
- See beyond their own personal experience

Many clinical microsystems and larger health care institutions have benefited from the unique skills and perspectives patients and families bring to local improvement projects, to program and policy development, and to system-wide strategic planning initiatives.

## CONCLUSION

The clinical microsystem model locates patients and families firmly at the center of sequentially nested systems of care, and the reach from this central position is extensive. Patients and families are not only final customers or end users in systems of value production (as Deming astutely describes), but also (in Wagner's chronic care model, in Lorig's paradigm of self-management, and in institutional programs of formal collaboration) active contributors to value production itself. As patients, as family members, as students of health care improvement, or as interdisciplinary professionals who deliver (or support delivery) of health care, we are all working together to preserve patients' healthy functioning and vitality for as long as possible. Embracing our partnership and our mutually supportive roles is the best, indeed the only, means of assuring success.

## SUMMARY

- Partnering with patients is an essential strategy for achieving the aim of health care, which is to preserve the health and well-being of patients.
- Powerful general models developed by Deming (systems of production) and Kano (typology of satisfaction), as well as health care models developed by Wagner (chronic care) and Lorig (self-management), frame the *patients as partners* discussion and provide a path forward to develop stronger, more meaningful partnerships.
- Techniques for partnering with patients can best be embedded in the flow of care, which includes the following: (1) assessing patients using patient-provided information on health status, risks, and perceptions; (2) setting health goals using patient contracting and motivational interviewing; (3) making decisions about treatment plans using shared decision making and shared medical appointments; and (4) executing the plan of care based on health coaching and educational information prescriptions.

## KEY TERMS

Chronic care model

Core concepts of patient-centered care

    Collaboration

    Dignity and respect

    Information sharing

    Participation

Deming model

Feed forward

Kano model of satisfaction

Fundamental aim of health care

Health assessment surveys

Health coaching

Informed decision making

Information prescriptions

Motivational interviewing

Partnering with patients

Patient contracting

Patient's current health status

Self-management education

Self-management model

Shared decision-making

Shared medical appointment

Value stream mapping

## REVIEW QUESTIONS

1. What are the IOM's ten aims? Define the process you would follow (including activities and examples) to achieve each aim.
2. How can Kano's framework of satisfaction inform redesign of health care systems? How might one gain patient and family insights based on this framework?
3. How might one apply Deming's system model to health care? What actions would you take to gain insight into planning, executing, and improving health care based on this model?
4. Where do tools, processes, and microsystem theory fit in Wagner's chronic care model?
5. How would you design self-management processes to enhance patient and clinician partnership to achieve health goals?
6. What tools and methods can be used to increase shared decision making?
7. How does value stream mapping enhance knowledge about the current processes of care?

## DISCUSSION QUESTIONS

1. Think about the different roles patients and families play in their own care and in relationship to health care teams. Select a particular kind of patient who is in a relationship with a specific type of health care team in a particular geographic location (microsystem). Then describe and explore the different roles patients and families might play in this microsystem. Some examples of roles patients might play include recipients, providers, beneficiaries, designers, members, co-designers, customers, and advisors. Some examples of roles families play might include chief safety officer, informant, advocate, and caregiver.
2. Now consider which most provocative roles patients and families might apply to this microsystem. How might the roles be leveraged to achieve best-designed care for patients in partnership with professionals?

## REFERENCES

1. Plsek, P., & Greenhalgh, T. The challenge of complexity in health care. *British Medical Journal*, 2001, *323*, 625–628.
2. Henderson, L. Physician and patient as a social system. *The New England Journal of Medicine*, 1935, *212*(18), 820.
3. Dubos, R. *Mirage of health: Utopias, progress and biological change*. Garden City, NY: Anchor Books. Doubleday and Company, 1959.
4. World Health Organization. Preamble to the Constitution of the World Health Organization as adopted by the International Health Conference. *Official Records of the World Health Organization, signed on 22 July 1946 by the representatives of 61 States and entered into force on 7 April 1948*, Vol. 2, p. 100. New York, 1946.
5. Institute of Medicine Committee on Assuring the Health of the Public in the 21st Century. *The future of the public's health in the 21st century*. Washington, DC: National Academy Press,1988.
6. U.S. Department of Health and Human Services. *The power of prevention: Steps to a healthier US*. Report issued 2003. Retrieved January 31, 2010, from www.healthierus.gov/STEPS/summit/prevportfolio/power/index.html

7. Institute for Family-Centered Care. Advancing the practice of patient- and family-centered care in primary care and other ambulatory settings: How to get started. Retrieved June 10, 2009, from www.Familycenteredcare.Org/Tools/Downloads.HTML

8. Kano, N., Seraku, N., Takahashi, F., & Tsuji, S. Attractive quality and must-be quality. *The Journal of the Japanese Society for Quality Control*, 1984, *14*(2), 39–48.

9. Deming, W. *The new economics: For industry, government, education.* (2nd ed.) Cambridge, MA: MIT Press, 1994.

10. Etzwiler, D. D. The contract for health care. *Journal of the American Medical Association*, 1973, *224*(7).

11. Wagner, E., Austin, B. T., & Von Korf, F. M. Organizing care for patients with chronic illness. *Milbank Quarterly*, 1996, *74*, 511–544.

12. Bodenheimer, T., Wagner, E. H., & Grumbach, K. Improving primary care for patients with chronic illness. *Journal of the American Medical Association*, 2002, *288*(14).

13. Bodenheimer, T., Wagner, E. H., & Grumbach, K. Improving primary care for patients with chronic illness—part two. *Journal of the American Medical Association*, 2002, *288*(15), 1909–1914.

14. Wagner, E. *Improving chronic care.* Retrieved June 6, 2009, from www .improvingchroniccare.org/index.php?p=The_Chronic_Care_Model&s=2

15. Lorig, K., Ritter, P. L., Laurent, D. D., & Plant, K. Internet-based chronic disease self-management: A randomized trial. *Medical Care*, 2006, *44*(11), 964–971.

16. Lorig, K., Bodenheimer, T., Holman, H., & Grumbach, K. Patient self-management of chronic disease in primary care. *Journal of the American Medical Association*, 2002, *288*(19), 2469–2475.

17. Lorig, K., Ritter, P. L., Laurent, D. D., & Plant, K. The Internet-based arthritis self-management program: A one-year randomized trial for patients with arthritis or fibromyalgia. *Arthritis Care and Research*, 2008, *59*(7), 1009–1017.

18. Rosenthal, T. The medical home: Growing evidence to support a new approach to primary care. *Journal of the American Board of Family Medicine*, 2008, *21*, 427–440.

19. Iglehart, J. No place like home—testing a new model of care delivery. *The New England Journal of Medicine*, 2008, *359*(12), 1200–1202.

20. Center for Shared Decision Marking. Breast cancer decision aids. Center for Shared Decision Making. Dartmouth-Hitchcock Medical Center. Retrieved June 10, 2009, from www.dhmc.org/webpage.cfm?site_id=2&org_id=108&morg_id=0&sec_id=0&gsec_id= 39685&item_id=39687

21. Foundation for Informed Medical Decision Making. Retrieved June 10, 2009, from www.fimdm.org/about.php

22. Nelson et al. Data and measurement in clinical microsystems: Part 2. Creating a rich information environment. *Joint Commission Journal on Quality and Safety*, 2003, *29*(1), 5–15.

23. Hvitfeldt et al. Feed forward systems for patient participation and provider support: Adoption results from the original US context to Sweden and beyond. *Quality Management in Health Care*, 2009, *18*(4), 247–256.

24. Wasson, J. *How's your health.* Retrieved November 16, 2009, from www.howsyourhealth.org/ idbox.html

25. Grossman, D., & Reid, R. *Group health profile.* Retrieved November 17, 2009, from www.ghc.org/about_gh/2007AnnualReport/PDF/2007AnnualReport.pdf

26. Weinstein, J., Brown, P. W., Hanscom, B., Walsh, T., & Nelson, E. C. Designing an ambulatory clinical practice for outcomes improvement: From vision to reality—the Spine Center at Dartmouth-Hitchcock, year one. *Quality Management in Health Care*, 2000, *8*(2), 1–20.

27. Dynamic Clinical Systems. Retrieved November 17, 2009, from www.dynamicclinical.com

28. Lindblad, S., personal communication delivered to E. Nelson in April 2007.

29. McKinley, K., Delivered to M. Godfrey and students in PowerPoint presentation given to Dartmouth master's degree class on the design of clinical microsystems, April 2005.

30. Nelson, E., Fisher, E. S., & Weinstein, J. N. Information knowledge and development: A perspective on patient-centric, feed forward "collaboratories." Paper prepared for Engineering a learning healthcare system: A look at the future, *Institute of Medicine,* Washington, DC, April 29, 2008.

31. Miller, W., & Rollnick, S. *Motivational interviewing: Preparing people for change.* New York: Guilford Press, 2002.

32. Becker, M., & Maiman, L. A. Strategies for enhancing patient compliance. *Journal of Community Health,* 1980, *6*(2), 113–135.

33. Herje, P. Hows and whys of patient contracting. *Nurse Educator,* 1980, *5*(1).

34. Kasper, J., Mulley, A., & Wennberg, J. Developing shared decision-making programs to improve the quality of health care. *Quality Review Bulletin,* 1992, *18*(6), 183–190.

35. O'Connor, A. The Ottawa Health Decision Centre. Retrieved November 17, 2009, from www.ohri.ca/programs/clinical_epidemiology/OHDEC/default.asp

36. Charles, C., Gafni, A., & Whelan, T. Shared decision-making in the medical encounter: What does it mean? (Or it takes at least two to tango). *Social Science and Medicine,* 1997, *44*(5), 681–692.

37. Charles, C., & DeMaio, S. Lay participation in health care decision-making: A conceptual framework. *Journal of Health Politics, Policy and Law,* 1993, *18*, 881.

38. Frosch, D., & Kaplan, R. Shared decision making in clinical medicine: Past research and future directions. *American Journal of Preventive Medicine,* 1999, *17*(4), 285–294.

39. Noffsigner, E. Use of group visits in the treatment of the chronically ill. In J. Nuovo (Ed.), *Chronic disease management.* Secaucus, NJ: Springer, 2007, pp. 32–86.

40. Kirsh et al. Shared medical appointments based on the chronic care model: A quality improvement project to address the challenges of patients with diabetes with high cardiovascular risk. *Quality and Safety in Health Care,* 2007, *16*, 349–353.

41. Kuiken, S., & Seiffert, D. Thinking outside the box!! Enhance patient education by using shared medical appointments. *Plastic Surgical Nursing,* 2005, *25*(4), 191–195.

42. Vale et al. Coaching patients on achieving cardiovascular health. A multicenter randomized trial in patients with coronary heart disease. *Archives of Internal Medicine,* 2003, *163*(22), 2775–2783.

43. Palmer, S., Tubbs, I., & Whybrow, A. Health coaching to facilitate the promotion of healthy behaviour and achievement of health-related goals. *International Journal of Health Promotion & Education,* 2003, *41*(3), 91–93.

44. Robert, H. *Masterful coaching fieldbook.* San Francisco: Jossey-Bass/Pfeiffer, 2000.

45. D'Alessandro, D. M., Kreiter, C. D., Kinzer, S. L., & Peterson, M. W. A randomized controlled trial of an information prescription for pediatric patient education on the Internet. *Archives of Pediatrics & Adolescent Medicine,* 2004, *158*(9), 857–862.

46. Leisey, M. R., & Shipman, J. P. Information prescriptions: A barrier to fulfillment. *Journal of the Medical Library Association,* 2007, *95*(4), 435–438.

47. Siegel et al. Information RX: Evaluation of a new informatics tool for physicians, patients, and libraries. *Information Services & Use,* 2006, *26*(1), 1–10.

48. Nelson, E., Batalden, P. B., & Lazar, J. S. *Practice-based learning and improvement: A clinical improvement action guide.* (2nd ed.) Oak Brook, IL: Joint Commission Resources, 2007.

49. Simmons, S. F. Continuous quality improvement for nutritional care services in nursing homes: The importance of direct observation. *Journal of the American Medical Association,* 2006, *7*(1), 61–62.

50. Coulter, A., & Cleary, P. D. Patients' experiences with hospital care in five countries. *Health Affairs (Millwood),* 2001, *20*(3), 244–252.

51. Fitzpatrick, R. Surveys of patients' satisfaction: Important general considerations. *British Medical Journal,* 1991, *302*(6781), 887–889.

52. Laine et al. Important elements of outpatient care: A comparison of patients' and physicians' opinions. *Annals of Internal Medicine,* 1996, *125*(8), 640–645.

53. Rother, M., & Shook, J. *Learning to see: Value stream mapping to add value and eliminate MUDA. Version 1.1.* Brookline, MA: The Lean Enterprise Institute, 1998.

Chapter Two Action Guide provides tools and methods to encourage your study of patients and their perspectives in your clinical microsystem, research value, and non-value-added activities in the processes of care and consider how to engage patients and families with their unique insights in improving the delivery of care and services.

## GAINING CUSTOMER KNOWLEDGE

Gaining customer knowledge can use a naturalistic approach or a structured approach to learn what is important in the delivery of care and services to your patients along with what actions, processes, and structures add value to the patient-care experience from their perspective.

Increasingly, health care professionals are realizing the benefits of partnering with patients and families to gain deeper insights into the delivery of care. The following materials support the beginning of the journey to learn what matters to the patient (a customer) in the delivery of care and services, and will help guide interdisciplinary health care professionals in delivering this care.

As depicted in Figure AG2.1, gaining customer knowledge can range from naturalistic to structured methods and processes.

The naturalistic approach uses the staff eyes (watching), ears (listening), and inquiry (asking) to gain insights into customer or patient knowledge, whereas a structured approach is more systematic. Methods employed by the naturalist approach are as follows:

1. Staff can be coached to listen to and watch patients and families and inquire, "Is anything bothering you today?"
2. Staff can track the number of patients who wait more than ten minutes or patients who want to be seen earlier in an ambulatory practice.
3. The microsystem can offer comment or suggestion cards with a return box to capture positive feedback and improvement suggestions.

In addition, the microsystem can offer a hot line for feedback and an ombudsman or patient advocate to gather and record insights. Unsolicited letters from patients and families should also be reviewed for clues to what patients and families are looking for in the delivery of care and services and what they expect.

The *structured approach* gathers customer insights more systematically. Examples of structural methods are as follows:

FIGURE AG2.1    Continuum of Methods for Gaining Customer Knowledge.

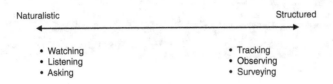

**Methods to Gain Customer Knowledge
(Naturalistic to Structured Continuum)**

Naturalistic                                    Structured

• Watching                    • Tracking
• Listening                   • Observing
• Asking                      • Surveying

1. Use of trackers who perform directed observation and document the journey of the patient in the health care process to gain deeper understanding of the process of care from the patient and family perspective. (The story of Amy in Chapter Two serves as an example of the benefits of this approach.). Amy was approached at her first appointment for care of a breast lump to inquire if a designated quality improvement staff member could follow Amy at each and every encounter she had with the health care system to observe and document Amy's journey to inform improvement activities in the system of care. Amy generously agreed. The observational experience was documented and shared with the interdisciplinary care team to review and identify improvement opportunities.

2. Mystery shoppers (secret agent patients) can be used to move through the health care system and note what delights them as patients and what needs improvement.

3. Staff can role play and assume the role of the patient and or family. Role playing helps staff increase knowledge of the customer, the current health care delivery system, and connect directly with other staff involved in the process of care.

A basic tool that supports the observation process or role playing in gaining customer knowledge is to experience or see the patients' health care journey as they experience it. "Through the Patient's Eyes" is a helpful tool for learning about the patient experience (see Figure AG2.2). The form can be found at www.clinicalmicrosystem.org in the *Assess, Diagnose and Treat Workbooks* also known as the *Greenbooks*. Many microsystem members have elected to follow a patient through his or her experience and document observations using this worksheet; others have assumed the role of the patient and traveled the patient care course as a patient might. Capturing patients' experiences with video or digital photography has been helpful for sharing information with other members of the microsystem. (It is important to determine your organization's policy on the use of video or digital photography for the purpose of health care improvement before you start your observation process.)

## Observational Skills and Ethnography

The science of *ethnography*, which is derived from Greek-ethos/folk or people and graphein/writing is aimed at gaining deeper understanding about the context and the people where care and services are delivered. Members of the microsystem can conduct direct firsthand observation of the daily activities and life to describe the context, people, physical layout, social structures, rituals, and traditions of the care setting. The result of the direct observation enables the interdisciplinary group to have a clearer

FIGURE AG2.2   Through the Eyes of Your Patients.

## Through the Eyes of Your Patients

**Tips for making the walk through most productive:**

1. Determine with your staff where the starting point and ending points should be, taking into consideration making the appointment, the actual office visit process, follow-up, and other processes.

2. Two members of the staff should role play with each playing a role: patient and partner/family member.

3. Set aside a reasonable amount of time to experience the patient journey. Consider doing multiple experiences along the patient journey at different times.

4. Make it real. Include time with registration, lab tests, new patient, follow-up, and physicals. Sit where the patient sits. Wear what the patient wears. Make a realistic paper trail including chart, lab reports, and follow-up.

5. During the experience note both positive and negative experiences, as well as any surprises. What was frustrating? What was gratifying? What was confusing? Again, an audio or video tape can be helpful.

6. Debrief your staff on what you did and what you learned.

Date: _____          Staff Members: _____  _____

Walk Through Begins: _____        Ends When: _____

| Positives | Negatives | Surprises | Frustrating/Confusing | Gratifying |
|---|---|---|---|---|
|  |  |  |  |  |

understanding of the microsystem setting and culture and to better plan improvement opportunities and strategies. Observation, keen listening, and recording through the use of video, digital photography, pen and note pad, and an observation worksheet are helpful. Beyond note taking, drawing flowcharts and diagrams of the context of the care and services helps build knowledge of the patient experience.

Before starting this structured work, it is essential to obtain permission and access to the care setting and to ask permission of staff and patients to observe their experience. Observers must commit to honesty, doing no harm, and remembering they are a guest in the lives of those receiving and giving care. The last step in the process of observation is to thank those one had the privilege to observe.

The *Gaining Customer Knowledge* worksheets can be found at www.clinical microsystem.org. The worksheets use an orderly process to gain initial knowledge and insights through observation and then deepen the knowledge with additional interviews and surveys.

**FIGURE AG2.3  Observation Skills Worksheet.**

**Context**

Aim: Build customer knowledge through observation

- 1. Outcomes → select a patient population

_____
*Specify patient population*

2. Aim → What's the general aim? Given our wish to limit or reduce the illness burden for this type of patient, what are the desired results?

Structured Aim Statement → We aim to improve the
_____ for_____
*(Insert process name)*     *(insert patient population)*

_____
*(Insert start of process boundary)*

_____
*(Insert end of process boundary)*

By working on this process we hope to achieve:

_____
*(Insert benefits)*

_____

It is important to work on this now because:

_____
*(List compelling reasons)*

_____

3. Microsystems → Given the process boundaries, the clinical microsystem(s) that serve this patient population for this process are:

_____
*(List microsystem(s) serving patients)*
_____

Observation # _____ : Facts
Today's Date
Patient Name/Initials
Family Member Name/Initials
Microsystem Name
Provider Name/Initials
Permission Obtained
Time Observation Started
Time Observation Ended
Name of Process Observed

**Tips. Process Observation Watch and Listen for**

Who did what, when? — Did anything disappoint or upset the patient?

What did the patient want? — Did the patient experience any problems?

What did the patient need? — What was the patient saying? Thinking?

Did anything delight the patient? — What did body language say?

Observer:_____ Date:_____

Person being observed: _____

Observation begins with:_____

**Activities Observed**

| When | Where | What | Who | Saying What |
|------|-------|------|-----|-------------|

Observation ends with _____

One might consider evaluating and increasing microsystem awareness by applying different "lenses" or perspectives to the clinical microsystem. Figures AG2.4 and AG2.5 are examples of different lenses that allow us to see, ask more questions, and begin to understand different elements in a microsystem.

An optional *Observation* worksheet provides space for creating diagrams and flowcharts (see Figure AG2.5). It uses the *Clinical Microsystem Lenses Model* to gain new perspectives based in ethnography when observing a microsystem. The microsystem lenses provide different vantage points for observing and studying the health care and have been included in this observational tool. The diagram and the annotated descriptions provide fresh ways to see people, processes, and patterns in your microsystem.

The experience of observing should inform the interview and survey processes to deepen your customer knowledge. Individual interviews of patients or staff, group interviews, or focus groups can be conducted to create surveys for current, new, old, and former patients.

Patient viewpoint surveys can then be created using the observation database insights and summaries. Patient viewpoint surveys deepen your knowledge of patients' attitudes, practices, and perceptions through development of key survey questions based on the direct observation experiences.

FIGURE AG2.4    Microsystem Lenses Model.

**Biologic System**
• Emergence
• Coordination/
  Synergy
• Structure,
  Process, Pattern
• Vitality

**Economic System**
• Inputs/Outputs
• Cost/Waste/Value/Benefits
• Customer/Suppliers

**Political System**
• Power
• Governance
• Citizenship
• Equity

**Sociologic System**
• Relationships
• Conversations
• Interdependence
• Loose-tight Coupling
• Meaning/Sense

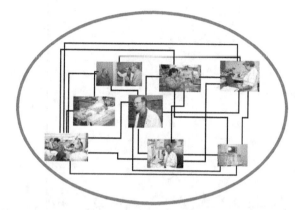

**Anthropologic System**
•Values
•Culture/Milieu

**Information System**
• Access
• Speed
• Fidelity/Utility
• Privacy/Security
• Storage

**Mechanical / Physical System**
• Flow
• Temporal Sequencing
• Spatial Proximities
• Logistics
• Information

**Psychological**
• Organizing
• Forces Field
• Ecological/Behavior Settings

Microsurveys can be used to measure the goodness of the patient journey; such surveys are attached to specific steps in the patient's journey in a specific care process. The microsurvey can identify key quality and value characteristics from the patient perspective to result in redesigned and improved processes of care based on what matters from the patient perspective.

## Tips for Writing Survey Items

Determine if there are experts in your organization who have experience writing surveys. Once you identify them, connect with them to ensure your surveys are well-written and to explore if similar surveys already exist in the organization. Some tips for writing good survey questions follow.

1. Use short sentences, simple sentence structure, and short words.
2. Avoid double-barreled questions where more than one question is being asked.
3. Avoid leading questions.
4. Create a visually clean layout of the survey.
5. Use logical response choices that match the question.
6. Always do a pretest to see how the questions work with real people.

FIGURE AG2.5  Tips and Lenses Worksheet.

# Observation Worksheet

**Date/Time:**

**Location:**

**Key Process:**

(starts)

(ends)

**Flowchart the Process:**

**Questions/Surprises:**

**Tips:**

Ask permission

Watch and listen for the following:

➤ What is the goal?

➤ Who did what when?

➤ What were the roles of patient, family, staff?

➤ Notice materials, supplies, documentation

➤ How might you adapt to your setting?

➤ Express appreciation

**Lenses:**

➤ *Biologic*
(Structure, process, pattern, emergence, vitality coordination/synergy)

➤ *Sociologic*
(Relationships, conversations, interdependence, meaning/sense)

➤ *Mechanical, Physical*
(Flow, sequencing, spatial proximities, logistics, information)

➤ *Psychological*
(Organizing, force fields, behaviors)

➤ *Information*
(Access, speed, fidelity, utility, privacy, security, storage)

➤ *Anthropologic*
(Values, culture, milieu)

➤ *Political*
(Power, governance, citizenship, equity)

➤ *Economic*
(Inputs/outputs, cost, waste, value, benefits, customer, suppliers)

## Different Types of Survey Questions

Survey items can be written as ratings, opinions, or reports. Patients' comments can also be recorded verbatim.

### Ratings

Some examples of how to ask patients to rate their evaluative judgments are shown in the sidebar.

### Opinions

Statements of an opinion where the respondent is asked to agree or disagree follow. These are often written as Likert-type items with four or five choices (see Table AG2.1).

### Reports

Declarative statements representing a person's understanding of what happened are shown in the sidebar.

### Verbatim

Open-ended questions that patients answer in their own words include the ones shown in the sidebar.

## Steps for Conducting a Written Survey

Some steps to plan and conduct a survey are as follow.

*Define your aim.* What is the AIM and what are the key questions to answer?

*Define your survey strategy and audience.* Determine who will be surveyed and how they will be invited to participate. Will Institutional Review Board (IRB) approval be needed? Will the survey be anonymous and confidential? Who will sponsor and champion the survey from the organization?

*Define your data collection methodology.* How will the survey be distributed and returned? Will it be handed out and handed back, mailed out and mailed back, or completed online?

*Design your layout.* How will the survey be designed so that it is clean, attractive, and easy to analyze?

*Analyze your results.* How will you analyze the results to provide answers to your key questions? Always make dummy data displays as part of the planning process. (A dummy data display is a make-believe figure or table showing the kind of results you might get.) A dummy data display helps you find relationships between data, discover what variables you will need to answer your questions, and decide how you will analyze data and display results.

*Summarize your results.* Reflect on your analysis and summarize the results. Consider doing this by stating major results as headlines that are linked to graphical data displays or to data tables.

---

Thinking about your own health care, how would you rate the following?
Length of time spent waiting at the office to see your provider: Poor, Fair, Good, Very Good, Excellent
Thoroughness of treatment: Poor, Fair, Good, Very Good, Excellent
Overall quality of care and services: Poor, Fair, Good, Very Good, Excellent

---

How long did you have to wait between the time you made the appointment for care and the day you actually saw the provider?
Same day, 2–3 days, 4–7 days, 1–2 weeks, 3–4 weeks, 5–6 weeks, more than 6 weeks

---

What, if anything, could be done to improve care and services?
Please list anything that happened during your hospital stay that delighted you or surprised you.

Table AG2.1    Opinion Survey

| Surgery and First Twenty-Four Hours After Surgery | Strongly Agree | Agree | Neutral or No Opinion | Disagree | Strongly Disagree | Does Not Apply |
|---|---|---|---|---|---|---|
| 1. The intensive care unit staff were sensitive to my needs and feelings. | 1 | 2 | 3 | 4 | 5 | N/A |
| 2. I received satisfactory pain relief while in the intensive care unit. | 1 | 2 | 3 | 4 | 5 | N/A |
| 3. I received adequate attention and comfort from the intensive care unit staff when I felt disoriented after my surgery. | 1 | 2 | 3 | 4 | 5 | N/A |
| 4. I had no problems communicating with the intensive care unit staff immediately after my surgery. | 1 | 2 | 3 | 4 | 5 | N/A |

## Structure of a Written Survey

A survey usually adheres to the following structure:

1. *Introduction*—Purpose of survey, uses, sponsor, type (confidential or anonymous), and clear instructions.
2. *Opening question(s)*—Initial questions should be short, simple, and relate to the aim of the survey. Once respondents become clear on the purpose of the survey with the opening questions, they are more likely to provide useful responses to more detailed questions later in the survey.
    Think about your overall hospital experience. How satisfied are you with your experience?
3. *Main body of questions*—The main body of the questions should be specific, in logical flow, and build on each other. For example:
    Think about the admission process to the medical/surgical unit. How satisfied were you with your experience?
    Think about the discharge to home process from the medical/surgical unit. How satisfied were you with your experience?
    How was your preparation for your discharge to home?
4. *Closing question(s)*—General summative questions and additional information the respondent may wish to share
5. *Thank you* and information about how to return the survey

After your observations, you can conduct interviews using individual, semi-structured interviews, or focus groups to gain the next level of deep knowledge about patient and family experiences. The information and insights you gain through your observations should inform your interview.

The phases of the interview process are described using a metaphor related to flying (see Figure AG2.6).

The worksheets that follow provide structured tools to support your interview process and to achieve the results you are hoping to obtain (see Figures AG2.7 and AG2.8).

## FIGURE AG2.6   Flying a Plane and Conducting an Interview.

**Flying**
Work your way through the interview guide, covering the main topics and exploring promising leads with clarifying questions.

**Taking Off**
Establish purpose and rapport with respondents, and express appreciation for their participation. Seek permission to record if desired.

**Preflight**
Review your aim and interview guide.

**Landing**
Ask your final question and remind respondents of how results will be used; thank them for participating.

**Debriefing**
Reflect on how the interview went and on what might be improved in the process and method before the next interview. Review notes and recordings to finalize documentation of the interview.

## FIGURE AG2.7   Interview Worksheet 1.

Aim: Continue to build customer knowledge to lead to improvements in health care.

### Interview # _____ : Facts

Today's Date: _____
Patient Name/Initials: _____
Family Member Name/Initials: _____
Microsystem Name: _____
Provider Name/Initials: _____
Permission Obtained: _____
Time Interview Started: _____
Time Interview Ended: _____
Aim of Interview: _____
_____
_____

### Tips
1. Use eye contact.
2. Use comfortable environment.
3. Consider audio/video taping.
4. Follow clues: for instance, "high quality" — what would that look like? How would you describe quality?
5. Observe body language and facial expressions.

### Notetaking Tips
1. Discuss notetaking with interviewee.
2. Take notes regularly and promptly.
3. Try close to verbatim notetaking.
4. Don't let notetaking interfere with ability to listen and ask questions.

### Steps for Doing Interviews
1. **Aim**: Set the aim and frame the key question(s).
2. **Who**: Determine who will be interviewed and how they will be invited to participate.
3. **Plan**: Who will conduct the interviews, in what setting, and with what tools and training? How will the results be recorded and analyzed?
4. **Interviews:** Conduct the interviews using an interview guide.
5. **Analysis:** Analyze the content of the results to identify the response patterns that provide answers to your key questions.
6. **Summarize:** Reflect on your analysis and summarize the results. Consider doing this using major results that are linked to actual verbatim statements contained in the interview notes.

### Steps for an Individual Interview
- **Preflight**
  - Review your aim and interview guide.
- **Taking Off:**
  - Establish purpose with respondent and rapport and appreciation for their participation.
- **Flying:**
  - Work your way through the interview guide covering the main topics and exploring the promising leads and asking questions to clarify and to probe.
- **Landing**
  - Ask your final question and remind the respondent of how results will be used and thank him for participating.
- **Debriefing:**
  - Reflect on how the interview went.
  - What might be done to improve the process and the method before conducting the next interview?

FIGURE AG2.8   Interview Worksheet 2.

---

**Interview Guide Template**

**Preflight**
- Interview who, where, under what auspices, with what guide, for what purpose.

**Taking Off**
- Introduce self, purpose of interview, how information is to be used, assure confidentiality, ask any questions, and ask permission to proceed with the interview.
- First question: Write an open-ended question that invites the respondent to tell his/her story re: topic of interest.
  My first question is:_____

**Flying**
- Frame several core questions to achieve your aim and answer key questions.
  1. _____
  2. _____
  3. _____
  4. _____
  5. _____

**Landing**
- Last question: write summative last question.

  My last question is:_____
- Thank respondent and say goodbye.

**Debriefing**
- If taking notes: review notes and add to them to make as complete a record as possible.
- Consider what new is learned by this interview.
- Consider refinements to interview guide based on what is learned.

---

The observations, interviews, and surveys will provide you with rich new perspectives on the patient and family experience. The *Analysis and Interpretation* worksheet can help pull all your information together to help you draw conclusions and guide improvement (see Figure AG2.9).

How might the new knowledge of patients and customers be built into the clinical microsystem and emphasized in the usual processes of care delivery? What measures from the patient perspective and the process perspective might be tracked to monitor the desired processes in care discovered through gaining customer knowledge? Once you have completed your analysis and interpretation, consider the following focus areas to create a patient- and family-centered environment.

- *Guidance:* create patient-centered mission, vision, and principles; that is, *say it, do it, live it.*
- *Stories:* tell stories about extraordinary patient care and service that include *above* and *beyond* examples.
- *Governance:* form patient advisory councils.
- *Education:* build patient-mindedness (a natural inclination to consider patient perspective), education, and training into staff development and evaluation process.
- *Feedback:* build data walls and provide direct feedback to staff.
- *Reports:* provide patient feedback data and comments to staff and display such input in public places.

# FIGURE AG2.9 Analysis and Interpretation.

Aim: Based on your observations and interviews (and other information), use value compass thinking to summarize the patients' and familys' view of the features of care and service that contribute to the goodness (or badness) of outcomes and process.

Tips. Value Compass
Purpose: To identify features of care that contribute most to the patients' perception of overall 'goodness.'
1  Select a clinically significant population.
2  Conduct observations of patients receiving care.
3  Start with east (satisfaction) on the compass and go counterclockwise around the compass.
4  List features that contribute to perception of goodness.

OUTCOMES ➜ Identify features of care that patients' perceive as contributing to its "goodness" in meeting their wants and needs.

**Functional**
- Physical function
- Mental health
- Social/role
- Other (health risk)
- Perceived well-being

**Clinical**
_____ -Morbidity
_____ -Complications
_____ -Signs
_____ -Symptoms
_____ -Side effects

**Satisfaction Versus Wants /Needs**
- Health care delivery
- Perceived health benefit
- Delights
- Disappointments
- Problems

**Costs**
- Direct medical
- Indirect
- .   .

Tips. Process Map
Purpose: To map patients' view of steps in process
1  Start by listing basic steps in patients' journey.
2  List features of care at each step that drive perception of goodness. List the key quality characteristics for each step.

**Process Map**

Patients with Needs

Patients with Needs Met

- *Ideal*: work with staff to map the ideal visit. Attach patient key quality characteristics to steps in the process flow.
- *Just-in-time reviews*: hold regular huddles with interdisciplinary staff during usual work hours to evaluate patient-centered performance and to identify improvements.
- *Rounds*: hold patient-needs rounds and then evaluate if the needs were met or how they could be met in an ideal system.
- *Lunches*: hold lunch-and-learn facilitated discussions about patient or customer knowledge and education.
- *Engagement*: put patients and families on your improvement teams.

## INSTITUTE FOR PATIENT AND FAMILY-CENTERED CARE MATRIX

The Institute for Patient and Family-Centered Care (previously known as The Institute for Family-Centered Care) offers a framework for patient and family involvement in quality improvement that can be used to analyze and strengthen your microsystem's level of patient and family engagement. Many organizations have benefited from formally including patients and families on advisory boards, developing family and patients as faculty to teach orientation to new health care professionals, embedding patients and families in structured interdisciplinary improvement groups, and identifying other formal roles in the organization such as *care innovator* or *patient and family advisors* to keep patient and family perspectives included in improving health care.

Figure AG2.10 can be viewed as a place to start your clinical microsystem assessment and methods to include patients and families more fully in the processes of care delivery.

The Institute for Patient and Family-Centered Care www.ipfcc.org continues to evolve and through their Web site offers many helpful publications, tools, and processes

**FIGURE AG2.10    Framework for Family Involvement in Quality Improvement.**

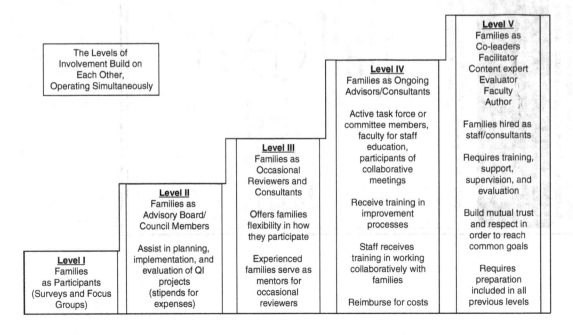

to "advance the understanding and practice of patient-and family-centered care in hospitals and other health care settings."

## VALUE STREAM MAPPING

Gaining customer knowledge can further be enhanced through the use of value stream mapping. The value stream map is an essential technique for redesigning processes to meet patient or customer requirements and be efficient, effective, and timely. The value stream map is a visual tool to show workflow, including information, data, communication, handoffs, and value added versus non-value added activities from the patient and family perspective. Metrics associated with value stream maps often include process time, wait time, lead time, first time quality, 100-percent accurate, 100-percent complete, and first time completed. Value stream maps focus on the patient or customer requirements and link work activities with information and data flow. As such, they are able to represent complex processes and show which activities add or do not add value for the patient or customer.

The goals of value stream mapping are as follows:

1. Focus on value for the patient or customer.
2. Reduce waste.
3. Design simple and clear forms of communication.
4. Instill quality in each step of the process.
5. Align resources to meet demands.
6. Improve flow of patient, information, and data.
7. Ensure caregivers have what they need when they need it to provide services.
8. Increase interdisciplinary understanding of roles and processes of providing care.

The six basic steps to create a value stream map follow. Use the *Value Stream Map* worksheets at www.clinicalmicrosystem.org (see Figure AG2.11) to complete the detailed measures of each of these basic steps:

**FIGURE AG2.11   Value Stream Map Worksheet.**

1. Clarify the beginning and the end of the process.
2. Create a flowchart of the current state that describes flow of information, documents, supplies, and communications.
3. Identify the customer for each step of the process.
4. Perform an observational walk (once the process is mapped initially) to observe, document, and validate the detail of each step in the process and understand the customer or supplier relationships and handoffs.
5. Measure the time of each step, note delays, and total the time for the entire process or *cycle time*. (Cycle time is the amount of time it takes to complete one step of the process from the end of the previous step to the end of the current step.)
6. Review the value stream map to identify value added and non-value added steps in the process. (For more information, refer to the *Value Stream Mapping* worksheet at www.clinicalmicrosystem.org.)

## DEFINITIONS OF SELECTED VALUE STREAM MAPPING TERMS

Figure AG 2.12 is used to map each current step of the selected process including the key measures of value. Each completed worksheet is then posted in order of occurrence on a wall to show the full process.

*Value added:* Any activity that improves the outcome of the patient or process or that increases or changes the form or function of the product or service. These are outcomes the patient would be willing to pay for.

*Non-value added:* Any activity that does not improve the outcome of the patient or process and is not necessary. These activities should be eliminated, simplified, reduced, or integrated with value added activities.

*Change over:* The amount of time it takes to change over or set up the room, patient, paperwork, machine, or program from the last operation (or patient) of the previous setup to the first operation (or patient) of the current setup. Examples include cleaning and changing a bed for a new patient and preparing an operating room for the next operation.

*First time quality or first-pass yield:* The percentage of time quality standards are met the first time through and the task is done accurately and completely.

*Touch time:* The amount of time the patient, document, or task is actually being worked on, not including non-value added items like travel, searching, and setup. For example, if you could do this task without interruptions and with everything you need to get it done, how long would it take you to do it?

*Up time:* The amount of time the machine, person, or program is available compared to the amount of time the machine, person, or program is expected to be available, expressed as a percentage. For example, if the echo machine is unavailable 4 times out of 10 when you need it, the up time is 60 percent.

*Work in process:* Amount of inventory before the next step of the process. For example, the number of patients, components, files, or forms waiting to be processed.

Once the current process is mapped and measured using the value stream mapping process, the next step is to develop the ideal or future state of the process through elimination of waste in the process, redesign of flow, optimization of roles, and continuing to measure and monitor the process to ensure highest value steps and outcomes.

**Aim:** Create a picture of the system of processes from beginning to end to improve the "value added" process through step-by-step review and identification of connections, activities, information, and flow.

**What is a value stream map?**

A hands-on visual tool to show workflow, information flow, and value using process cycle time and first time quality metrics. Supports identification of system waste and builds common perspective for interdisciplinary teams.

COMPLETE THIS PROCESS WITH AN INTERDISCIPLINARY TEAM CLOSEST TO THE PROCESS

**Interdisciplinary Team Members**

1. _____   7. _____
2. _____   8. _____
3. _____   9. _____
4. _____   10. _____
5. _____   11. _____
6. _____   12. _____

Clarify process to improve
We aim to improve the process of _____
Beginning
of process _____
End of
process _____

**Checklist:**

A. Clarify aim

B. Create high-level flowchart of process

C. Add information and data flows

D. Identify customer and supply handoffs

E. Perform observational walk
   1. Note customer/supplier,
   2. Measure time of each step and total cycle time of process

F. Determine delivery and quality requirements

G. Design LEAN/improved process

| | Name of the Step | |
|---|---|---|
| | # of People Doing This Step at the Same Time | Notations About Special Needs, Training, Limitations, and so on |
| C-T Cycle Time | The amount of time it takes to complete this step measured from the end of the previous step to the end of this step, including the wait time, walk time, search time, and change over time | |
| V-A Value Added | An estimate of the percentage of value added time in the total cycle time | |
| C-O Change Over or Setup | The amount of time it takes to change over or set up a room, patient, paperwork, machine, or program from the last good piece (operation) of the previous setup to the first good piece (operation) of the current setup | |
| U-T Up Time | The amount of time the machine, person, program, and so on are available compared to the time they are expected to be available, expressed as a percentage | |
| FPY First Pass Yield | The percentage of time that quality standards are met (it is done correctly) | |
| Inventory | The amount of inventory (patients) before next step | The amount of time associated with the inventory |
| T-T Touch Time | The amount of time the task by itself takes | |
| Notes | State other information about the process that is important but not captured | |

# IMPROVING SAFETY AND ANTICIPATING HAZARDS IN CLINICAL MICROSYSTEMS

Gautham K. Suresh

Marjorie M. Godfrey

Eugene C. Nelson

Paul B. Batalden

## LEARNING OBJECTIVES

- Describe the frequency and scope of medical errors in health care systems.
- Differentiate between medical errors and adverse events.
- Compare and contrast the person approach versus the systems approach to patient safety in microsystems.
- List four methods to identify medical errors and adverse events.
- Discuss work conditions, human conditions, and organizational factors that affect patient safety.
- Describe how microsystem members should respond to medical errors and adverse events within their microsystem.
- Describe the five hallmarks that constitute *mindfulness* in a clinical microsystem.

Patient safety is one of the six aims for health system improvement described in the Institute of Medicine (IOM) report *Crossing the Quality Chasm,*[1] the others being effectiveness, patient centeredness, timeliness, efficiency, and equity. Although patient safety problems (medical errors and preventable adverse events) have been sporadically described in the medical literature and in the lay press, it was only after a landmark report in 1999 from the IOM, *To Err Is Human,*[2] that widespread attention was paid to the high frequency of medical errors and to the importance of reducing them. The IOM report emphasized that medical errors were a leading cause of death in the United States and that these errors were responsible for the deaths of 44,000 to 98,000 patients each year in U.S. hospitals. Yet, there was little social agreement about how to proceed. Emphasizing that the status quo was intolerable, the report called for an urgent and comprehensive approach to improving patient safety. Currently, much regulatory, administrative, research, media, and public attention is focused upon patient safety as a distinct and important topic that falls under the umbrella of improvement in health care.[3]

Ideally, within clinical microsystems, the building blocks of health care, safety should be a precondition, and should exist before the patient and family even enter the microsystem. A patient entering a clinical microsystem to receive health care arrives with some expectations about the type of care and services he or she is going to receive and about desired results of this care and services. Chapter Two is a review of *patients as partners.* Patients arrive with an unstated, implicit trust that the health care system will help them and not harm them. Unfortunately, numerous studies have shown that patients are often harmed by medical errors that occur within clinical microsystems. To create the precondition of safety it is necessary to assess and improve processes at the microsystem, mesosystem, and macrosystem levels of the organization to ensure vigilance about safety hazards, tracking of near misses and medical errors, and also ensure immediate and subsequent responses to errors.

Before moving into the heart of this chapter on safety, which provides definitions, principles, concepts, and methods that are helpful for promoting safety in microsystems, we first offer a case study. The case discusses how one clinical program, a neonatal intensive care nursery, has worked for more than a decade to build a culture of safety, to take specific actions to reduce medical errors, and to avoid harming the infants they care for.

## CASE STUDY OF ORGANIZATIONAL FACTORS TO PROMOTE A CULTURE OF SAFETY

Early in the process of improving patient safety in the Intensive Care Nursery (ICN) at Dartmouth, the leaders of this microsystem realized the importance of creating a non-punitive culture that would encourage staff to report errors and discuss patient safety hazards without fear of retribution. To achieve this, the nurse and physician leaders encouraged the ICN staff in meetings and through notices on bulletin boards to speak up if they noticed another health care provider in the ICN not following a recommended safety practice.

For example, as a standardized infection-prevention safety practice, all health care providers entering the ICN are expected to remove their white coats, remove wrist jewelry and watches, and roll up their sleeves to the elbow. Many of the providers entering the ICN for consultation are from hospital units (microsystems) other than the ICN, and it was essential to communicate with them to ensure *all* providers followed the infection-prevention process. A letter was sent by the ICN medical director to other

# CASE STUDY CONTEXT: THE INTENSIVE CARE NURSERY AT THE CHILDREN'S HOSPITAL AT DARTMOUTH

The Intensive Care Nursery (ICN) at the Children's Hospital at Dartmouth is a clinical microsystem that cares for about four hundred neonates a year. These fragile, critically ill neonates (most of whom are premature infants), and their families are cared for by health professionals from multiple disciplines who work collaboratively under conditions of high intensity and stress. Caregivers use a variety of interventions, including cardiopulmonary monitoring, medications, invasive devices, computer information systems, and other technologies. Because of the complexity of the setting, there are multiple opportunities for error to occur, and because of the fragility of the patients, there is only a narrow margin of tolerance for error. Most of the neonates are born at Dartmouth-Hitchcock Medical Center and are cared for by the interdisciplinary ICN team immediately from birth. This requires close collaboration and good communication between the microsystem that cares for the babies (the intensive care nursery) and the microsystem that cares for the mothers of the babies (the obstetrics department).

Patient safety has been an important focus of the ICN since 2002, primarily guided by its participation in a national collaborative quality improvement project organized by the Vermont Oxford Network, called Neonatal Intensive Care Quality (NICQ). The physician and nurse leaders of the microsystem meet once a week to review overall ICN performance and issues. Patient safety topics are prominent in the meeting agenda and discussions. In addition, the Medication Error Reduction Improvement Team (MERIT) committee focuses on patient safety. A multidisciplinary nosocomial sepsis task force also meets periodically.

## Identification of, and Learning from Near Misses, Errors, and Adverse Events

Near misses, errors, and adverse events are identified in the ICN through voluntary reporting by ICN health professionals using a computerized hospital reporting system. This system informs the microsystem leaders electronically whenever any serious incident occurs and allows the leaders to identify trends and patterns in reported incidents. The reporting system data is reviewed monthly at MERIT meetings, and the multidisciplinary team decides what actions are required in response to these reports. This group also regularly reviews safety alerts from organizations such as the Joint Commission and the Institute for Safe Medication Practices; the reviews help the group identify whether the safety hazards described in the alert might exist in the ICN as well. In addition, actual or potential errors may also be identified in real time during nursing or safety rounds.

The ICN uses time trend charts to closely track the rate of nosocomial bloodstream infections, both as a percentage of babies with a birth weight of 401 to 1,500 grams (*runchart*) and of the number of days in between infections (*gchart*). (Chapter Four provides more details about displaying data over time.) The nosocomial data is displayed on a data wall near the nurses' lounge to inform staff of progress in nosocomial infection reduction. When a serious error or adverse event occurs, physician and nurse leaders perform a broad-based investigation into work conditions, human conditions, and organizational conditions (the *WHO framework*) that potentially contributed to the causation of the incident. Based on the factors identified in this investigation, interventions to prevent future incidents are developed and implemented within the microsystem.

## Implementation of Practices to Promote Patient Safety (WHO)

During the past many years, several safety interventions have been implemented in the ICN. Some of these were driven by the Joint Commission's National Patient Safety Goals. Others were put in place based on risk factors locally identified within the microsystem (see Table 3.1).

Table 3.1    Workplace and Human Factors (WHO) Examples

| Intervention | Explanation |
|---|---|
| 1. Preprinted medication order entry sheet. | • Increases legibility.<br>• Contains reference doses of the medication.<br>• Clearly defines fields to prompt prescribers to correctly and completely complete prescription requirements. |
| 2. Mechanically designed oral medication syringe and enteral feeding tubes that do not fit into intravenous catheters. | • Prevents inadvertent intravenous administration of medications or enteral feeds. |
| 3. Universal protocol[4] prior to the performance of any invasive procedure. | • Prevents procedures from being performed on the wrong patient, the wrong site, or the wrong side of the body. |
| 4. TALL man lettering for a portion of the medication when prescribing similarly named medications. (Example: "cefoTAXime" instead of "cefotaxime" to avoid confusion with "ceftriaxone.") | • Prevents one medication from being confused with a similarly named medication. (Change stimulated by identification of near misses in which similarly sounding cephalosporin medications were confused for each other and the wrong one was dispensed by the pharmacy.) |
| 5. Random safety audits. | • Monitors compliance with safety practices. (Audits performed using a deck of cards, each with a safety or quality-related question that is randomly picked from the deck and is either answered by the staff or by direct observation or chart review. An example is, "Have the positions of the current central venous lines and surgical drains or tubes been verified by radiographs and repositioned if necessary?") |
| 6. Standardization of fentanyl administration for mechanically ventilated infants. | • Prevents adverse drug events by using standard reference doses. |
| 7. Golden hour project. | • Improves team performance during the resuscitation and stabilization of high risk newborn infants immediately after the golden hour (birth). Principles of Crew Resource Management, a method widely used in aviation to promote safety, are applied to improve team performance during neonatal resuscitation.[5] |
| 8. High risk preventive practices such as those used to prevent heparin overdoses. | • In response to reported serious and sometimes lethal heparin overdoses in other NICUs, builds awareness of preventive practices, including the following: elimination of heparin to flush peripheral IV catheters or umbilical catheters; inventory of single concentration of heparin 10 unit/ml in an automated dispensing machine; preparation of all IV fluids containing heparin in the pharmacy. |
| 9. Standardization of handoff communication. | • Use of SBAR (situation, background, assessment, response) format to standardize the handoff process communication.[6] |
| 10. Elimination of all verbal orders except in urgent or emergent situations. | • Increases clarity and reliability of ordering process. |

hospital unit staffs to notify them of this practice and ask for cooperation in protecting the neonates. All ICN staff, including the unit secretaries who sit at the reception desk and the ICN nurses, are vigilant in enforcing these practices and will ask others to do the same. If a provider refuses to comply with the safety practice or is rude when approached, the ICN staff sends a note to the medical director, who then follows up on the incident.

For many years, data about nosocomial infections and other patient safety events has been posted prominently on a *data wall* near the nurses' lounge to raise staff awareness of these events and to continually and visually remind staff of the intention to create a safe ICN (see Chapter Four on creating a rich information environment for more information).

Recently the ICN instituted *Executive Walk Rounds* where the Patient Safety and Quality Officer of the Children's Hospital and the ICN leaders walk through the ICN and talk to staff and to parents of the hospitalized neonates to identify patient safety concerns. This provides a visible display of leadership commitment and support for patient safety in the microsystem.

When new nurses join the unit, they undergo a special educational session on patient safety facilitated by a neonatologist interested in this topic. Before any equipment is purchased for the ICN, a careful evaluation is made of the various options available from different manufacturers to identify potential safety problems that can arise from the use of that equipment and to prioritize makes of equipment that have embedded safety features (for example, *smart* infusion pumps that have preprogrammed safeguards to prevent inadvertently high infusion rates).

Finally, an explicit sign of the ICN's commitment to a safety culture is its policy of transparent disclosure when a significant error or adverse event occurs. When such an event occurs, the MERIT committee members investigate it. Then the attending physician, other health care team members, and sometimes the senior microsystem leaders meet with the infant's family to disclose known facts about the event. Apologizing to the family if there was an error is an essential part of this disclosure practice. The health care team also holds follow-up meetings with the family to provide emotional support and to keep lines of communication open.

## Prevention of Nosocomial Infections

Prevention of nosocomial infections has been an important focus of the ICN since 1995. Faced with a high nosocomial infection rate that was above the 75th percentile for similar units in the Vermont Oxford Network (VON), a multidisciplinary ICN team performed an in-depth analysis of processes relevant to nosocomial infections. They also collaborated with other hospitals through VON and performed benchmarking site visits to neonatal intensive care units that had low nosocomial infection rates to discover how units were achieving superior results. Through these efforts, a significant discovery was made: the ICN team found the mental model of the microsystem staff toward infection was an important contributing factor to that microsystem's infection rate (see Chapter One, Luan research). ICNs that had low infection rates treated infections as a *preventable event* the staff had the capacity to prevent, whereas microsystems with a high infection rate had an attitude that babies undergoing neonatal intensive care were inevitably going to get infected; the latter view has been described as an *entitlement mental model*.

Attempts to reduce nosocomial infections in the ICN over the years have focused on the following actions:

- Improving hand hygiene by unit staff
- Ensuring adequate barrier precautions during insertion of central venous catheters
- Standardizing IV line setup to minimize the number of connections
- Ensuring scrupulous alcohol prepping of intravenous tubing entry sites prior to entry for blood draws and administration of medications
- Promoting the use of breast milk
- Minimizing the use of central venous lines
- Minimizing the number of times the tubing lumen is entered for blood sampling or for administering medications or fluids
- Ensuring that parenteral nutrition solution is prepared under a laminar flow hood in the pharmacy
- Constantly educating the staff about infection prevention practices

Every time a baby develops a nosocomial infection, the Clinical Nurse Specialist performs an immediate chart review and e-mails all care providers who were involved in the infant's care during the previous ninety-six hours to identify factors that might have contributed to that baby developing an infection.

In recent years, the following standardized practices to prevent Ventilator Associated Pneumonia (VAP) have also been implemented:

- Elevate the head end of the bed.
- Perform routine oral care.
- Limit ventilator disconnections.
- Drain circuit condensate away from the infant.
- Place suction catheter device in a clear plastic bag (and not in the bed with the infant).
- Place flow-inflating bags on flow meters.
- Reassess the need for extubation on a daily basis.

Implementation of these practices has resulted in a substantial and statistically significant decrease in the rate of nosocomial infections. However, there are periodic resurgences of infection that are likely the result of hand hygiene becoming less meticulous, slippage of compliance with standardized processes of care, new staff entering the ICN, and other unidentified factors.

Each time there is an increase in the infection rate, the nosocomial sepsis task force rigorously ensures infection control practices are being implemented with high reliability and decides what new practices need to be adopted. These renewed efforts are usually effective in decreasing infection rates again. It is apparent that decreasing nosocomial infection rates requires constant vigilance and constant maintenance of infection control practices at high levels.

## DISCUSSION

This case study describes how a microsystem can set in place formal programs, allocate resources, and attempt to change its culture to promote patient safety. The WHO factors are depicted clearly to create a safe environment, practice, and culture. It becomes abundantly clear that patient safety cannot be achieved with a single intervention or technique that is installed into the microsystem. Instead, multiple facets must be in place, monitored, and improved over time. The experience of periodic resurgences of nosocomial infections within this microsystem also emphasizes the need for constant vigilance and sustained efforts to pursue the precondition of patient safety in the ICN.

## DEFINITIONS

It is helpful to define the following terms used in this chapter to discuss safety practices.

*Medical error:* Failure of a planned action to be completed as intended, or the use of a wrong plan to achieve an aim.[3]

*Adverse event:* An injury resulting from a medical intervention.[3,7] Not all errors lead to adverse events. Sometimes, even when an error occurs, it does not result in harm to the patient because the error is detected and intercepted before it reaches the patient. For example, a nurse may check a doctor's prescription for a medication and detect a dosage error in the prescription. In other cases, an error may be made, yet appropriate action is taken to neutralize the harmful effect of the error. (For example, an antidote may be administered after a medication overdose occurs.) Another reason errors may not result in harm to patients is that some patients are intrinsically resilient. For example, some patients may not suffer any harm even when they receive a tenfold overdose of a medication.[8] Thus, only a certain proportion of errors lead to adverse events.

Even when a patient is cared for without any errors, there may still be unavoidable adverse events. For example, even when a medication is administered in the right dosage to the right patient at the right interval through the right route, the patient may suffer from a rash or from renal toxicity due to effects of the medication. Such adverse events are not yet preventable and are commonly called *complications*. Therefore, when analyzing an adverse event, it is important to determine whether or not it was a *preventable* adverse event (one that resulted from a medical error) or a *non-preventable* one. A small proportion of preventable adverse events are also due to gross deviation from the *accepted* standard of care, and these are considered to be the result of *negligence*. Figure 3.1 depicts the relationship between medical errors and adverse events.

*Near miss:* Errors that do not result in patient harm are known as near misses or as close calls.[3] An error that could have caused harm but that was intercepted before it reached the patient to cause harm may also be labeled as a near miss.[9]

*Diagnostic error:* A diagnosis that is missed, wrong, or delayed, as detected by subsequent definitive tests or findings.[10]

*Patient safety:* Freedom from accidental injury. Ensuring patient safety involves establishing operational systems and processes that minimize the likelihood of errors and maximize the likelihood of intercepting errors when they occur.[3] Cincinnati Children's Hospital Medical Center's (CCHMC) Pediatric Early Warning Systems is an excellent example of an operational system designed to intercept potential errors and harm (see Cincinnati Children's Hospital Medical Center Sidebar).

*Negligent adverse event:* preventable adverse events that satisfy legal criteria used in determining whether the care provided failed to meet the standard of care reasonably expected of a physician qualified to take care of the patient in question.[3]

FIGURE 3.1    Terms Related to Patient Safety.

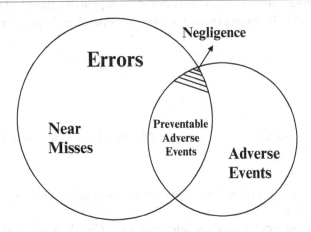

*Source:* Adapted from Hofer, T. P., Kerr, E. A., & Hayward, R. A. What is an error? *Effective Clinical Practice*, 2000, *3*(6), 261–269.

*Sentinel event:* an adverse event in which death or serious harm to a patient has occurred. It usually refers to events that are not expected or acceptable, such as an operation on the wrong patient or body part. The choice of the word sentinel reflects the egregiousness of the injury (for example, amputation of the wrong leg) and the likelihood that investigation of such events will reveal serious problems in current policies or procedures. A well-known sentinel event is the death of an 18-month-old child Josie King from medical errors, which led to establishment of The Josie King Foundation, www.josieking.org. This foundation, whose mission is to prevent others from being harmed by medical errors, provides resources and programs to design safer health care practices and systems. By uniting health care providers and consumers and funding innovative safety programs, the foundation hopes to create a culture of patient safety.

*Potential safety event:* an event that, when first identified, appears to have the potential to be a medical error or an adverse event that is the result of a medical error. After further investigation, a potential safety event can be categorized as an error (with or without a resulting adverse event) or as a non-error.

## IDENTIFICATION OF MEDICAL ERRORS AND ADVERSE EVENTS

A variety of methods have been used to detect and monitor medical errors and adverse events. Some of these are listed in Table 3.2, along with relevant advantages and disadvantages. Which method is used to measure patient safety depends on the intended purpose of the measurement, the resources available, and the accessibility of data sources. Some methods (such as prospective surveillance) can yield reliable and valid data but may be expensive and time-consuming, whereas others (such as voluntary reporting by health professionals) require fewer resources but do not yield an accurate incidence or prevalence of the measured events; they are also vulnerable to bias.

## CINCINNATI CHILDREN'S HOSPITAL MEDICAL CENTER

Cincinnati Children's Hospital Medical Center (CCHMC) has sharpened its focus on improving patient safety and has achieved early results that reflect their intentional actions. Some of the operational systems and processes that have resulted in safety improvements include the following:

1. An early warning system to detect clinical deterioration, including a decision algorithm for action by all staff

2. Charge nurses' and senior residents' focus attention on children at risk for deterioration

3. Unit-level leader walk rounds and real-time analysis of all key outcome failures

4. Evidence-based care reviewed and when it isn't in place, nurses mitigate the situation by implementing the evidence-based care

5. Systematically approaching of patients to elicit concerns and complaints that need to be addressed immediately

6. Simulation training at the unit level with nurses and physicians[1]

1. Godfrey, M., Melin, C. N., & Muething, S. E. Clinical microsystems, part 3. Transformation of two hospitals using microsystem, mesosystem and macrosystem strategies. *Joint Commission Journal*, October 2008, *34*(10), 591–603.

## FREQUENCY OF ADVERSE EVENTS AND MEDICAL ERRORS

A systematic review by de Vries and colleagues[11] of eight studies found the median incidence of in-hospital adverse events was 9 percent. (The range was 5 percent to 12 percent.) Of these adverse events, a median of 44 percent were preventable. Of these preventable events, 26 percent resulted in moderate to severe disability and 7 percent were lethal. Numerous other studies have also described the frequency of specific types of errors and adverse events in specific types of patients. For example, in a systematic review, the incidence of medication errors in hospitalized children was found to range from 5 to 27 percent, with 3 to 37 percent occurring during the prescribing process, 5 to 58 percent during dispensing, 72 to 75 percent during administration, and 17 to 21 percent during documentation.[12] Using ethnographic methods that included direct observation, one study[13] found that as many as 46 percent of hospitalized patients suffered from adverse events. The exact incidence of medical errors (including those that do not lead to patient harm) is unknown, but is likely to be high.

Recently it has been recognized that *nosocomial infections*, also known as health care acquired infections, make up one of the most common types of medical errors.[14] Health care–associated infections occur in 5 to 30 percent of hospitalized patients[15,16] and are responsible for annual direct medical costs to U.S. hospitals of $28 billion to $45 billion.[17,18]

Errors related to the use of medications are also very common. Medical errors have huge economic consequences to the U.S. health care system, and amount to several billion dollars a year.[7,19,20,21]

Table 3.2    Methods to Identify Medical Errors and Adverse Events

| Method | Advantages | Disadvantages |
|---|---|---|
| 1. Prospective surveillance | Can yield accurate estimates of numerators and denominators of events and true incidence of events. | Can be expensive; not good for detecting latent errors. |
| 2. Chart review | Data sources may be easy to access, especially if electronic records are used. | Judgments about adverse events may be unreliable and expensive; judgments may require trained abstractors who are subject to hindsight bias and unable to detect events not documented in the record. |
| 3. Observation (direct visual or videotaped) | Potentially accurate and precise; detects more active errors than other methods; used to detect errors in real time. | Can be expensive; requires trained observers or reviewers; may threaten staff or patient confidentiality; subject to potential hindsight bias; not effective at detecting latent errors; results in voluminous information. |
| 4. Interviews or questioning of providers | Easy to conduct; can identify events and latent errors that are not reported or documented elsewhere. | Does not identify events if providers do not recognize them as errors; subject to hindsight bias; may seem punitive to providers; may discourage providers from reporting errors by colleagues. |
| 5. Automated methods, including trigger tools | Can search a large volume of patient records with minimal effort; can provide periodic reports automatically; can potentially generate real-time alerts. | Unlikely to detect all events; do not detect latent errors; require resources for initial setup; may be expensive; may still require chart review to confirm errors and adverse events. |
| 6. Administrative data (Patient Safety Indicators, ICD-9 codes) | Data are readily available and easy to analyze. | Subject to vagaries of coding; may rely on incomplete and inaccurate data that are divorced from clinical context. |
| 7. Malpractice claims data | Provides multiple perspectives (patients, providers, lawyers) and can detect latent errors. | Subject to hindsight and reporting bias; sources of data are non-standardized. |
| 8. Autopsy | Familiar to providers; data are relatively easy to obtain. | Conducted infrequently and non-randomly; subject to hindsight and reporting bias; focused on diagnostic errors. |
| 9. Mortality and morbidity conferences | Familiar to providers; cases selected are more likely to have errors and adverse events. | Errors are rarely acknowledged or discussed explicitly; subject to hindsight and reporting bias. |
| 10. Reporting by providers, patients, and families | Can detect latent errors, provide multiple perspectives over time, and be part of routine operations; requires few resources. | Subject to reporting and hindsight bias. |

*Source:* Adapted from Thomas, E. J., & Petersen, L. A. Measuring errors and adverse events in health care. *Journal of General Internal Medicine.* January 2003, *18*(1), 61–67.

Diagnostic errors are now increasingly being recognized as a problem in the health care system,[22] with the reported rates of diagnostic error in radiology and pathology (the two specialties that rely heavily on visual interpretation for diagnosis) ranging from 2 to 5 percent and the rates in clinical specialties commonly in the range of 10 to 15 percent, and sometimes higher, depending on the specialty and on the specific conditions being studied.[23] In some autopsy studies of specific conditions, as many as 55 percent of diagnoses were missed before death. Additionally, 69 percent of patients with bipolar disorder had an incorrect initial diagnosis.[23] Diagnostic errors also are reported to make up anywhere from 7 to 17 percent of adverse events.[23]

## Causation of Medical Errors

Traditionally, when a medical error occurred and was called to the attention of others, the nurse, physician, or other health professional involved in caring for the patient was likely to be blamed for causing the error. This person would then be subjected to punitive measures or disciplinary action, perhaps forced to undergo retraining, and in severe cases terminated from the job. This has been called the *person approach* by Reason.[24] Recently, there has been increasing awareness among most health care institutions that: (1) errors are usually caused by multiple factors related to the overall systems of care (including working conditions, human factors, and organizational culture); (2) individuals are not solely responsible for causing errors; and (3) blaming or punishing individuals for causing errors actually prevents identification of the true set of underlying causes of errors. This *systems approach*[24] encourages a broad investigation of the multiple contributing factors to an error and looks beyond the immediately obvious causes. The basic premise in the systems approach is that humans are fallible, and errors are to be expected, even in the best organizations staffed by the best people. Human fallibility contributing to error causation is the result of intrinsic and unavoidable imperfections of human cognitive processes such as memory, vigilance, attention, concentration, and reasoning, as well as the tendency of human performance to degrade with fatigue, sleep-deprivation, distractions, excessive task demands, stress, and anxiety. Several types of these cognitive attributes can generate errors.

Using a systems approach, the list of causal factors that might have contributed to a particular error is classified into three main categories that are easily remembered with the acronym *WHO*, which stands for *W*ork conditions, *H*uman conditions, and *O*rganizational conditions. WHO conditions are listed in "Conditions That Contribute to Errors and Adverse Events as Seen Through the WHO Framework." When an error occurs, instead of asking "who committed the error?" institutions should look for a broad range of WHO conditions that might have contributed to the causation of the error. These factors, which are often the result of strategic, economic, policy, human resource, architectural, and equipment-purchase decisions, may lie dormant within a system for years and contribute to the causation of an error on one unpredictable day when the *perfect storm,* or combination of circumstances, is present. Such factors that lie dormant but contribute to error causation under certain circumstances are known as *latent conditions,* or *latent errors.*[24]

One method to assess and improve work factors in microsystems is to apply the *5S method* to gain deep insight into the workplace conditions. The 5S process aims to create standardized, value added conditions in the workplace to promote improved safety. Chapter Three Action Guide further explains the 5S approach and offers a 5S worksheet to evaluate and improve the setup of the workplace. The development and implementation of checklists can also improve work conditions and human performance in microsystems. Chapter Three Action Guide offers additional information about checklists.

## The Swiss Cheese Model

The *Swiss cheese model*[24] shows simply but powerfully how errors can reach patients and harm them in spite of existing defense mechanisms and barriers. Health care systems

---

# CONDITIONS THAT CONTRIBUTE TO ERRORS AND ADVERSE EVENTS AS SEEN THROUGH THE WHO FRAMEWORK

## Work Conditions: W

- Inadequate staffing, excessive patient-nurse ratio, excessive workloads
- Undesirable shift patterns and work schedules that promote fatigue
- Equipment poorly designed, not available, or poorly maintained
- Poor ergonomic design of work area
- Lack of administrative and managerial support
- Protocols and standard procedures not available or hard to access
- Use of unclear written communication and verbal communication methods that are prone to misinterpretation; unclear task design and lack of clarity of the organizational structure and about when and how to seek help
- Inadequate supervision or backup
- Poor team structure, functioning, and leadership

## Human Conditions: H

- Mismatch between skills of health care worker and requirements of the job
- Health care worker lacks knowledge, is in poor physical or mental health, is in a highly emotional state, is under stress, or does not consistently adhere to safety standards
- Patient's condition is very complex or serious
- Patient has language problems or hearing impairments that make effective communication more difficult
- Patient personality and social factors make care more difficult

## Organizational Conditions: O

- Financial constraints and economic pressures encourage production and efficiency over safety
- Equipment, personnel, or other resources are either lacking or are not allocated to patient safety
- Lack of policies, standards, goals, and regulations make it difficult to work safely
- Excessively stringent regulations encourage violations
- Medical-legal environment

*Source:* Adapted from Vincent et al. How to investigate and analyze clinical incidents: Clinical risk unit and association of litigation and risk management protocol. *British Medical Journal*, 2000, *320*, 777–781.

**FIGURE 3.2** The Swiss Cheese Model of How Defenses, Barriers, and Safeguards May Be Penetrated by an Accident Trajectory.

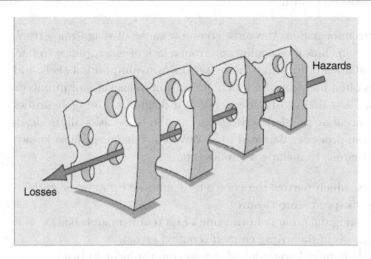

*Source:* Reason, J. Human error: Models and management. *Western Journal of Medicine,* 2000, *172*(6), 394.

of all shapes and sizes have defenses in place that are intended to prevent errors from occurring or to prevent the error from being propagated downstream and reaching the patient. According to the Swiss cheese model shown in Figure 3.2, each of these defenses, like a slice of Swiss cheese, contains holes. For example, error prevention strategies are not always effective and do not intercept the error every time. When multiple defenses are in place, an error that passes through one defense is usually intercepted by the next defense. (An error that passes through a hole in one layer of Swiss cheese is caught by the intact portion of the next layer of Swiss cheese). However, on occasion, an error may pass through all existing defenses because all of them fail. This results in the error reaching the patient and potentially causing harm.

Although the systems approach is recommended for understanding the causes of medical errors, this framework does not completely absolve individuals from their involvement in errors. Systems require certain contributions from people involved in patient care. A statement such as "it was the system" should not be used to hide underlying human failures to perform expected work. Ultimately, patient safety depends significantly on optimal human performance as well as on optimal system design and performance. The *just culture* school of thought emphasizes the interplay between individual factors and system factors in creating and sustaining safe practices and high reliability.[24,25]

## Diagnostic Errors

The following mechanisms underlying diagnostic errors have recently received much attention:[23,26,27]

- lack of necessary data (for example, incomplete records may have been provided by a referring provider)
- failure to recognize the significance of the data (for example, misinterpretation of laboratory test results)

- lack of intrinsic knowledge (for example, when the provider encounters a disease he or she has never seen before)
- failure to synthesize existing information[23,27]

Failure to synthesize information, the most common cause of diagnostic errors, typically results from flaws in clinical reasoning and from a lack of *metacognition* (reflection and critical examination of one's own thinking processes, assumptions, beliefs, and conclusions). Clinicians often use *heuristics,* which are subconscious rules of thumb or cognitive shortcuts that allow them to rapidly arrive at a diagnosis. Use of heuristics often leads to rapid and accurate problem solving, but can also be occasionally misleading. Examples of cognitive processes that lead to an erroneous diagnosis (also known as *cognitive dispositions to respond*)[28] include the following:

- Using faulty heuristics, which narrow the choice of diagnostic options too early in the process of diagnosis (premature closure)
- Seeking out and accepting data that confirms one's bias (confirmation bias)
- Formulating the diagnosis in the wrong context (context error)
- Assessing past events in light of knowledge of the outcome (hindsight bias)
- Perceiving data differently, depending on how it is presented (framing effect)
- Neglecting base rates of an illness
- Believing diagnostic test results or an expert recommendation without question (blind obedience)[23,26,29]

Clinicians who fall prey to these cognitive errors are often overconfident about their diagnoses. Clinicians who are unaware of the true frequency of their own diagnostic errors or who believe errors are inevitable are often complacent.[23,26]

## Prevention of Medical Errors to Ensure Patient Safety

To ensure patient safety, a microsystem can adopt three strategies:

1. Proactively identify and mitigate for error risks (design)
2. Implement and monitor safety practices (measurement system)
3. Learn from errors (reflection)

The foundations laid down by these three strategies promote safety (which is the precondition for health care work as described by Paul O'Neill[30]) and at the same time foster a culture of safety. The CCHMC sidebar provides an excellent example of application of the three strategies.

## Proactive Identification and Mitigation of Error Risks

In addition to learning from actual errors and adverse events, microsystems can attempt to improve patient safety by proactively analyzing their risks for errors and mitigating these risks before an error occurs. The best-known method for this is called *Failure Mode and Effects Analysis* (FMEA).[31,32] (Additional information and an example can be found in Chapter Three Action Guide.)

In this method, a multidisciplinary team is created, a discrete process is selected (for example, therapy with a medication), and the sequential steps in this process are identified (for example, medication therapy relies upon prescription, transcription, dispensing, administration, and monitoring). Using methods such as process performance rehearsals, brainstorming, expert opinion, and review of available data on errors and adverse events it is possible to identify ways something could go wrong at each of these steps. Unwanted outcomes are called *failure modes*. Next, the likely frequency with which these failure modes could occur, the likelihood of the failure mode being propagated downstream (without being detected and intercepted by existing safety mechanisms), and the seriousness of the potential resulting error are each identified and quantified on a scale, such as from one to ten. By multiplying the values on each of these three scales, a *risk priority number* (RPN) is calculated. This provides information about the *criticality* of the failure mode, which includes a relative measure of the importance of the failure mode (based on its consequences), its frequency of occurrence, and other factors.[32] Another method for assessing criticality is to use a hazard scoring matrix to calculate a hazard score.[31] Failure modes with the highest RPNs (or hazard scores) then constitute the priority failure modes most in need of safety interventions and process redesign efforts. The potential causes and contributing factors for the high-criticality failure modes are then identified and potential preventive measures, such as redesign of the process, are developed and implemented. The proactive use of FMEA has the potential to improve safety without an error actually occurring within the microsystem.

## Implementation and Monitoring of Safety Practices

*Safety practices* can be defined as changes or interventions that, when implemented, are expected to prevent medical errors or the harm resulting from medical errors. These can be identified through analysis of errors that occurred within a microsystem, through FMEA, from empirical research, and from expert recommendations. Currently many of the safety practices recommended by experts and by authoritative organizations are based not on high-level evidence,[12,33,34] but are derived from reasoning based on mechanistic principles, knowledge of cognitive psychology, and from extrapolation of interventions believed to be effective in fields other than health care, such as aviation. For example, in a systematic review of medication errors in pediatric patients, twenty-six unique recommendations for strategies to reduce medication errors were identified, of which the majority were based on expert opinion only.[12] Before discussing specific safety interventions, it is worth discussing some general principles for improving patient safety that have been described in various forms by multiple authors[35,36,37] and that have been depicted in Figure 3.3.

In general, it makes sense to place a safety intervention as far upstream as possible (as close as possible to the influential causes) in the cascade of events leading to a medical error. The first category of safety intervention to consider should be *elimination* of the activity that generates the risk of the error. Is the medication, the invasive procedure, or the surgery really necessary? If the error-generating activity can itself be eliminated, then the opportunities for these errors to occur are eliminated.

○ Examples of error elimination are abolishing verbal orders in hospitals, not storing concentrated potassium chloride solution on the ward or on the patient floor, and avoiding unnecessary diagnostic tests and therapies. In addition, it should be a high priority to also eliminate latent (WHO) factors that predispose medical professionals to err.

The second category of safety interventions is *replacement*, where an error-prone step in a process (or an entire error-prone process) is replaced by one that is less error-prone.

FIGURE 3.3    Principles of Developing and Implementing
Patient Safety Interventions.

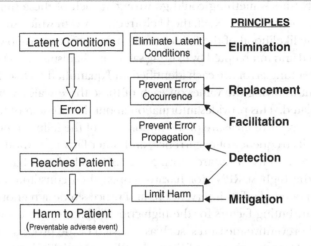

*Sources:* Based on Grout, J. R. Mistake proofing: Changing designs to reduce error. *Quality and Safety in Health Care,* 2006, *15 Suppl 1,* i44–49. Nolan, T. W. System changes to improve patient safety. *British Medical Journal,* 2000, *320*(7237), 771–773. Norman, D. A. *The design of everyday things.* New York: Doubleday, 1989.

- Examples of this include replacement of free text handwritten provider orders by preprinted order sheets, use of computerized provider order entry,[38,39] and use of barcoding instead of visual checking to dispense and administer medication.

The third category of safety interventions to consider is *facilitation,* where human performance is made less error-prone by the use of cognitive or physical facilitators. For example, different colors, fonts, shapes, and sizes can be used to distinguish between two medications, devices, labels, syringes, or tubes that might be confused with each other.

- A good example of this concept comes from the field of anesthesiology, where the risk of oxygen tubing being inadvertently plugged into a nitrous oxide outlet is reduced by designing the nozzles and wall outlets of the two gases in such a way that the oxygen nozzle only fits in the oxygen outlet and not in a nitrous oxide outlet. Similarly, the outlets on the anesthesia machine for different anesthetic gases each have a unique shape and will only accept the nozzle of the correct gas. The nozzle and the outlet are also color-coded. These are examples of the use of physical constraints[40] to prevent error.

The fourth category of safety interventions to consider is *detection,* where an attempt is made to identify an error as soon as possible after it occurs so it can be intercepted and prevented from reaching the patient.

- Examples of detection include the triggering of alarms on patient monitors, infusion pumps, ventilators and incubators when monitored parameters are outside the desired range or when there is a situation that might harm the patient. Other examples include performing radiographs after placement of an indwelling device (such as a central venous catheter or an endotracheal tube) to detect misplacement of the device, or performing radiographs after surgery to identify retained surgical instruments.

The fifth category of safety interventions is *mitigation,* where an attempt is made to prevent or limit patient harm from an error after it has occurred.

- Examples of this include using an antidote for a medication, escalating the intensity of patient monitoring, initiating respiratory support, performing dialysis, or performing repeat surgery to correct a surgical error (for example, to retrieve a retained surgical instrument).

In manufacturing, software design, construction, and other industries, a method called *mistake-proofing* is widely used to improve the safety of operations. Mistake-proofing, also known as *error-proofing* or *Poka-Yoke,* is the use of process or design features to prevent errors or the negative impact of errors.[41] It consists of devices or methods to prevent defects, either by preventing errors from occurring or by detecting an error soon after it happens. The principles of error-proofing can be applied to develop patient safety interventions. A variety of examples of mistake-proofing in health care have been compiled.[41]

## Learning from Errors

Each microsystem should have methods in place to (1) identify errors occurring within it, (2) investigate and learn from these incidents, and (3) redesign processes to prevent their recurrence. These systems can be paper-based or electronic. The most common method of identifying errors and adverse events within a microsystem is *voluntary reporting* by health care workers. Although voluntary reporting does not reveal the true incidence of errors, it requires few resources, may identify all or nearly all serious events (especially if health care workers are trained and encouraged to make reports), and can provide an adequate number and variety of reports to track patterns and to take a significant number of actions to improve patient safety. The other methods listed in "Conditions That Contribute to Errors and Adverse Events as Seen Through the WHO Framework" can also be used to identify errors.

Near misses, in particular, offer easy opportunities for microsystems to improve patient safety because, compared to errors that lead to patient harm, they are more frequent, easier to discuss (the staff involved are less defensive and less afraid), and share many of the same underlying causal mechanisms. By conducting a detailed analysis of near misses, microsystems can gain valuable insight into their safety vulnerabilities and put preventive measures in place before a patient is harmed. Therefore, near misses have been called *free lessons.*[24]

When a near miss is identified, it is best thought of as a potential safety event. When a potential safety event occurs, microsystem leaders should as soon as possible investigate the processes and factors leading to the event. Using the WHO acronym, leaders should investigate work conditions, human conditions, and organizational conditions.

### Work Conditions

- Inspection of the event location
- Examination of the equipment involved in the event
- Photographing of the physical location and equipment
- Review of assignments and staffing, including clinical support
- Review of the documentation and of patient vital signs, monitoring data, laboratory, and imaging data
- Preservation of physical artifacts, such as equipment, signs, medical samples, and infusion tubing
- Step-by-step mapping of process and events, if possible

## Human Conditions

- Interviews with the involved health care professionals
- Assessment of health care professional knowledge, skills, and abilities
- Evaluation of health care professionals' level of stress
- Review of patient acuity
- Interviews with the patient and the patient's family
- Assessment of successful communication skills of staff and patients to determine if any barriers exist

## Organizational Conditions

- Decreased resources due to financial constraints
- Missing or overly stringent safety policies, standards, and goals
- Legal and regulatory requirements that apply

After this initial investigation, one or more subsequent investigations may be required to identify further details and obtain clarifications. The people performing these investigations should take great care to reconstruct the situation leading to the event and to be non-judgmental, unbiased, and objective while gathering the facts.[42] Simulation of the situation can provide a safe time and place to reenact the events. A formal high technology simulation laboratory is not required. Many times an *in situ* simulation and/or rehearsal can be conducted in the actual microsystem setting (see Chapter Three Action Guide for simulation and rehearsal ideas).

In particular, when interviewing individuals involved in a safety event, the investigator should have a non-punitive, non-judgmental approach, ask open-ended questions, and allow the individual to tell the story of what happened. Investigators should not ask leading questions to confirm a hypothesis. The importance of conducting an investigation immediately after the event cannot be overemphasized. Often the investigation is conducted several days or weeks after the incident in a conference room with only some of the involved individuals present and with no review of the actual scene of the event or of the equipment. A delayed analysis usually results in a superficial understanding of the event.

When the investigation is complete, a hypothesized sequence of events and contributing factors should be constructed and should include a timeline of events. One useful technique to construct such a sequence of events is called the *Five Why's*.[43] For each identified variation from desired practice the investigator asks, "Why did this happen?" As additional causal factors are identified, the investigator inquires as to why those occurred, sequentially identifying the cascade of causal factors.

## Valuing a Culture of Safety

For any patient safety intervention to be successful, it is important for the right organizational culture to exist. A local culture of safety, where safety is valued above production and efficiency, is a key characteristic of industries where complex high risk activities are routinely undertaken under considerable time pressure with a very low frequency of errors and almost complete absence of catastrophic failures. Examples of such organizations are nuclear power plants, naval aircraft carriers, and air traffic control centers, all which are often referred to as high reliability organizations (HROs). The five hallmarks of HROs (collectively termed *mindfulness,* see Chapter Three Action Guide) are as follows:[44]

- Preoccupation with failure
- Reluctance to simplify interpretations
- Sensitivity to operations
- Commitment to resilience
- Deference to expertise

Using surveys for *Understanding Mindfulness* and *Understanding Vulnerability to Mindfulness* (within microsystems) can provide clear guidance and actions to create a culture of safety.

The safety culture of an organization has been defined as the product of individual and group values, attitudes, perceptions, competencies, and patterns of behavior that determine the commitment to and the style and proficiency of an organization's health and safety management.[45] The term *safety climate* refers to the measurable aspect of an organization's safety culture and focuses on perceptions and attitudes.[46] Safety climate is an aspect of *safety culture* (attitudes are part of both definitions)[37] although the two terms are sometimes used interchangeably.[46] The safety climate of a microsystem can be assessed and monitored by surveying its health care workers' attitudes[47,48] using questionnaires such as the *Safety Attitudes Questionnaire,* an adaptation of a survey used in commercial aviation.[49,50] Patient safety culture surveys are also available from the Agency for Healthcare Research and Quality.[35]

In an organization with a strong safety culture, the health care workers are willing to report errors and near misses, feel safe from punitive retaliation, willingly point out safety hazards, collaborate across different levels in the organization's hierarchy to reduce safety vulnerabilities, and consider protecting patient safety as an important part of their job.

High performing microsystems draw on principles of both personal and social ethics. The traditional biomedical ethical base is important but not sufficient. To own the work in systems, including owning the performance of the system, invites attention to the precepts of social ethics. Hannah Arendt[36] provides useful guidance. She believes individuals in a society must be able to make promises to one another. If we make promises, we must be able to seek forgiveness at times when our promises could not be kept. Applying these principles to the clinical microsystem and to the behavior of patients and providers, we need to be able to make good promises about the performance of the microsystem, about our own role(s) in the microsystem, and about the roles of others involved in the work; and when those promises cannot be kept we need to be able to seek forgiveness.

To create a culture of safety, leaders of microsystems and macrosystems should not just make safety a high priority; rather, patient safety should be a precondition. Leaders who stimulate conversations about safety, mindfulness, promise making and forgiveness, who allocate resources to patient safety, and who demonstrate their commitment to safety through activities such as executive walk rounds,[37] visibly demonstrate a deep commitment to creating a culture of safety. The case study entitled "The Intensive Care Nursery at the Children's Hospital at Dartmouth" illustrates how many of the ideas, concepts, and actions specific to safety can be designed into the real world of an intensive care nursery.

## Responding to Medical Errors

There are three victims of medical errors that cause adverse events: the patient, the patient's family, and the health care workers involved in the error. As described above, part of the immediate response to a medical error should include the performance of a rapid investigation to identify causal and contributing factors and to construct a hypothesized sequence of events. In responding to an error, especially one that resulted in an adverse event, health care workers should also take the following steps:

- Ensure the patient's health by stopping a harmful intervention, instituting necessary interventions, using antidotes, rescue therapy, and consulting other specialists if necessary.
- Provide the family with all assistance required during the crisis.
- Inform risk management and discuss with them how to approach the patient involved in the error and the patient's family. The institution's disclosure policies should be reviewed before taking any action in the case of a specific patient.
- Disclose the error to the patient and the patient's family.

### Communicating with the Patient and the Patient's Family After an Error

A prevalent philosophy in health care, primarily driven by fear of litigation, has been to *deny and* defend in response to a medical error. In contrast, the current recommended approach is aptly summarized as *disclose, apologize, and compensate.*

Disclosure of the error should be performed openly, transparently, and empathetically.[9] The Joint Commission standards now call for open disclosure, which should be restricted to just the known facts and should not involve conjecture. Health care workers performing the disclosure should not speculate about the causes and contributing factors or about the potential consequences. They should avoid loose language. They should prepare for the disclosure session by having a discussion with the rest of the health care team and with risk management experts to decide on what exactly should and should not be said during the conversation with the patient and the family. The same general principles of communication that apply to communicating other types of bad news in medicine should be used. In the hospital setting, the attending physician (or other high-ranking administrator) should take primary responsibility for disclosure. Above all, the health care professionals performing the disclosure should listen carefully to the family. Disclosure is preferred by patients, may reduce the risk of lawsuits (but not if serious harm results from the error), and has not resulted in a flood of lawsuits. If a lawsuit is filed, effective disclosure can hasten the settlement time and reduce legal fees.

Patients and their families often wish to know how recurrences of the same error will be prevented in the future. Providing this information along with follow-up reports about implementation of preventive interventions are essential components of the disclosure process (see Josie King story, www.josieking.org).

Apology is an important component of disclosure.[51] Apology, when properly performed, consists of (1) acknowledgement of the error, (2) explanation about why the error occurred, (3) expression of remorse, and (4) reparation.[51] *Pseudo-apology*, or *apologia*, where one expresses sympathy and regret but does not admit blame, is considered to be worse than not apologizing. Apology is often disliked by both defendant's and plaintiff's attorneys, and can be interpreted as an admission of guilt during litigation. Therefore, health care workers should confer with their institution's risk management department to discuss how the apology should be phrased. Some states provide legal immunity for physician apology, but usually not for admissions of fault.

Financial or other compensation and waiver of hospital charges should be decided upon by risk management and insurers. Follow-up sessions should be scheduled and communication maintained with the family after the initial event. Contact information should be provided in case patients and their families have questions. Finally, good documentation of the event and of the communication with the family should be maintained.

## Care of Involved Health Professionals

The effects of medical errors on the health professionals involved can be significant and long-lasting.[9,52,53,54] Most health professionals operate under a *perfectionist* model and blame themselves severely when they are involved in an error. They may not be aware of, or accept the possibility, that factors other than their own performance may have contributed to (or caused) the error; they may not understand their performance could have been affected by extraneous factors. Feelings of shock, guilt, depression, and self-recrimination are common and can lead to inability to function. In the long term, providers can become gun-shy, develop post-traumatic stress, develop adversarial attitudes toward all patients, become substance or alcohol abusers, or even leave the profession. Health care workers involved in errors should be treated with sympathy and understanding and should be emotionally supported, especially in the immediate aftermath of the event. They should not be blamed, humiliated, or punished for the error, unless there was obvious negligence or an unjustifiable violation of procedures.

## CONCLUSION

Large numbers of patients are being harmed by the same health care systems they trust in and depend on for care. Leape offers the analogy of three jumbo jets crashing every two days to dramatize the enormity of the situation.[55] Microsystems should aim to prevent harm from medical errors. Patient safety should be a precondition for care and should be built into the structure, processes, and culture of each microsystem. Every microsystem should have an active safety program founded on a systems approach, with leadership behavior that fosters a culture of safety. Patient safety should be emphasized during the education and training of health professionals. Mindfulness, promise making, and forgiveness should be discussed, and patients should be encouraged to participate in their own health care to make it safer. Finally, rigorous research is required to identify effective patient safety interventions and the best methods of implementing them at all levels of the health care system.

## SUMMARY

- Patient safety, one of the six aims for improvement recommended by the Institute of Medicine, should not be a priority but rather it should be a precondition for microsystems as they aim to provide the highest quality care possible.
- Errors and adverse events can be identified through a variety of methods, such as voluntary reporting, chart review, use of trigger tools, and prospective surveillance systems. Each of these methods has strengths and weaknesses and requires different levels of resources.

- To prevent medical errors and promote patient safety, a *systems approach* is recommended, rather than the *person approach*, which blames individuals.
- A search for causal mechanisms and preventive interventions should focus on **W**ork conditions, **H**uman conditions, and **O**rganizational conditions that predispose health care workers to errors.
- Microsystems should have mechanisms in place to learn from errors, to proactively identify and mitigate risks for errors, and to monitor safety practices.
- General principles to enhance patient safety consist of eliminating error-prone activities, replacing an error-prone step in a process by one that is less error-prone, facilitating human performance through use of cognitive or physical facilitators, detecting errors early, and mitigating for harm to patients involved in errors.
- When an error leads to an adverse event, a health care professional should openly disclose the known facts to the patient and the patient's family and apologize.
- Health care staff involved in an error (the *second victims*) should be treated in a sensitive, compassionate, and supportive manner.

## KEY TERMS

Adverse event

Detection

Diagnostic error

Elimination

Executive walk rounds

Facilitation

Failure mode and effects analysis
   (FMEA)

Five whys

Heuristics

Medical error

Mitigation

Near miss

Negligent adverse event

Nosocomial infections

Patient safety

Person approach

Poka-yoke

Potential safety event

Replacement

Safety practices

Sentinel event

Systems approach

WHO

## REVIEW QUESTIONS

1. What is the frequency and scope of medical errors in health care systems?
2. What is the difference between medical error and adverse events?
3. How would you describe the difference between the *person approach* versus the *systems approach* to patient safety in microsystems? Can you offer examples of each approach?
4. What are the methods used to identify medical errors and adverse events in a microsystem?
5. How should microsystem members respond to medical errors and adverse events within their microsystem?
6. How might you promote discussion about mindfulness, promise making, and apologies in your microsystem?
7. What are the five hallmarks of safety mindfulness in a clinical microsystem?

## DISCUSSION QUESTIONS

1. Discuss the various safety activities, processes, and operational systems within a microsystem that you are aware of. What activities, processes, and operational systems might you develop to further increase safety and reliability?
2. How might you keep safety awareness alive and active in your microsystem?
3. Discuss medical errors and adverse events and cite clear examples of their differences.
4. Once you design a new process in your microsystem, what proactive tool could you use to identify potential errors before incorporating your process into daily practice?

## REFERENCES

1. Institute of Medicine, Committee on Quality Health Care in America. *Crossing the quality chasm: A new health system for the 21st century.* Washington, DC: National Academy Press, 2001.
2. Institute of Medicine, Committee on Quality Health Care in America. *To err is human: Building a safer health system.* Washington, DC: National Academy Press, 2000.
3. Leape, L. L. Scope of problem and history of patient safety. *Obstetrics & Gynecology Clinics of North America,* March 2008, *35*(1), *vii*, 1–10.
4. The Joint Commission. *Universal protocol.* Retrieved February 2, 2010, from www .jointcommission.org/PatientSafety/UniversalProtocol/up_facts.htm
5. Thomas et al. Teaching teamwork during the neonatal resuscitation program: A randomized trial. *Journal of Perinatology,* 2007, *27*(7), 409–414.
6. Haig, K., Sutton, S., & Whittington, J. SBAR: A shared mental model for improving communication between clinicians. *Joint Commission Journal on Quality and Patient Safety,* 2006, *32*(3), 167–175.
7. Bates et al. The costs of adverse drug events in hospitalized patients. Adverse drug events prevention study group. *Journal of the American Medical Association,* 1997, *277*(4), 307–311.
8. Narayanan, M., Schlueter, M., & Clyman, R. Incidence and outcome of a 10-fold indomethacin overdose in premature infants. *Journal of Pediatrics,* 1999, *135*(1), 105–107.
9. Massachusetts Coalition for the Prevention of Medical Errors. *When things go wrong. Responding to adverse events. A consensus statement of the Harvard hospitals,* 2006. Retrieved February 28, 2010, from www.macoalition.org/documents/respondingToAdverseEvents .pdf
10. Graber, M. Diagnostic errors in medicine: A case of neglect. *Joint Commission Journal on Quality and Patient Safety,* 2005, *31*(2), 106–113.
11. de Vries et al. The incidence and nature of in-hospital adverse events: A systematic review. *Quality and Safety in Health Care,* 2008, *17*(3), 216–223.
12. Miller, M. et al. Medication errors in paediatric care: A systematic review of epidemiology and an evaluation of evidence supporting reduction strategy recommendations. *Quality and Safety in Health Care,* 2007, *16*(2), 116–126.
13. Andrews et al. An alternative strategy for studying adverse events in medical care. *Lancet,* 1997, *349*(9048), 309–313.
14. Gerberding, J. L. Hospital-onset infections: A patient safety issue. *Annals of Internal Medicine,* 2002, *137*(8), 665–670.
15. Stoll et al. National institute of child health and human development neonatal research network. Neurodevelopmental and growth impairment among extremely low-birth-

weight infants with neonatal infection. *Journal of the American Medical Association*, 2004, *292*(19), 2357–2365.

16. Weinstein, R. A. Nosocomial infection update. *Emerging Infectious Diseases*, 1998, *4*(3), 416–420.

17. Scott II, R. D. The direct medical costs of healthcare-associated infections in U.S. hospitals and the benefits of prevention, March 2009. Retrieved August 3, 2010, from www.cdc.gov/ncidod/dhqp/pdf/Scott_CostPaper.pdf

18. Stone, P. W. Economic burden of healthcare-associated infections: An American perspective. *Expert Review of Pharmacoeconomics and Outcomes Research*, October 2009, *9*(5), 417–422.

19. Brennan et al. Incidence of adverse events and negligence in hospitalized patients. Results of the Harvard Medical Practice Study. *New England Journal of Medicine*, 1991, *324*(6), 370–376.

20. Classen, D. C. et al. Adverse drug events in hospitalized patients. Excess length of stay, extra costs, and attributable mortality. *Journal of the American Medical Association*, 1997, *277*(4), 301–306.

21. Johnson, J. A., & Bootman, J. L. Drug-related morbidity and mortality. A cost-of-illness model. *Archives of Internal Medicine*, 1995, *155*(18), 1949–1956.

22. Newman-Toker, D. E., & Pronovost, P. J. Diagnostic errors—the next frontier for patient safety. *Journal of the American Medical Association*, 2009, *301*(10), 1060–1062.

23. Berner, E. S., & Graber, M. L. Overconfidence as a cause of diagnostic error in medicine. *American Journal of Medicine*, 2008, *121*(5 Suppl), S2–23.

24. Reason, J. Human error: Models and management. *Western Journal of Medicine*, 2000, *172*(6), 393–396.

25. Wachter, R., & Pronovost, P. J. Balancing "no blame" with accountability in patient safety. *New England Journal of Medicine*, 2009, *361*(14).

26. Croskerry, P., & Norman, G. Overconfidence in clinical decision making. *American Journal of Medicine*, 2008, *121*(5 Suppl), S24–29.

27. Singh, H., Petersen, L. A., & Thomas, E. J., Understanding diagnostic errors in medicine: A lesson from aviation. *Quality and Safety in Health Care*, 2006, *15*(3), 159–164.

28. Croskerry, P. The importance of cognitive errors in diagnosis and strategies to minimize them. *Academic Medicine*, 2003, *78*(8), 775–780.

29. Redelmeier, D. A. Improving patient care. The cognitive psychology of missed diagnoses. *Annals of Internal Medicine*, 2005, *142*(2), 115–120.

30. P. O'Neill, personal communication, delivered to M. Godfrey, Lake Morey, 2003.

31. DeRosier, J., Stalhandske, E., Bagian, J. P., & Nudell, T. Using health care failure mode and effect analysis: The VA National Center for Patient Safety's prospective risk analysis system. *Joint Commission Journal on Quality and Improvement*, 2002, *28*(5), 248–267, 209.

32. Joint Commission on Accreditation of Health Care Organizations. *Failure mode and effects analysis in health care. Proactive risk reduction.* Oakbrook Terrace, IL: Joint Commission Resources, 2002.

33. Ranji, S. R., & Shojania, K. G. Implementing patient safety interventions in your hospital: What to try and what to avoid. *Medical Clinics of North America*, 2008, *92*(2), *vii–viii*, 275–293.

34. Shojania, K. G., Duncan, B. W., McDonald, K. M., & Wachter, R. M. Safe but sound: Patient safety meets evidence-based medicine. *Journal of the American Medical Association*, 2002, *288*(4), 508–513.

35. Agency for Healthcare Research and Quality. *Patient safety culture surveys*. Retrieved February 28, 2010, from www.ahrq.gov/qual/patientsafetyculture

36. Arendt, H. *The human condition*. Cambridge England: Polity Press, 1998.

37. Thomas, E. J., Sexton, J. B., Neilands, T. B., Frankel, A., & Helmreich, R. L. The effect of executive walk rounds on nurse safety climate attitudes: A randomized trial of clinical units. *BMC Health Services Research*, 2005, *5*(1), 28.

38. Kozer, E., Scolnik, D., MacPherson, A., Rauchwerger, D., & Koren, G. Using a pre-printed order sheet to reduce prescription errors in a pediatric emergency department: A randomized, controlled trial. *Pediatrics*, 2005, *116*(6), 1299–1302.

39. Shamliyan, T. A., Duval, S., Du, J., & Kane, R. L. Just what the doctor ordered. Review of the evidence of the impact of computerized physician order entry system on medication errors. *Health Services Research*, 2008. *43*(1 Pt 1), 32–53.

40. Nolan, T. W. System changes to improve patient safety. *British Medical Journal*, 2000, *320*(7237), 771–773.

41. Grout, J. R. Mistake proofing: Changing designs to reduce error. *Quality and Safety in Health Care*, 2006, *15* (Supplement 1), i44–i49.

42. Dekker, S. *The field guide to understanding human error.* Burlington, VT: Ashgate Publishing Company, 2006.

43. Chalice, R. *Improving healthcare using Toyota lean production methods.* (2nd ed.) Milwaukee: ASQ Quality Press, 2007.

44. Weick, K., & Sutcliffe, K. *Managing the unexpected: Assuring high performance in an age of complexity.* Ann Arbor: University of Michigan Business School, 2001.

45. Health and Safety Commission (HSC). *Organizing for safety: Third report of the human factors study group of ACSNI.* Sudbury: HSE Books, 1993.

46. Kao, L. S., & Thomas, E. J. Navigating towards improved surgical safety using aviation-based strategies. *Journal of Surgical Research*, 2008, *145*(2), 327–335.

47. Colla, J. B., Bracken, A. C., Kinney, L. M., & Weeks, W. B. Measuring patient safety climate: A review of surveys. *Quality and Safety in Health Care*, 2005, *14*(5), 364–366.

48. Flin, R., Burns, C., Mearns, K., Yule, S., & Robertson, E. M. Measuring safety climate in health care. *Quality and Safety in Health Care*, 2006, *15*(2), 109–115.

49. Sexton et al. The safety attitudes questionnaire: Psychometric properties, benchmarking data, and emerging research. *BMC Health Services Research*, 2006, *6*, 44.

50. Center for Healthcare Quality and Safety. Retrieved August 3, 2010, from www.uth.tmc.edu/schools/med/imed/patient_safety/products.html

51. Lazare, A. Apology in medical practice: An emerging clinical skill. *Journal of the American Medical Association*, 2006, *296*(11), 1401–1404.

52. Rowe, M. Doctors' responses to medical errors. *Critical Reviews in Oncology/Hematology*, 2004, *52*(3), 147–163.

53. Waterman et al. The emotional impact of medical errors on practicing physicians in the United States and Canada. *Joint Commission Journal on Quality and Patient Safety*, 2007, *33*(8), 467–476.

54. Wu, A. W. Medical error: The second victim. The doctor who makes the mistake needs help too. *British Medical Journal*, 2000, *320*(7237), 726–727.

55. Leape, L. Error in medicine. *Journal of the American Medical Association*, 1994, *272*(23).

Chapter Three Action Guide provides tools and methods to encourage your study and design of high reliability and safety in your clinical microsystem.

Safety and reliability are related but different key characteristics of a high performing clinical microsystem. Safety is providing care and services in a manner that minimizes the risk of avoidable harms. Reliability is doing the right thing at the right time in the right place every time. Evidence-based care can tell us what is right but often there is no evidence-base to tell us what is right. The following variables and actions contribute to creating a highly reliable and safe clinical microsystem:

- *Values:* intending to be reliable as a core value.
- *General knowledge:* scanning to identify relevant evidence-based practice that is available in literature and in best practices repositories.
- *Specific adaptation:* adapting the evidence-based practice to be used in each unique microsystem.
- *Reflection and measurement:* observing the patterns of care and identifying opportunities to improve reliability and breaches in consistency; developing metrics and monitors to gauge reliability.

Most clinical microsystems offer many opportunities for improving safety and reliability. The following suggestions intend to offer basic support and guidance to improve reliability and safety for your consideration.

The following specific methods and tools can be used to increase reliability and safety in microsystems:

1. *Setting it up right:* (work environment) 5S
2. *Doing it right:* (processes) checklists
3. *Analyzing it:* (results) failure mode and effects analysis
4. *Practicing it:* (process) rehearsals and simulations

## 5S METHOD

5S is a method to organize the workplace to reduce staff time and motion (for example, to reduce searching, hunting, and gathering what is needed to provide care and services) and at the same time reveal problems in the workplace more readily. Originating from the Toyota Production System LEAN principles, 5S focuses on the setup of the workplace.[1] The aim is to make the workplace more organized and to use visual management to spot problems. (For examples of visual management through 5S, see www.clinicalmicrosystem.org.) The benefits of 5S include the following:

- Organizing the workplace for improved productivity and efficiency
- Cleaning the workplace for improved safety
- Reducing inventory and supply costs by matching inventory to need and by removing infrequently used items
- Recapturing valuable floor space and minimizing overhead costs by removing unused equipment and clutter, thereby providing more floor space for needed equipment storage
- Contributing to pride in work
- Providing an always-ready customer showcase to promote business

5S comes from five Japanese words—Seiri, Seiton, Seiso, Seiketsu, and Shitsuke—which are described in the following section. Figure AG3.1 illustrates the five categories of 5S.

## Sort/Seiri (Organization)

A messy workplace where drawers, cabinets, and storage areas are not well organized or labeled, is hard to work in; wastes time due to increased need to search for misplaced items; and is costly to maintain.

FIGURE AG3.1    5S Method.

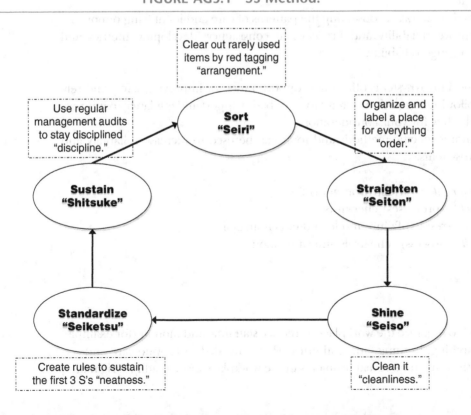

Sort through items and keep only what is needed while disposing of what is not. Be honest about what is not being used anymore. Create permanent locations for remaining equipment or supplies, and organize by how frequently the item is used to support patient care. You should be able to reach items immediately.

### Straighten/Seiton (Orderliness)

To ensure materials can be easily retrieved, ask yourself the following questions:

1. Is there a place for everything?
2. Is everything in its place?
3. Are items labeled and inventoried so they are easy to see and use?
4. Are the most frequently used items closest to the point of use?

### Shine/Seiso (Cleanliness)

Cleanliness is essential in maintaining patients' and employees' health. The cleaning process often exposes abnormal and prefailure conditions that could hurt quality or cause machine failure. Examples include storage space in an intensive care unit where monitoring equipment sits that isn't regularly cleaned and could harbor microorganisms or electrical plugs that might be exposed to liquid spills. To assess your general unit cleanliness, ask yourself and the interdisciplinary members of the microsystem the following questions:

- What is the cleaning schedule for the selected work areas?
- What staff are responsible for cleaning and ensuring cleanliness?
- Who cleans and how?
- Are work areas neat and clean?
- Are the cleaning materials easily available if there is an accident or if additional cleanliness is needed?
- How do you contact someone if something needs to be cleaned?

### Standardize/Seiketsu (Adherence)

Develop systems and procedures to maintain and sort, straighten, and shine. For example, use tape and signs to label each item's location to help remind staff where supplies belong. You could also outline an item's place on the shelf so when the item is removed, the shadowed outline remains to remind staff where the item should be placed upon return.

Ask yourself the following questions as you develop systems to maintain the standard way:

- Are the visual data and information sources easily visible and up-to-date?
- Are the standard processes clearly understood and can they be performed in a standardized fashion?
- Are standardized forms readily available and do members of your team consistently use them?

### Sustain/Shitsuke (Self-Discipline)

Shitsuke helps prevent the 5S approach from being a one-time event or spring cleaning. Maintaining a stabilized workplace is an ongoing process of continuous improvement that involves everyone. A formal audit process done in a scheduled manner helps ensure standardization is being maintained. Questions you can ask yourself to help sustain are as follows:

- Are procedures being followed with minimal (or no) variation?
- How do you know if standardized procedures are being followed?
- What processes of sort, straighten, shine, and standardize do you measure and track?
- How and at what frequency do you do your 5S audit?
- How do members of the microsystem get feedback about the standardization and 5S process?
- How do members of the microsystem improve the 5S processes?

The 5S *Evaluation and Improvement* worksheet (see Figure AG3.2) can be used for completing a baseline assessment in the workplace to determine what to focus improvement on. The worksheet can be used to audit the workplace throughout the year as 5S is sustained.

## CHECKLISTS

Atul Gawande writes in *The Checklist Manifesto*, "we need a different strategy for overcoming failure, one that builds on experience and takes advantage of the knowledge people have but somehow also makes up for our inevitable human inadequacies. . . . It is a checklist."[2]

Checklists provide two main benefits. First, they help with memory recall. Second, checklists make explicit the minimum expected steps in complex processes.

### How to Make a Checklist

The steps for making a checklist are as follows.

1. Identify a process that can be improved through standardization and result in higher reliability and safety.
2. Study the best-known process that consistently produces the best results. Examples of best known processes can be found at the Institute for Healthcare Improvement, www.ihi.org. Search specific topics, for example, central venous catheter infections.
3. Identify what steps are done in what order.
4. Place steps on a form in the correct order.
4. Educate staff to use the checklist as part of their standard work process.
5. Monitor checklist use and improve the checklist as experience is gained.

An example of an ICU Central Line Checklist is shown in Figure AG3.3. The aim of the ICU Central Line Checklist is to ensure all processes related to central line placement are executed for each line placement, thereby leading to a reliable process.

Nurses should be empowered to supervise central line preparations using the checklist prior to line insertion and to stop the process if necessary.

This checklist includes a list of activities that are considered standard work before, during, and after the procedure. It also includes items that ensure safety.

# FIGURE AG3.2   5S Evaluation and Improvement Worksheet.

## 5S Evaluation and Improvement Worksheet

**Evaluators Name(s):**

Name the WORK AREA:

Scoring:
0= No problems
1= One to two problems
2= More than two problems

| | | Before | After |
|---|---|---|---|
| **Sort** (Organization) | **Distinguish between what is needed and not needed** | | |
| | Have all unnecessary items been removed? | | |
| | Are walkways, work areas, locations clearly identified? | | |
| | Does a procedure exist for removing unneeded items? | | |
| **Straighten** (Orderliness) | **A place for everything and everything in its place** | | |
| | Is there a place for everything? | | |
| | Is everything in its place? | | |
| | Are locations obvious and easy to identify? | | |
| **Shine** (Cleanliness) | **Cleaning and looking for ways to keep it clean** | | |
| | Are work areas, equipment, tools, desks clean and free of debris, and so on? | | |
| | Are cleaning materials available and accessible? | | |
| | Is there contact number to call if cleaning is needed? | | |
| | Cleaning schedules exist and are posted? | | |
| **Standardize** (Adherence) | **Maintain and Monitor for adherence** | | |
| | Is all necessary information visible? | | |
| | Are all standards known and visible? | | |
| | Are all visual displays current and up to date? | | |
| | Is there adherence to existing standards? | | |
| **Sustain** (Self-Discipline) | **Following the rules to sustain** | | |
| | Are procedures being followed? | | |
| | Does an on-going audit and feedback system exist? | | |
| | Does a system exist to respond to audit feedback? | | |
| | **Total Score** | | |

*Source:* 5S worksheet adapted from Vital Enterprises. www.vitalentusa.com.

## FIGURE AG3.3   Procedure Checklist.

Patient Label

Indication: To document procedural practices in the CCU related to insertion technique for CVP lines, dialysis access ports, and central lines, including PICC

| Type of Catheter: | ☐ Central Line | Location: _____ |
| | ☐ CVP | Location: _____ |
| | ☐ Dialysis Catheter | Location: _____ |
| | ☐ PICC Line | Location: _____ |
| **Is this a NEW line?** | ☐ Yes | ☐ No |
| **Is the procedure:** | ☐ Elective | ☐ Emergent    ☐ _____ |
| | ☐ Rewire | ☐ Reposition |

### Procedural Checklist

| Safety Practice | Yes | Yes (after reminder) |
|---|:---:|:---:|
| **Before Procedure,** did the provider: | | |
| • **Perform** Procedural Pause | | |
|     Perform patient ID x 2 | ☐ | ☐ |
|     Announce the procedure to be performed | ☐ | ☐ |
|     Mark/assess site | ☐ | ☐ |
|     Position patient correctly for procedure | ☐ | ☐ |
|     Assemble equipment/verify supplies | ☐ | ☐ |
|     Use relevant documents (chart/forms) | ☐ | ☐ |
|     Order follow-up radiology images (PRN) | ☐ | ☐ |
| • Cleanse hands (ASK if unsure) | ☐ | ☐ |
| • Prep procedure site with ChloraPrep<br>*30 seconds for dry site*<br>*2 minutes for moist site (especially femoral)* | ☐ | ☐ |
| • Use large drape to cover patient in sterile fashion | ☐ | ☐ |
| **During Procedure,** did the provider: | | |
| • Wear sterile gloves during catheter insertion? | ☐ | ☐ |
| • Wear hat, mask, and sterile gown? | ☐ | ☐ |
| • Maintain sterile field? | ☐ | ☐ |
| • Use ultrasound if appropriate? | ☐ | ☐ |
| • Assist physician follow same precautions (hand washing, mask, gloves, gown)? | ☐ | ☐ |
| • All staff and patient in room wear mask? | ☐ | ☐ |
| **After Procedure:** | | |
| • Was sterile technique maintained when applying dressing? | ☐ | ☐ |
| • Was dressing dated? | ☐ | ☐ |

**Name of Intensivist:**_____

**Name of Procedure MD:**_____

**Name of Assisting MD:**_____

**Name of RN (auditor):**_____ **Today's Date:**_____

**Unit:**_____ **Room:** _____

**Please return completed form to:**_____

# FAILURE MODE AND EFFECTS ANALYSIS

Failure Mode and Effects Analysis (FMEA) is a team-based structured, proactive approach to identifying and prioritizing errors that could occur in a process. The FMEA is usually built using a spreadsheet while those who work in the process are brainstorming about what could go wrong with the process. FMEA is usually used before beginning detailed final design and rollout of a new process. Its specific uses are as follows:

- Identify ways a product, service, or process can fail. Estimate risk associated with specific failure causes.
- Prioritize actions to reduce the risk of failure.
- Evaluate design validation plan. Ensure the end product and or process meets customer needs.
- Design new systems, products, and processes.
- Change existing designs or processes.
- Evaluate a new design and new processes before rollout to understand how the design could fail.
- Evaluate and improve existing processes to understand how people, materials, equipment, methods, and environment cause process problems.

## How to Conduct the FMEA Process

Use the following steps when conducting your FMEA process:

1. Start with the steps that contribute the *most* value.
2. Brainstorm possible failure modes.
3. List one or more potential effects for each failure mode.
4. Assign ratings for severity and occurrence.
   Severity = 1–10, with 10 having the most severe impact on customers and patients.
   Likeliness failure will occur = 1–10, with 10 representing most likely to occur.
5. List current monitoring and controls for each failure.
   Detectability of failure = 1–10, with 10 representing the least likely to be noticed with the current control methods.
6. Calculate risk priority number (RPN) for each effect by multiplying the scores for severity, occurrence, and detection.
7. Use the RPN to select high priority failure modes. The highest RPNs are the top priorities.
   NOTE: Any failure with a severity rating of 10 must be immediately addressed by the clinical microsystem to minimize risk to safety or reliability.
8. Plan to reduce or eliminate the risk associated with the high priority failure modes.
   Identify potential causes of selected failure modes.
   Develop recommended actions and assign responsible persons.
   Look for preventive actions and contingent actions to take to prevent failure.
9. Carry out the plan and document your team's actions.
10. Recompute RPN.

Table AG3.1 provides an example of a failure mode and effects analysis with regard to anticoagulant drug use. Because there are many potential errors and risks of patients having their blood clotting function minimized with anticoagulants, this FMEA example illustrates the potential risks of an inappropriate patient receiving anticoagulation, the risks of drug and food interactions, and reasons why the risks might not be identified. This assessment will inform a future process design with built-in steps to ensure risk is minimized.

Additional information and helpful resources can be found at www.jointcommission .org.

Table AG3.1   Failure Mode and Effects Analysis

| Steps | Failure Mode | Failure Causes | Failure Effects |
|---|---|---|---|
| 1 | Is anticoagulant indicated? | | |
| | | | Anticoagulant administered when not indicated |
| | Is diagnosis correct? | Diagnostic tests not performed | No treatment given when indicated |
| | | | Failure of test to diagnose |
| | | Doesn't meet standards of practice Clinicians unaware of standards | Inappropriate prescribing of anticoagulants |
| 1B | Are there contraindications or disease interactions? | No or incomplete patient information Not evaluated Diagnosis inconclusive Didn't know patient had a given contraindication (for example, epidural) Interpretation biases | Bleeding Death Thrombosis |
| 1C | Are there drug or food interactions? Can they be managed? | Incomplete medication history No computer alerts Skipped alert Incomplete alert Herbal or supplement interactions not considered Didn't check | Bleeding Death Thrombosis |
| | | | (Severity can range from 1–10) |

## REHEARSALS OR SIMULATIONS

Rehearsals or simulations offer participants the chance to practice a clinical process, technique, interaction, and scenario to learn how to do it right or to learn how to do it better. Rehearsals or simulations are powerful teaching tools and can be as simple or as complex as you need them to be.

The level of technology required for rehearsals or simulations can also range from simple to complex. Technology should not be perceived as a barrier to rehearsals and simulations.

Rehearsals or simulations can take any of the following forms: (1) as a role play in an appropriate setting like your microsystem, without special technology; (2) with live actors serving as programmed patients' prerehearsed actions and reactions according to script; and (3) in a simulation lab using computerized dummies and mannequins to model the physiological response to treatment actions.

| Likelihood of Occurrence (1–10) | Likelihood of Detection (1–10) | Severity (1–10) | Risk Priority Number (RPN) | Actions to Reduce Occurrence of Failure |
|---|---|---|---|---|
|  |  |  |  |  |
|  |  |  | 0 | • All caregivers double-check diagnosis. |
|  |  |  | 0 |  |
|  |  |  | 0 | • Use two tests to diagnose when possible.<br>• Repeat inconclusive tests. |
|  |  |  | 0 | • Pharmacists check indication.<br>• Educate prescribers.<br>• Establish treatment guidelines. |
|  |  |  | 0 | • Pharmacists double-check indication.<br>• Establish treatment guidelines that include information on contraindications. |
|  |  |  | 0 | • Use pharmacy computer system that screens for drug interactions.<br>• Take a complete medication history including herbal or supplement information. |
|  |  |  | 0 |  |

The process to plan a rehearsal or simulation is as follows:

1. Set up a clinical *scenario* that is important to master by establishing learning objectives, a setting, and necessary equipment.
2. *Gather* the learners. This is often done with an interdisciplinary team.
3. *Brief* the learners on the clinical situation and on what their objective is.
4. *Run* the rehearsal to respond to the clinical scenario.
5. Have expert(s) *observe* the learner's performance in the rehearsal.
6. Videotape the rehearsal if desired and if equipment and personnel are readily available.
7. *Debrief* the learners on their performance and highlight those areas (for example, knowledge, skills, attitudes, communications, and interactions) that went well and those areas that could be improved upon. Review the videotape of the performance if available.
8. *Repeat* the process until competency is achieved.

Rehearsals and simulations are most often used in situations involving technical skills and processes, or in communications between staff and patients and their families. Rehearsals and simulations can also be used in situations that need improvement or when team members need to develop any number of competencies.

## DESIGNING PATIENT SAFETY INTO THE MICROSYSTEM

(Contribution of Julie Johnson and Paul Barach)

Safety is a property of the microsystem. It can only be achieved through thoughtful and systematic application of a broad array of process, equipment, organization, supervision, training, simulation, and teamwork changes. Characteristics of high performing microsystems (as discussed in Chapter One—leadership, organizational support, staff focus, education and training, interdependence, patient focus, community and market focus, performance results, process improvement, and information technology) can be linked to specific design concepts and actions to enhance patient safety in microsystems.

### Background

In 2000, the release of the IOM report *To err is human: Building a safer health system*[3] was a landmark event in that it estimated that 44,000 to 98,000 people die each year from medical errors. Even the lower estimate was higher than the annual mortality from motor vehicle accidents (43,458), breast cancer (42,297), or AIDS (16,516), and medical errors were the eighth leading cause of death in the United States. Patient harm from medical error isn't unique to the United States. Across the world, people seeking care in hospitals are harmed 9.2 percent of the time, with death occurring in 7.4 percent of these events. Furthermore, it is estimated that 43.5 percent of these harm events are preventable.[4] The rates could be debated as they depend on the methods used in the studies as well as unknown levels of underreporting, in addition to the difficulty of determining retrospectively whether an error actually occurred. However, most significantly, the study of patient safety has identified a problem that needs to be addressed and the focus quickly shifted from quantifying errors to the more complex issue of how to prevent errors from causing patient harm.

Evidence suggests medical errors may result more frequently from the organization of health care delivery. For example, Leape and colleagues discovered that failures at the system level were the real culprits in more than 75 percent of adverse drug events.[5]

A 2003 report from the Agency for Healthcare Research and Quality found that the most common causes of errors are (1) communication problems, (2) inadequate information flow, (3) human (or performance) problems, (4) patient-related issues, (5) organizational transfer of knowledge, (6) staffing patterns and work flow, (6) technical failures, (7) inadequate policies and procedures.[6]

James Reason suggested that some systems are more vulnerable and therefore more likely to experience adverse events.[7] The following organizational pathologies can contribute to what Reason refers to as *vulnerable system syndrome:* blaming frontline individuals, denying the existence of systemic weaknesses, and single-mindedly pursuing the wrong type of performance measures (for example, pursuing financial and production indicators instead of the balanced set of measures espoused by the clinical value compass).

The recommendations contained in the IOM report emerged from a four-tiered strategy:

1. Establish a national focus on patient safety by creating a center for patient safety within the Agency for Healthcare Research and Quality (AHRQ).[8]
2. Identify and learn from errors by establishing nationwide mandatory and voluntary reporting systems.
3. Raise standards and expectations for improvement in safety through the actions of oversight organizations, group purchasers, and professional groups.
4. Create safety systems inside healthcare organizations through the implementation of safe practices at the delivery level.

Research in managing safety has focused on the culture and structure of the organization. Perrow advanced the theory that accidents are inevitable in complex, tightly coupled systems such as chemical plants and nuclear power plants.[9] These accidents occur irrespective of the skill of the designers and operators; hence, they are normal and are difficult to prevent. Perrow further argues that, as the system gets more complex, it becomes opaque to its users so that people are less likely to recognize and be afraid of potential adverse occurrences.

Organizational models view human error more as a consequence than as a cause. Such models stress the need for proactive measures to ensure safety and health, with constant reform of the system's processes. For an organization to remain sufficiently flexible to adapt to changing demands, its culture must value flexibility.

High reliability organizations (HROs) are an example of highly complex, technology-sensitive organizations that must operate to a failure-free standard. Examples include naval aircraft carriers and air traffic controllers. HROs carry out demanding activities with a very low error rate and an almost complete absence of catastrophic failure over many years.

## THE LINK BETWEEN SAFETY, THE MICROSYSTEM, AND MINDFULNESS

Initiating the improvement of the safety of care for patients and populations in clinical microsystems involves increasing the work unit's awareness of its functioning as a microsystem and its mindfulness of its reliability. Weick and Sutcliffe offer the idea that HROs have become reliable by virtue of their *mindfulness*.[10] By mindfulness they mean these organizations exhibit the following qualities.

A *preoccupation with failure:* they "treat any lapse as a symptom that something is wrong with the system, something that could have severe consequences if separate small errors happen to coincide at one awful moment."[10]

A *reluctance to simplify interpretations:* in general, there is a temptation to oversimplify key issues related to our work. Instead of giving into the temptation to oversimplify, high reliability organizations deliberately simplify less often so that they can see more of the complex and unpredictable nature of their work.

A *sensitivity to operations:* HROs recognize that unexpected events usually stem from what James Reason called *latent failures*—system failures that result because of loopholes in the system's defenses, barriers, and safeguards. Loopholes are essentially imperfections in system properties, for example, loopholes in supervision, error reporting mechanisms, safety training, and so on. Latent failures are often discovered after an accident occurs; the potential for failure isn't obvious until there is a problem. HROs pay more attention to the frontline operations, where the real work is accomplished, which allows them to make small corrections before errors accumulate into an accident.

*A commitment to resilience:* HROs recognize that they will never be completely free from error, so they develop capabilities to detect, contain, and bounce back from errors instead of being disabled by errors.

*A deference to expertise:* HROs encourage decisions to be made at the front line and migrate authority to the people with the most expertise, regardless of rank.

According to Weick and Sutcliffe, becoming more mindful means practicing more of these behaviors. Mindfulness implies a radical state of being present by exhibiting situational awareness of one's current surroundings and the actual requirements of the current situation, and at the same time not letting go of a chronic sense of unease that something catastrophic might occur at any moment. Mindfulness, as a property of the HRO, is inculcated in all members of the unit, from the leaders to the most junior professionals on the team.

A foundational idea of HROs suggests that team as well as individual performance depends on the development of certain organizational norms such as mindfulness. Therefore, translating these principles to the microsystem requires attention to the individual within the microsystem as well as to the microsystems as a whole. Often we think of characteristics of HROs existing at a larger system level—for example, at the organizational level instead of a microsystem level. We propose that individual microsystem can strive for and achieve mindfulness. It may therefore be possible for mindful microsystems to exist in an organization that is not mindful throughout or that is dysfunctional. In considering this possible relationship between a mindful microsystem and a dysfunctional organization, it is important to recognize the importance of the larger system to the success or failure of the microsystem. The importance of the larger system's support of the microsystem is explained as noted in the sidebar by an interviewee at a geriatric unit.

> The administration has continued to support the geriatric unit by providing both staffing and general resources. Getting a *yes* for a request from the administration depends on how they feel about you and your department. On the converse, rarely do units exist in a vacuum. So, where there is a larger structure, there are always potential negatives.

As pointed out by this interviewee, the microsystem is to some extent dependent on the larger organizational structure for resources. It isn't possible to completely uncouple the relationship. Some organizations have recognized the need to support the functioning of the microsystem. Furthermore, a focus at the microsystem level changes the role of senior leadership, which is not a minor detail. The Health Care Advisory Board reported a common ingredient in successful organizations is a "tight, loose, tight" deployment strategy.[11] If a microsystem were striving to provide safer care, a *tight, loose, tight* deployment strategy would involve senior leaders mandating that each microsystem should have a "tight" alignment of its mission, vision, and strategies with the organization's mission, vision, and strategies. Senior leadership would also give each microsystem the flexibility needed to achieve its mission. At the same time, senior leaders would hold the microsystems accountable to achieve its strategic mission to provide safer care. Figure AG3.4 illustrates a hypothetical scenario we have used to connect patient safety principles with clinical microsystem thinking. In this scenario the patient is Allison, a 5-year-old preschooler, with a history of wheezy bronchitis. As

FIGURE AG3.4 Patient Safety Scenario.

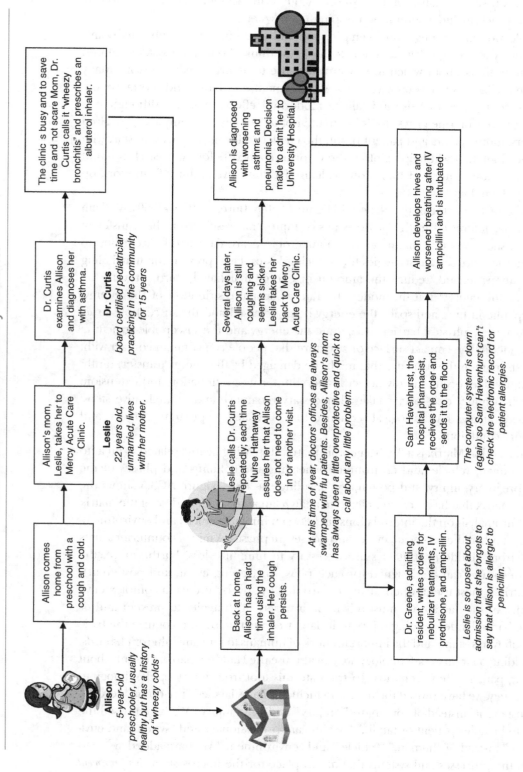

Allison
5-year-old preschooler, usually healthy but has a history of "wheezy colds"

Allison comes home from preschool with a cough and cold.

Allison's mom, Leslie, takes her to Mercy Acute Care Clinic.

Leslie
22 years old, unmarried, lives with her mother.

Dr. Curtis examines Allison and diagnoses her with asthma.

Dr. Curtis
board certified pediatrician practicing in the community for 15 years

The clinic's busy and to save time and not scare Mom, Dr. Curtis calls it "wheezy bronchitis" and prescribes an albuterol inhaler.

Back at home, Allison has a hard time using the inhaler. Her cough persists.

Leslie calls Dr. Curtis repeatedly; each time Nurse Hathaway assures her that Allison does not need to come in for another visit.

At this time of year, doctors' offices are always swamped with flu patients. Besides, Allison's mom has always been a little overprotective and quick to call about any little problem.

Several days later, Allison is still coughing and seems sicker. Leslie takes her back to Mercy Acute Care Clinic.

Allison is diagnosed with worsening asthma and pneumonia. Decision made to admit her to University Hospital.

Dr. Greene, admitting resident, writes orders for nebulizer treatments, IV prednisone, and ampicillin.

Leslie is so upset about admission that she forgets to say that Allison is allergic to penicillin.

Sam Havenhurst, the hospital pharmacist, receives the order and sends it to the floor.

The computer system is down (again) so Sam Havenhurst can't check the electronic record for patient allergies.

Allison develops hives and worsened breathing after IV ampicillin and is intubated.

we follow the scenario, it is clear that Allison and her mother interact with several microsystems in an attempt to address Allison's illness. There is the hypothetical community-based pediatric clinic (Mercy Acute Care Clinic) and the University Hospital, which includes several overlapping microsystems.

While working through the scenario, you will encounter many obvious points where the system failed. Pay attention to how you think about these system failures. In addition, think about which tools you would use to analyze medical errors. Many tools are available, such as crew resource management, morbidity and mortality conferences, root cause analysis, and failure mode and effects analysis. Although it is tempting to rely on one or two tools in an attempt to simplify the complexity involved in understanding errors and patient harm, the challenge for most of us is to start with a broader look that will help us place the error in context before we search for root causes. One useful method builds on William Haddon's overarching framework on injury epidemiology.

As the first Director of the National Highway Safety Bureau (1966–1969), William Haddon was interested in the broad issues of injury that result from the transfer of energy in such ways that inanimate or animate objects are damaged.[12] According to Haddon, there are several strategies for reducing losses. First, prevent the marshaling of the energy; second, reduce the amount of energy marshaled; third, prevent the release of the energy; fourth, modify the rate or spatial distribution of the energy; fifth, separate in time and space the energy being released and the susceptible structure; sixth, use a physical barrier to separate the energy and the susceptible structure; seventh, modify the contact surface or structure that people can come in contact with; eighth, strengthen the structure that might be damaged by the energy transfer; ninth, when injury does occur, rapidly detect it and counter its continuation and extension; tenth, when injury does occur, take all necessary reparative and rehabilitative steps. All these strategies have a logical sequence that is related to pre-injury, injury, and post-injury conditions.

The Haddon Matrix is a $3 \times 3$ algebraic matrix displaying factors related to an auto injury (human, vehicle, and environment) heading the columns and phases of the event (pre-injury, injury, and post-injury) heading the rows. Figure AG3.5 shows the Haddon Matrix that has been completed to analyze an auto accident. Use of the matrix focuses the analysis on the interrelationship between human, vehicle, and environmental factors and on the pre-event, event, and post-event phases. A mix of countermeasures derived from Haddon's strategies are necessary to minimize loss. Furthermore, the countermeasures can be designed for each phase (pre-event, event, and post-event). The matrix is most useful when we are confronted by adverse events in complex environments; in such a case we must rely upon a variety of strategies to prevent and or mitigate harm. Understanding injury in its larger context helps us recognize the basic lack of safety in systems and the important work of humans to mitigate inherent hazards.

Building on injury epidemiology, we can also use the Haddon matrix to think about analyzing patient safety scenarios. To translate this tool from injury epidemiology to patient safety, we have revised the matrix to include phases labeled "pre-event," "event," and "post-event" instead of "pre-injury," "injury," and "post-injury." We have revised the factors to include "patient or family," "health care professional," and "system and environment," instead of "human," "vehicle," and "environment." We have added *system* to refer to the processes and systems that are in place for the microsystem. *Environment* refers to the context the microsystem exists within. The addition of system recognizes the significant contribution systems make toward harm and error in the microsystem.

## FIGURE AG3.5   Haddon Matrix.

| | Factors | | |
|---|---|---|---|
| **Phases** | Human | Vehicle | Environment |
| Pre-injury | Alcohol intoxication | Braking capacity of motor vehicles | Visibility of hazards |
| Injury | Resistance to energy insults | Sharp or pointed edges and surfaces | Flammable building materials |
| Post-injury | Hemorrhage | Rapidity of energy reduction | Emergency medical response |

*Source:* Haddon, W. J. A logical framework for categorizing highway safety phenomena and activity. *Journal of Trauma,* 1972, *12*(197).

## FIGURE AG3.6   Patient Safety Matrix.

| | Factors | | |
|---|---|---|---|
| **Phases** | Provider | Patient or Family | System and Environment |
| Pre-event | • Physician decision about diagnosis | • Child with history of wheezy colds | • Busy primary care clinic<br>• University hospital |
| Event | • IV ampicillin | • Allergy to penicillin | • Computer systems down |
| Post-event | • Intubation | • Hives, difficulty breathing | • Hospital (team response to allergic reaction) |

Figure AG3.6 shows a completed matrix using Allison's scenario. The next step in learning from errors and adverse events is to develop countermeasures to address the issues in each cell of the matrix.

Based on the authors' experience with multiple microsystems across diverse settings and with the authors' understanding and interpretation of the safety literature, we offer several safety principles that can be used as a framework for embedding patient safety concepts within clinical microsystems.

## Principle 1. Humans Are Error-Prone by Nature and so Errors Will Occur

Errors are not synonymous with negligence. Medicine's ethos of infallibility leads wrongly to a culture that sees mistakes as an individual problem or weakness and remedies them with blame and punishment. Instead, we should look for the multiple factors that contributed to the error and then improve our systems.

## Principle 2. The Microsystem Is the Unit of Analysis and Training

We can train microsystem staff to include safety principles in their daily work through rehearsing scenarios, through simulation, and through role playing. The goal is for the microsystem to behave like a robust high reliability organization (HRO), which is defined as an organization that is preoccupied with the possibility for failure or chronic unease about safety breaches.[13]

## Principle 3. Design Systems to Identify, Prevent, Absorb, and Mitigate Errors

Identify errors by establishing effective, sustainable reporting systems that encourage and support transparency, freedom from punitive actions, and empowerment of workers to feel comfortable to speak up, even if speaking up means they will challenge the authority gradient. Design work, technology, and work practices to uncover, mitigate, or attenuate the consequences of error.

There are many ways to reduce the impact of errors by simplifying the systems and processes people use. For example, tools such as checklists, flow sheets, and ticklers reduce reliance on memory. You can also improve access to information and information technology and design systems that are able to absorb a certain amount of error without harm to patients. You might also include key buffers in your system, such as time lapses (built-in delays) to verify information before proceeding, redundancy, and forcing functions such as intentional removal of potassium chloride from a microsystem forcing a deliberate action to order the medication to minimize inadvertent use.

## Principle 4. Create a Culture of Safety

A culture of safety recognizes that the cornerstone to making health care safer is a transparent climate that supports reporting errors, near misses, and adverse events and that recognizes these events as opportunities for learning and improving. Embrace and celebrate storytelling by patients and clinicians. Storytelling is where safety is made and breached and much learning occurs.

## Principle 5. Talk to and Listen to Patients

Patients have much to say about safety. When a patient is harmed by health care, all details of the event pertaining to the patient should be disclosed to the patient and or family. Elements of disclosure should include the following:

- A prompt and compassionate explanation of what is understood about what happened and the probable effects
- Assurance that a full analysis will take place to reduce the likelihood of a similar event happening to another patient

- Follow-up based on the analysis
- An apology

## Principle 6. Integrate Practices from Human Factors Engineering into Microsystem Functioning

Design patient-centered health care environments that are based on human factor principles that include usability and ergonomics. Design for human cognitive failings and for the impact of performance-shaping factors such as fatigue, poor lighting, and noisy settings. New limitations on medical resident hours of duty have been designed to counter fatigue and signs have been created to alert staff to shift report processes to discourage interruptions, which can result in errors and incomplete information sharing.

## CONCLUSION

Our discussion of patient safety within clinical microsystems would not be complete without acknowledging how characteristics of high performing microsystems could be used to help shape a microsystem's response to the challenge to embed safety into the daily work of patient care. Table AG3.2 lists several characteristics of high performing

### Table AG3.2   Linkages to Safety

| Microsytem Characteristics | What This Means for Patient Safety |
|---|---|
| 1. Leadership | <ul><li>Define the safety vision of the organization.</li><li>Identify existing constraints within the organization.</li><li>Allocate resources for plan development, implementation, and ongoing monitoring and evaluation.</li><li>Build in microsystem participation and input to plan development.</li><li>Align organizational quality and safety goals.</li><li>Provide updates to board of trustees.</li></ul> |
| 2. Organizational Support | <ul><li>Work with clinical microsystems to identify patient safety issues and make relevant local changes.</li><li>Put necessary resources and tools into the hands of individuals without making organizational support superficial.</li></ul> |
| 3. Staff Focus | <ul><li>Assess current safety culture.</li><li>Identify gap between current culture and safety vision.</li><li>Plan cultural interventions.</li><li>Conduct periodic assessments of culture.</li></ul> |
| 4. Education and Training | <ul><li>Develop patient safety curriculum.</li><li>Provide training and education of key clinical and management leadership.</li><li>Develop a core of people with patient safety skills (as a resource) who can work across microsytems.</li></ul> |
| 5. Interdependence of the Care Team | <ul><li>Build plan-do-study-act (PDSA) into debriefings.</li><li>Use daily huddles for after action reviews (AARs) and celebrate identifying errors.</li></ul> |
| 6. Patient Focus | <ul><li>Establish patient and family partnerships.</li><li>Support disclosure and truth around medical error.</li></ul> |

*(Continued)*

### Table AG3.2   Linkages to Safety (Continued)

| Microsystem Characteristics | What This Means for Patient Safety |
|---|---|
| 7. Community and Market Focus | • Analyze safety issues in community and partner with external groups to reduce risk to population. |
| 8. Performance Results | • Develop key safety measures.<br>• Create the business case for safety. |
| 9. Process Improvement | • Identify patient safety priorities based on assessment of key safety measures.<br>• Address the work that will be required at the microsystem level.<br>• Establish patient safety demonstration sites.<br>• Transfer the learning. |
| 10. Information and Information Technology | • Enhance error reporting system.<br>• Build safety concepts into information flow (checklists, reminder systems). |

microsytems and describes specific actions that can be further explored in your microsystem. The list of actions is not intended to be exhaustive, but offers a place to start and an organizing framework for applying patient safety concepts to the microsystem.

Safety is a dynamic property of the microsystem. It can only be achieved through thoughtful and systematic application of a broad array of changes to process, equipment, organization, supervision, training, simulation, and interdisciplinary health care professional working structures.

## REFERENCES

1. Liker, J. *The Toyota way.* New York: McGraw Hill, 2003.
2. Gawande, A. *The checklist manifesto.* New York: Metropolitan Books, 2009, p. 13.
3. Institute of Medicine Committee on Quality Health Care in America. *To err is human: Building a safer health system.* Washington, DC: National Academy Press, 2000.
4. de Vries, E., Ramrattan, M., Smorenburg, S., Gouma, D. J., & Boermeester, M. A. The incidence and nature of in-hospital adverse events: A systematic review. *Quality and Safety in Health Care,* 2008, *17,* 216–223.
5. Leape, L. Error in medicine. *Journal of the American Medical Association,* 1994, *272*(23).
6. Agency for Healthcare Research and Quality. Patient safety initiative: Building foundations, reducing risk. *Interim Report to the Senate Committee on Appropriations,* 2003. Rockville, MD: Agency for Healthcare Research and Quality.
7. Reason, J. Human error: Models and management. *Western Journal of Medicine,* 2000, *172*(6), 393–396.
8. Agency for Healthcare Research and Quality. Patient safety culture surveys accessed at http://www.ahrq.gov/qual/patientsafetyculture.
9. Perrow, C. *Normal accidents.* New York: Basic Books, 1984.
10. Weick, K., & Sutcliffe, K. *Managing the unexpected: Assuring high performance in an age of complexity.* Ann Arbor: University of Michigan Business School, 2001.
11. Health and Safety Commission (HSC). *Organizing for safety: Third report of the human factors study group of ACSNI.* Sudbury: HSE Books, 1993.
12. Haddon, W. J. A logical framework for categorizing highway safety phenomena and activity. *Journal of Trauma,* 1972, *12*(197).
13. Dekker, S. *The field guide to human error investigations.* Aldershot: Ashgate Publishing Limited, 2002.

# USING MEASUREMENT TO IMPROVE HEALTH CARE VALUE

Eugene C. Nelson

Joel S. Lazar

Marjorie M. Godfrey

Paul B. Batalden

## LEARNING OBJECTIVES

- Describe measuring, monitoring, evaluating, and improving health care outcomes and efficiency within the context of the microsystem.
- Compare and contrast the patient value compass with the balanced scorecard.
- Demonstrate how to develop and use the patient value compass and balanced score-card frameworks to measure and improve microsystem performance.
- Discuss feed forward and feedback systems and their benefits to the clinical microsystem.
- Describe principles for designing rich information environments so data may be used to answer critical questions in microsystems.
- Design a rich information environment that uses cascading measures to align work and dashboards to show trends.

Leading, executing, learning, and measuring are the *big four* activities that support clinical microsystems' creation of high value care. In this chapter we focus specifically on measurement. We begin with three case studies that illustrate how exemplary microsystems use measures and build rich information environments at the front line of care. We reflect on these cases and generate useful principles for intelligent design of such environments, with attention to *measuring what matters* for multiple health care stakeholders. We discuss data flow and the use of feed forward and feedback methods, and we introduce two powerful frameworks, the patient value compass and the balanced scorecard, which together permit measurement and improvement of both health care value and operating performance. We conclude with a discussion of clinical dashboards and data cascades, and address their application in real-world clinical programs and health systems.

## MEASURING WHAT MATTERS AT ALL LEVELS OF THE SYSTEM

The design, delivery, and improvement of high value health care require thoughtful and continuous attention to the *measurement* of meaningful outcomes. In patient-clinician dyads, in organizational macrosystems, and especially in clinical microsystems at the value-generating interface of patients, health professionals, and larger health care institutions, a robust *information environment* supports best clinical practices and best system performance. High functioning clinical practices and programs ask themselves repeatedly: "How do we know if specific care processes and entire clinical services add genuine value?" "How do we know if planned changes to those processes and services represent actual improvement?" Measurement provides answers to these questions and also facilitates improvement.

We have observed in prior chapters that health care value is created within sequentially embedded and mutually supportive systems of care. Let us now consider the extent to which measuring what matters can support participants and stakeholders at every level of these interacting systems (see Figure 4.1). Individual clinicians, in partnership with patients and families, use real-time data to monitor response to focused interventions, and then to adjust these interventions as necessary to achieve health goals. Clinical microsystems aggregate these same data at the level of well-defined practice populations to evaluate the impact of specific care processes and to improve these processes on a continuous basis. Organizations employ balanced scorecards to manage institutional imperatives, which include practice innovation, key processes, customer satisfaction, finance, and growth. External stakeholders (such as insurers and government regulators) rely upon macrosystems to report performance, which in turn guides reimbursement and future programmatic support.

In well-functioning health care systems, measurement-supported activities of *monitoring, evaluating, improving, managing,* and *reporting* are all tightly linked, and the measures themselves are designed to cascade from one level of the organization to the next. Creation of a rich information environment requires alignment of resources and processes both within discrete system levels and across them. In this chapter we focus especially upon the design of measurement infrastructure at the front line of clinical care, that is, within clinical microsystems where patient-centered value is actually generated. But we suggest as well the manner and the extent to which measurement within the microsystem aligns with cascading organizational, regional, and even national health care priorities.

## FIGURE 4.1   Multiple Functions of Measurement Within Embedded Levels of a Health System.

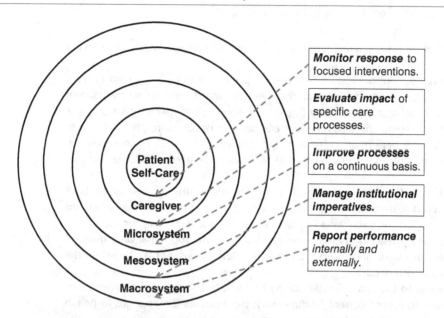

We first present three case studies of clinical microsystems that use data in everyday practice to provide high-quality, cost-effective care. Next we offer principles for display and use of data and discuss concepts and frameworks that facilitate intelligent design of rich information environments. We conclude with one final case that integrates several of these principles and that illustrates their application in the continuous improvement of clinical care.

## SPECIALTY CARE CASE STUDY: DARTMOUTH-HITCHCOCK SPINE CENTER

*We needed a language to work with our patients. The value compass provides the language that helps our multidisciplinary team work with our patients to get them back to work, back to play, one back at a time.*

—James Weinstein, Spine Center founder

### A Typical Illness Episode: Health Outcomes Tracking and More

A patient arrives for his first visit to the Dartmouth-Hitchcock Spine Center in Lebanon, New Hampshire. He is greeted by the receptionist, given a touchscreen computer, and asked to use the computer to answer a set of important questions about his health before seeing the physician. He takes less than twenty minutes to answer questions about his back problem, functional status, expectations for treatment, and working status. When the patient finishes, he hands the computer back to the receptionist. The receptionist transfers the survey data to the reception desk computer, which has a custom-designed database application for processing and printing a *patient value compass* (PVC) in the form of a one-page summary report (see Figure 4.2). The PVC provides a balanced view of clinical and functional status, patient expectations for and

*(Continued)*

# SPECIALTY CARE CASE STUDY: DARTMOUTH-HITCHCOCK SPINE CENTER (Continued)

satisfaction with his clinical care management, as well as other data on work status and costs of care.

The PVC is used to enhance communication between the provider and patient to better meet the patient's needs. It is placed on the front of the medical record, and when the patient sees the physician for an initial assessment, they together review the PVC, which describes the health status of the patient's spine and also related areas, such as bodily pain, physical health, mental health, and social role performance (such as capacity to go to work or to engage in normal activities around the house), compared to that of an average person of his or her age and sex.

The sample PVC in Figure 4.2 shows not only that the patient is suffering from acute back pain, but also that he has an extreme sleeping problem, may be suffering from depression, has been unable to work at his job for three weeks, and has had chronic back pain for more than three years. The patient and physician discuss these results, generate additional data through history taking and a physical examination, and then together develop a care plan based on the patient's preferences and health needs.

On each subsequent visit to the Spine Center during the next two months, the patient uses the touchscreen computer to record current health status; this updates the changes in health outcomes including back pain, physical functioning, and mental health. After six months the patient is back on the job, is free from depression, and has only slightly more pain than the average adult his age.[1]

## Other Facts About the Spine Center Information Environment

Here are further features of data flow and utilization within the Spine Center:

- The Spine Center uses a *data wall* to display important indicators of clinical outcomes, patient satisfaction, and business performance. (A data wall displays key measures for use by the clinical team; these measures show current performance and trends over time.) The various data displays create a *story* about practice performance, which can be viewed by the entire practice staff.
- The Spine Center views statistical process control charts and measures of processes and outcomes as essential keys to management and improvement.
- The Spine Center creates an outcomes-based annual report and uses it as a key document during the center's all-staff annual retreat, where staff review past improvements and set up small teams to work on needed improvements for the coming year.
- The Spine Center is the lead organization for a $24 million, thirteen-site, National Institutes of Health–sponsored, randomized clinical trial on the value of spine surgery for the three most common diagnoses for which spine surgery is performed.
- Many patients are delighted with the care they receive, but the Spine Center still has important improvements to make because caregivers who embrace modern improvement continuously assess and refine processes to better meet patient needs and to remove all forms of waste.
- The Spine Center has embraced the IOM's call for making quality data transparent and posts its outcomes, quality, and cost data on the Dartmouth-Hitchcock Medical Center Web site www.dhmc.org/qualityreports.

FIGURE 4.2   Patient Value Compass for a Typical Spine Patient.

Patient:
Patient A-Number: _ _ _ _ _ _ _ _ _
Date of Birth:
Visit Type: Initial visit
Clinician: Thom Walsh, PT

DHMC          10/10/01

## Initial Visit Summary

Age: 20
Gender: male
Race: white
Weight: 190
Height: 5'11"

### HISTORY

Current Problem Areas: shoulder, neck, middle back, lower back, and knee
Had Spine-Related Problems for: more than three years
Most Recent Episode Began: 9/4/01
Previous Providers: none of the listed care providers
Previous Treatments: medication
Daily Physical Requirements Prior to Problems: moderately strenuous
Reason for Visit: for a second opinion and because another doctor recommended it

### FUNCTIONAL STATUS

**Pain and Daily Activities**

*Activity: Impact of pain*
Dressing:   2 - slight
Lifting:    2 - slight
Walking:    5 - severe
Sitting:    5 - severe
Standing:   5 - severe
Sleeping:   6 - extreme
Social life: 4 - substantial
Traveling:  3 - moderate
Sex life:   3 - moderate
*Oswestry Disability Index (0-100)*
ODI:  42

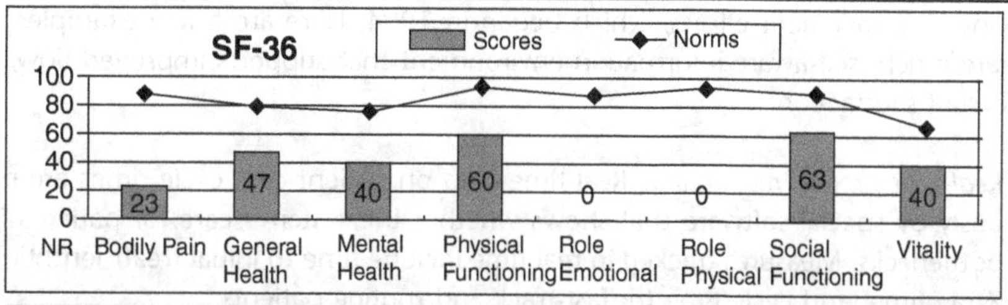

**SF-36** — Scores / Norms

NR / Bodily Pain 23 / General Health 47 / Mental Health 40 / Physical Functioning 60 / Role Emotional 0 / Role Physical 0 / Social Functioning 63 / Vitality 40

**Work Status:** on leave of absence (not due to ill health)
Hours/Week Before: 40 or more
Hours/Week Now: does not apply
Stopped Work: 9/16/01
Back to Work:
Date Back:

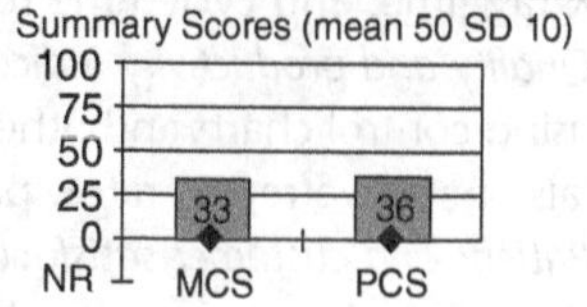

Summary Scores (mean 50 SD 10)
NR / MCS 33 / PCS 36

### CLINICAL STATUS

Comorbidities: depression and back pain

**Smoking:** never smoked
Duration: no response
Frequency: no response
**Symptoms:**

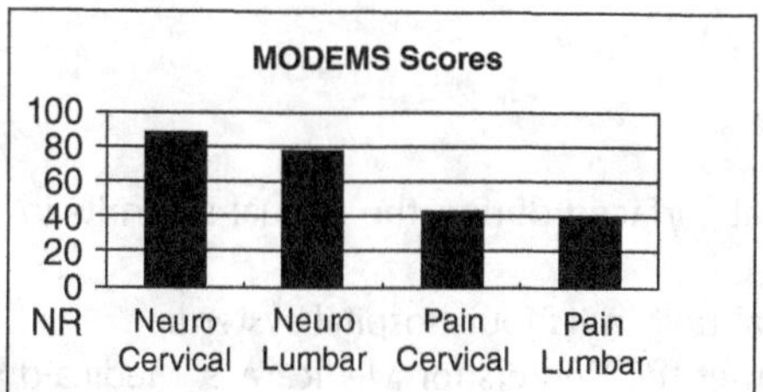

**MODEMS Scores**
NR / Neuro Cervical / Neuro Lumbar / Pain Cervical / Pain Lumbar

**Medications:**
Current medications over-the-counter

Frequence in past week not at all
Effect of meds: no response

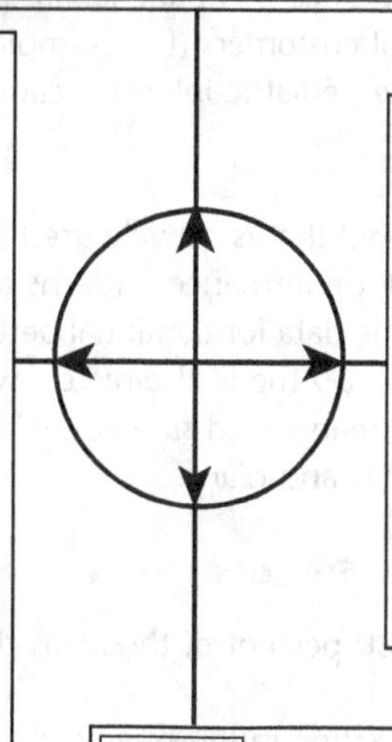

### EXPECTATIONS

**Expect from treatment:**

Symptom Relief: not sure
More Activities: not sure
Sleep Better: probably yes
Return to Job: not sure
Exercise and Recreation: not sure

**Satisfaction:**

If rest of life with
current symptoms: somewhat dissatisfied

### COSTS

**Work Lost**
Missed: 3 weeks

**Financial Assistance:**
Social Security: (not applicable)
Disability: (not applicable)
Worker's Compensation: (not applicable)

**Provider Signature:**

*Note:* The patient's value compass provides a balanced view of clinical and functional status, patient expectations, and satisfaction with the clinical care management and other data on the patient related to work status and costs of care.

# OVERLOOK HOSPITAL EMERGENCY
# DEPARTMENT CASE STUDY

We have a culture of change right here that goes back many years to our first work with the reduction of thrombolytic cycle time. The ED [Emergency Department] moved to understanding how to use industrial quality improvement methods and microsystems thinking to be safer, more reliable, and better able to meet customer needs and expectations.

—James Espinosa, former ED medical director

## A Glimpse at the Uses of Data, Real-Time Flow Monitoring, and More

The Emergency Department of Overlook Hospital in Summit, New Jersey, has made data a critical part of its continuous improvement efforts, which began in 1994. Here are a few examples of the ways the ED uses data to create a rich, self-aware information environment that supports improved flow, quality, productivity, and patient and staff satisfaction:

- *Real-time process monitoring.* Real-time data on patient care cycle times are monitored and displayed continuously by special software that shows whether the system's care for patients is flowing well or is experiencing bottlenecks. Measures tracked in real time include time to initial treatment, time to transfer to an inpatient unit, X-ray time, and cycle time for fast-track and routine patients.
- *Quality and productivity indicator tracking.* A system of process and outcome metrics is compiled and displayed using control charts and other graphical displays. Process indicators monitor trends in many areas, such as X-ray false-negative report rates, patient fall rates, and other indicators of growth and safety.
- *Patient and customer satisfaction tracking.* The Overlook ED uses several formats to gain knowledge of its customers. It uses a national comparative database on patient satisfaction, as well as locally developed customer satisfaction surveys for key internal customers (for example, residents in training and ED staff) and for peer microsystems (for example, the pediatric intensive care unit, radiology area, and emergency medical technician [EMT] squads).

These *data streams* create an information pool that is actively used in this ED microsystem (minute by minute, hourly, daily, weekly, and annually) to analyze performance patterns and to spot flaws that require action. Two regularly scheduled forums in which staff use the data for continual betterment are: (1) the dynamic and energetic monthly microsystem meetings chaired by the ED medical director, which are freewheeling exchanges of data, dialogue, and ideas; and (2) full-day annual retreats called *summits,* which look back to review progress and problems and also look forward to establish priorities and plans.

## Other Facts About the Overlook ED's Success

- The Overlook ED implemented more than 80 percent of the ideas that surfaced during the annual summits in the past several years.
- The Overlook ED has the highest staff satisfaction rating of any clinical unit in its four-hospital system.
- The Overlook ED has been recognized nationally. For example, it has met the Centers for Medicare & Medicaid Services (CMS) best-practice standards for *time to thrombolytics,* the evidence-based standard of care for acute myocardial infarction patients to receive the first dose of thrombolytics, and it has received the American Hospital Association's Quality Quest Award.
- The Overlook ED served as an important source of best-practice change concepts that the Institute for Healthcare Improvement has promoted in various programs and in its Breakthrough Collaborative, which is a national learning program to facilitate best practice adaptation in clinical practice.

# INTERMOUNTAIN HEALTH CARE SHOCK TRAUMA UNIT CASE STUDY

The data system allows us to monitor the patient remotely and share information at any time in real time. I get to see and use data and information to help me take better care of the patient.

—A STRICU clinician

## The Wired Patient and Real-Time Monitoring and Management

At the Shock Trauma Intensive Care Unit (STRICU) of Intermountain Health Care (IHC) in Salt Lake City, Utah, the data system is built around the patient and the clinical care team, and it is used every minute of every day with every patient. The injured patient is *wired* so staff can monitor clinical parameters, such as vital signs, intake and output, blood gases and infusions, in real time. Each room has a bedside computer for entering all relevant information into the patient's electronic medical record (EMR). Every day starts with formal, interdisciplinary rounds, which take two or more hours and involve reviewing and planning care for the eight to twelve patients who are in the unit at any one time. During rounds the patient's clinical team members (intensivist, nurse, technician, medical resident, primary physician, respiratory therapist, social worker, and family) review all aspects of the patient's status, with the assistance of the EMR projected on a large screen.

Using these data and a discussion of alternatives, the team adjusts the care plan and then tracks the impact of the changes on the patient's clinical parameters such as blood pressure and respiratory rate. Despite the complexity of each patient's condition, the information technology environment makes it possible for staff to complete shift reports in ten minutes. Physicians can dial into the information system from home to monitor the patient remotely at any time of the day or night and can communicate with everyone on the care team at any time, from any place. Current data, based on the local epidemiological profile, are available on the most common types of nosocomial infections, and decision support is built into the information system to guide cost-effective selection of medications for patients who acquire infections.

Statistics that track trends over time are a way of life in the STRICU. Time-trended data on key performance indicators, such as medication error rates, protocol use rates, complication rates, and costs, are compiled and reviewed at monthly staff meetings by the unit's coordinating council and at annual all-staff retreats to monitor, manage, and improve performance.

## Other Facts About the Environment

Additional information on this intensive care unit provides a broader understanding of this high performing clinical microsystem.

- Protocols that address topics such as heparin use, prevention of deep vein thrombosis, and pain relief are developed and refined locally (by any member of the clinical team); each is typically less than one page long.
- Inflation-adjusted costs per patient day have been reduced over time.
- Safety is a primary concern; more than thirty types of errors are tracked.
- The EMR has been under development at IHC for decades, and the STRICU has a full-time staff member devoted to ongoing EMR and information system refinements.

# TIPS AND PRINCIPLES TO FOSTER A RICH INFORMATION ENVIRONMENT

The three cases just discussed give rise to a set of useful tips for leaders who are guiding microsystems, mesosystems, and macrosystems in their quests to provide great, cost-effective care with minimal delays. These tips are listed in Table 4.1.

In addition to the specific tips from the case studies, we have identified four principles concerning information, information technology, data, and performance results. These principles come from our detailed qualitative analysis of twenty high-performing clinical microsystems.[2]

## Principle 1: Design It—Provide Access to a Rich Information Environment

Information guides intelligent action. This is the primary principle among all these principles. Lack of information makes intelligent action difficult. Processes that support Principle 1 include the following:

- Design the information environment to support and inform daily work and to promote core competencies and core processes essential for care delivery.
- Establish multiple formal and informal communication channels to keep all the microsystem players (patients, families, staff) informed in a timely way.

### Table 4.1    Tips to Foster a Rich Information Environment

**Spine Center Specialty Practice**

- Use full assessment of patient's health status to match treatment plan to the patient's changing needs.
- Integrate data collection and information technology into the flow of patient care delivery.
- Use information technology to provide patients and staff with tailored health status.
- Use outcomes tracking over time to evaluate results of care for individual patients and for specific subpopulations of patients.
- Build a clinical research infrastructure on top of a rich clinical information environment that makes use of structured data collection from patients and staff.
- Use leadership, cultural patterns, and systems to make a firm foundation for technology.

**Overlook Emergency Department**

- Improve patient flow by visibly monitoring cycle times and key results in real time to promptly initiate needed actions.
- Use comparative data to stimulate improvements in clinical processes and in patient satisfaction.

**Shock Trauma Intensive Care Unit**

- Use biomedical monitoring (for patients with complex, critical problems) to provide ongoing information on the patient's status.
- Use graphical and visual data displays to connect staff to staff and staff to patients to develop optimal care plans.
- Build local epidemiological knowledge and use it to guide clinical decision making.

## Principle 2: Connect with It—Use Information to Connect Patients to Staff and Staff to Staff

The success of the clinical microsystem is contingent upon the interactions between the players, including patients, clinical staff, and support staff. The players must be connected for positive and productive interactions to take place and for the right things to be done in the right way at the right time. Processes that contribute to Principle 2 are as follows:

- Give everyone the right information at the right time to do the work.
- Invest in software, hardware, and expert staff to take full advantage of information technology to support medical care delivery.
- Hear everyone's ideas. Connect these ideas to benefit the patient and to improve the actions that support servicing the patient (for example, a staff observation about the inaccessibility of handwashing soap dispensers would result in the relocation of the soap dispenser to cause higher handwashing rates and thus lower infection rates).
- Provide multiple channels for patients to interact with and to receive information from the microsystem (for example, written materials, telephone calls, e-mails, Web-based information, and shared medical appointments).

## Principle 3: Measure It—Develop Performance Goals and Linked Measures That Reflect Primary Values and Core Competencies Essential for Providing Needed Patient Services

To improve performance or to maintain performance in the desired range of excellence, it is important to set goals that are aligned with critical values, competencies, and processes and to measure goal attainment over time. Processes that promote Principle 3 are as follows:

- Work with the microsystem team to set goals and link rewards and incentives to measured results.
- Use measures to gauge performance, ideally in real time, in both upstream processes and downstream outcomes.

## Principle 4: Use It for Betterment—Measure Processes and Outcomes, Collect Feedback Data, and Redesign Continuously Based on Data

This last overarching principle completes the loop. It emphasizes using the information being gathered to provide insight to all the players, to instigate actions to improve or innovate, and to use the information streams to determine the impact of design changes. Processes that promote Principle 4 are as follows:

- Build data collection into the daily work of clinical and support staff.
- Create and use *self-coding forms* and checklists as part of workflow.
- Turn the patient into an information source so that his or her interactions with the microsystem produce critical data elements in a standard or systematic way.
- Design work processes and supporting technology to automatically throw off or generate important results that show how the system is working.

# DESIGNING INFORMATION FLOW TO SUPPORT HIGH-VALUE CARE

To grow and to thrive in today's competitive marketplace, and to meet the needs of all stakeholders (including patients and families, clinical and support staff, organizational leaders and external payers), health systems must be able to answer *Yes* to three essential questions:

1. Are we improving patient or population outcomes?
2. Are we improving system performance?
3. Are we able to grow and develop our professional staff?

As discussed in Chapter One, and as illustrated in Figure 1.12, these questions are the core imperatives of Batalden and Davidoff's Improvement Triangle. The mutually supportive goals of better clinical outcomes, better system performance, and better professional development together create a virtuous cycle that engages everyone in improving the health care system and sustains the effort at improvement.[3] Achievement of these imperatives depends, in turn, upon a rich information environment that enables evaluation, integration, and improvement of value-based activities.

But an information environment does not simply happen; it must be designed and improved over time. It must be engineered to support an organization's frontline care processes, so its development requires deep understanding of those very processes. Measurement and monitoring must be embedded into the workflow itself. In this section we offer several useful frameworks and metaphors that facilitate the actual design of information systems and information flow and that support delivery of high-value care. The frameworks include *feed forward and feedback*, the *patient value compass*, and the *balanced scorecard*. The metaphors are *dashboards* and *cascades*. We explore each item, and then review how they combine to promote *measuring what matters*.

## Framework 1: Feed Forward and Feedback

Figure 4.3 portrays an information environment built by one microsystem to incorporate both feed forward and feedback data into its management and into its improvement of care. The general activity in feed forward processes is to collect data at an early stage of care delivery, to save this data, and to use it again at a later stage: that is, to manage and inform service delivery in a prospective manner and to do the right thing, in the right way, and in real time, for each patient. The complementary activity of feedback is to gather data about what has previously happened to a patient, or to a set of patients, and to use this information to improve care processes so *future* patients will get the right treatment in the right way, efficiently, safely, and effectively.

Both feed forward and feedback methods are commonly used in care delivery. For example, many medical practices caring for patients with hypertension have a nurse or medical assistant measure the patient's blood pressure level and *feed forward* this information to the physician, who uses it to guide decision making about appropriate treatments. In a complementary manner, many primary care practices monitor physician-specific outcomes for panels of hypertensive patients, and they offer this *feedback* to the clinicians themselves to identify successes and improvement opportunities.

The case studies presented at the beginning of this chapter offer examples of more advanced uses of feed forward data. Examples are as follows:

FIGURE 4.3   The Spine Center Design for Information Flow.

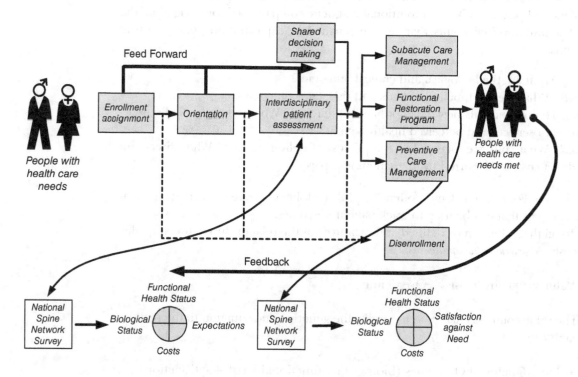

- The Spine Center uses touchscreen computers to collect information on the patient's general and disease-specific health status; this database provides a well-rounded basis for patient and clinician to engage in shared decision making to best match the patient's changing needs with the preferred treatment plan.
- The Overlook ED uses cycle time monitoring to determine if and when bottlenecks are occurring in patient flow; this provides a basis for taking immediate corrective action before a slowdown degenerates into a meltdown.
- The IHC STRICU uses real-time monitoring of each patient's clinical parameters to feed forward into daily rounds; this provides full-bandwidth data to the multidisciplinary team that assures care plans match patients' level of acuity.

Each of these three clinical microsystems uses feed forward data concepts to embed timely data collection and interpretation within frontline processes of care. In addition, all three microsystems use data feedback methods (such as graphical data displays; statistical process control charts; data walls; and weekly, monthly, quarterly, and annual reports) to *aggregate up* performance measures and to use resulting information to manage and improve care. It is possible and desirable to use advanced process flow analysis methods, such as value stream mapping and other lean-thinking methods and tools, to specify the flow of information that should accompany the flow of health care service delivery.[4]

## Framework 2: Patient Value Compass

Patient value compass (PVC) thinking can be used to determine whether the microsystem is providing care and services that meet patients' needs for high quality and high value. It is based on the Clinical Value Compass model designed for health care improvement.[5,6,7]

The PVC was designed to provide a balanced view of outcomes (such as health status, patient satisfaction, and patient care costs) for an individual patient or a defined population of patients. Like a conventional magnetic compass used for navigation, the PVC has four cardinal points that can be pursued in exploring answers to critical questions:

- *West:* What are the biological and clinical outcomes?
- *North:* What are the functional status and risk status outcomes?
- *East:* How do patients view the goodness of their care? What is their level of satisfaction with services and perceived health benefit?
- *South:* What costs are incurred in the process of delivering care? What direct and indirect costs are incurred by the patient and payer?

Chapter Four Action Guide offers helpful worksheets to create a useful patient value compass that can be used to track patient outcomes.

Recall that value can be defined and measured as the relationship between quality and costs. A *generic value equation* is:

Value = Quality/Costs ... Over Time

The value compass enables us to modify the generic value equation to the realities of health care:

Value = Quality of Outcomes (biological + functional + risk + satisfaction)

as well as Quality of the Process of Care (evidence-based care

+ patient experiences while receiving care)

Costs = Costs to Patient and/or Payer (medical costs + social costs)

... Over the relevant span of time for a patient or a population of patients

The PVC framework can be adapted to virtually any population of patients, including outpatients, inpatients, home health clients, and community residents.[8] The model assumes patient outcomes such as health status, satisfaction, and costs evolve over time and through illness episodes. For example, a person may be in generally good health at thirty-two years of age, and may then suffer a herniated disc, undergo short-term treatment for the disc problem, and regain full health. Then at age thirty-five he may reinjure his back, suffer from prolonged chronic back pain, lose his job, and become clinically depressed. At each point in the patient's illness journey it is possible, through data collection, to explore that individual's PVC for that point in time and to compare it to his PVC readings at earlier points in time. PVC data can be collected and analyzed to answer the question: *Is this patient improving or declining with respect to health status, functional status, and satisfaction with care, and at what cost?*

The patient value compass is thus dynamic. It invites a focus on *outcomes* (changes in states over time). Figure 4.4 depicts changes in value compass measures over an entire lifetime. The figure shows, for example, an infant who receives well-baby care to protect health, and then in childhood has a bloodstream infection, in adolescence breaks her arm, in middle age requires knee replacement for osteoarthritis, in later years develops

FIGURE 4.4    Value Compass Measures Over a Lifetime.

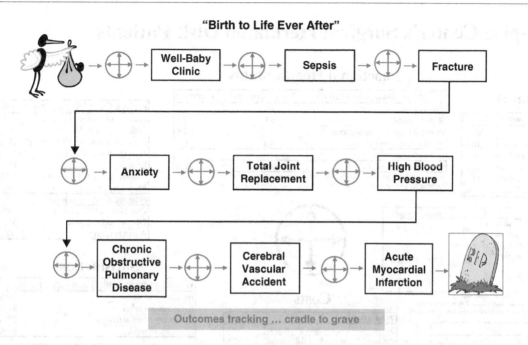

high blood pressure, and in old age succumbs to an acute myocardial infarction. After each health event it is possible to assess individual outcomes in relationship to costs using pertinent data to answer these questions: what is the clinical/biological status, functional status, risk status, and the satisfaction with care experiences, in relation to the costs for each illness episode?

The compass is also engaging: its different domains connect with the primary interests of different stakeholders. Doctors and nurses tend to focus on biological outcomes, patients and families key on functional and satisfaction results, whereas employers and purchasers fix their gaze on health care costs and lost productivity.

The Spine Center case illustrates the use of the PVC framework to design the information environment. First, feed forward data are used at each patient visit to create an up-to-date PVC, which is placed on the front of the patient's medical record and which launches the patient-clinician interaction (see again Figure 4.2). An individualized PVC puts the clinician in an excellent position to rapidly understand the patient's health strengths and health deficits, and this enables patient and clinician together to negotiate a plan of care that best matches evidence-based medicine with the patient's own preferences and needs. Second, feedback data are used to evaluate care for distinct subpopulations seen at the Spine Center, such as patients who underwent surgery for a herniated disk, as shown in Figure 4.5.

## Framework 3: Balanced Scorecard—Can We Use Data to Measure and Improve?

The balanced scorecard, developed by Kaplan and Norton, can be used to answer the question, "Is the microsystem making progress in areas that contribute to operating excellence?" It is a powerful approach that has gained popularity during the past decade.[9,10,11,12,13,14] In contrast to the PVC, in which the patient is the unit of analysis, the balanced scorecard examines the organization or a smaller operational unit within

FIGURE 4.5    Patient Value Compass: Herniated Disk Patients.

# Spine Center's Surgical Herniated Disk Patients

## Functional Health Status

### Clinical Status

| Common Health Problems | |
|---|---|
| Comorbidities Besides Spine Condition | 57% |
| Depression | 18% |
| Frequent Headaches | 18% |
| High Blood Pressure | 14% |
| Osteoarthritis | 11% |
| Heart Disease | 5% |

| SF-36 Norm-based (mean 50 SD 10) | Initial | Follow-up | Improved |
|---|---|---|---|
| Bodily Pain | 26 | 40 | 77% |
| Role Physical | 27 | 37 | 50% |
| Physical Component Summary | 28 | 38 | 62% |
| Mental Component Summary | 43 | 51 | 58% |
| General Health | | | |
| Excellent and Very Good | 40% | 43% | 26% |

Improved for SF-36 is a difference of 5 points or greater between Follow-up and Initial
Improved for General Health is a positive change category from Initial to Follow-up

| Patient Case Mix (July '98 to Mar. '02) | |
|---|---|
| Patients (have follow-up survey) | 170 |
| Follow-up rate (N=370) | 46% |
| Average follow-up (SD) days | 121 (47) |
| Average Age (SD) years | 44 (12) |
| Female | 42% |
| Chronic greater three years | 35% |
| Prior surgery | 14% |
| Hospital Surgery Indicators | |
| One-Day Length of Stay | 69% |
| Discharged to Home | 91% |
| Average Charges | $7,721 |

| Symptoms | Initial | Follow-up | Improved |
|---|---|---|---|
| Oswestry Disability Index How pain has affected your ability to perform activities | 46 | 71 | 70% |
| MODEMS: Degree of suffering and bothersome | | | |
| Numbness, tingling, and/or weakness i *lower* body | 41 | 70 | 69% |
| Numbness, tingling, and/or weakness i *upper* body | 77 | 89 | 43% |

Oswestry Disability Index (ODI): reported as lower is more disability
Improved for ODI is a difference of 10 points or greater between Follow-up and Initial
Improved for MODEMS is a difference of 5 points greater between Follow-up and Initial

### Costs

| Pain at Follow-up | |
|---|---|
| Experience pain in the neck, arms, lower back, and/or legs most or all of the time | 33% |
| Medications at Follow-up | |
| Taking medication(s) | 61% |

| Work Lost | |
|---|---|
| Missed work (28 weeks average) | 54% |
| On leave from work at follow-up | 6% |
| Financial | |
| Receiving Worker's Compensation | 17% |
| Litigation: Legal action pending | 6% |

### Satisfaction

| Results of treatment(s) met expectations: | |
|---|---|
| for ability to sleep | 66% |
| for symptom relief | 61% |
| for ability to do activities | 55% |
| to return to work | 54% |
| Satisfaction: | |
| Satisfied with treatment(s) | 85% |
| Would choose same treatment(s) | 85% |

| Charges: One year episode spine specific ICD-9 codes | | | | | |
|---|---|---|---|---|---|
| Spine Center | | Outpatient | | Inpatient | |
| Professional | $48,481 | Diagnostic Radiology | $63,498 | Surgical | $1,525,132 |
| Physical Therapist | $71,032 | Neurosurgery | $158,411 | Inpatient | $2,810,156 |
| | | Orthopaedics | $160,987 | Other | $737,737 |
| | | Pain Clinic | $34,769 | | |
| | | Office, urgent, other | $32,918 | | |
| Total | $119,513 | | $450,583 | | $5,073,025 | $5,643,121 |

Median per patient $13,330
Average $15,995 (SD $10,818)
Range $169 to $74,339

the organization. Just as the PVC can work at multiple levels (the individual patient or a discrete subpopulation), the balanced scorecard can work at the level of the clinical microsystem, mesosystem, or macrosystem.

The balanced scorecard is designed to provide a well-rounded view, specifying and assessing an organization's strategic progress from four critical perspectives: learning and growth, core processes, customer viewpoint, and financial results. The scorecard can be used to answer fundamental questions such as these:

- Are we learning and growing in business-critical areas?
- How are our core processes performing?
- How do we look in the eyes of our customers?
- Are we managing costs and making margins?

The *Strategic Performance Balanced Scorecard* worksheet in Chapter Four Action Guide enables working through the critical perspectives in knowing how the microsystem is performing using a balanced scorecard framework. The balanced scorecard approach can be adapted to virtually any type of organization, including a manufacturing plant, a service enterprise, or a health care system. Balanced scorecards offer a simple yet elegant way to link strategy and vision with the following:

- Objectives for strategic progress
- Measures of objectives
- Target values for measures
- Initiatives to improve and to innovate

Other positive features of the balanced scorecard framework are its capacity (1) to align different parts of a system toward common goals, (2) to deploy high-level themes to ground-level operating units that directly serve the patient or customer, and (3) to establish succinct methods for communicating results and for holding operating units accountable.

The scorecard (like a dashboard) is dynamic. It can depict a *virtuous cycle,* whereby innovation and learning produce better key processes and products, which in turn meet customer needs and expectations, which generate growth and stronger financial performance, which support further innovation and learning. The scorecard is also strategic and operational; it reflects the organization's overall strategy and its deployment to different operating units across the enterprise. The scorecard is tactical and practical. A well-designed scorecard can summarize overall strategic themes, can specify metrics and target values related to these themes, and can identify who will take what actions to achieve measured goals. Finally, the scorecard meets the requirements for successful execution in real-world organizations by linking strategy with operations and with people in a transparent and measurable way.[15]

Figure 4.6 shows a balanced scorecard for the Spine Center. This microsystem examines its scorecard at annual retreats, reviews its progress as revealed by measured results, and then sharpens its strategic focus for the upcoming year through analysis of improvement imperatives. The Spine Center's balanced scorecard emphasizes top-priority objectives in each of four dimensions. Participants recognize, for example, that the Spine Center had yet to meet its goal of inviting 80 percent of patients to view a shared decision-making video. Timely patient access is also targeted for improvement, and this is associated with the financial measure of physicians' clinic utilization time.

## Comparing the Compass and the Scorecard

The patient value compass was developed by clinicians and health services researchers seeking to measure and improve patient outcomes.[5,6,7] The scorecard was formulated by business school faculty and consultants attempting to measure and improve business performance.[9,10,11,12,13,14] As summarized in Table 4.2, the distinguishing features of these two instruments suggest complementary and mutually supportive functions. Although both models provide powerful information on whether or not strategic intent is being transformed into operating reality, each directs the microsystem's attention to different questions and activities, and each permits assessment within different units of analysis and levels of aggregation.

Together, the compass and the scorecard provide powerful information about whether the system's strategic intent is being transformed into operating reality. These models are especially useful when integrated with the feed forward and feedback framework discussed earlier in this chapter. Two additional measurement metaphors, dashboards and cascades, serve to combine the overlapping utilities of compass and

**FIGURE 4.6    Balanced Scorecard: Spine Center Business Unit.**

# Spine Center's Scorecard

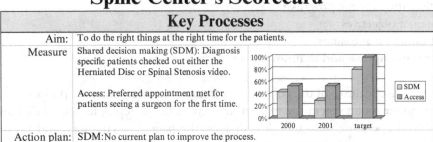

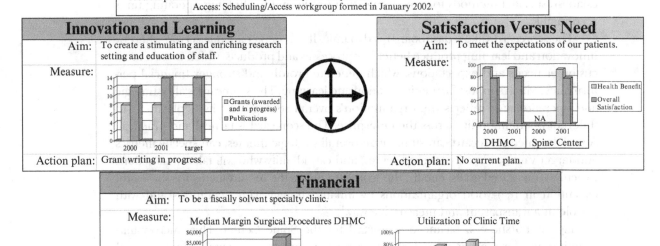

*Note:* The Spine Center examines its scorecard at its annual retreats to review progress based on measured results and to sharpen its strategic focus for the upcoming year based on an analysis of improvement imperatives.

scorecard and to foster alignment of strategic and operational priorities from macro-system planning to microsystem implementation of care.

## The Dashboard Metaphor

Consider the following thought experiment:

> Imagine you are a competent pilot flying a reliable airplane. You look at your air-craft's dashboard and at a glance you can read your gauges and dials to check on airspeed, altitude, orientation, heading, fuel level, and more. You can monitor your flight path versus flight plan, and can assess electrical systems and engine tempera-ture to ensure everything is in a safe performance zone. If a core system malfunctions, you will be warned by alarms and flashing lights. You are confident you will land safely at your desired destination.

Table 4.2    Some Distinguishing Characteristics of the Value Compass and the Balanced Scorecard

| Topic | Value Compass | Balanced Scorecard |
|-------|---------------|--------------------|
| Question | Is our health care system providing high-quality, high-value care to patients and populations? | Is our health care business producing results needed to thrive in a competitive environment? |
| Dimensions | Biological, health risk, functional, satisfaction, costs | Learning and innovation, core processes, customer satisfaction, finance and growth |
| Unit of Analysis | The patient (can be aggregated up to form a population) | The business unit (can be aggregated up to form an organization) |
| Levels of Aggregation | Patient, physician, microsystem, mesosystem, macrosystem, community, region | Microsystem, mesosystem, macrosystem, whole enterprise |
| Special Features | Can be used to (1) clarify and quantify the aims of a health system, (2) measure the value of what is produced, and (3) represent the main interests of different stakeholders | Can be used to (1) convert strategy into measurable operational goals, into current data values relative to goals, and into actions to take to reach goals; (2) promote accountability throughout the organization; (3) illustrate leadership's theory about what must be done to grow and thrive in a challenging climate |

Now imagine you are flying this same plane, but it is night, gale winds are blowing, snow is falling, and visibility is poor. You must land in a small airstrip that is nestled between two mountains . . . and suddenly, your dashboard goes dark. All your usual gauges are inaccessible. How confident are you now of finding your airport and landing safely?

The dashboard metaphor invites us to consider what vital information we need in real time to do our work well and to safely and efficiently perform all activities related to clinical care and system support. Unlike airplane pilots, most health care professionals (and health systems of all sizes) have never had a working dashboard, and they may find themselves flying blind all too often. A good health care system needs to manage many critical processes simultaneously for the following reasons: to provide care for patients, to manage the health of populations, to get an early warning of impending problems, and to run the system in a manner that optimizes safety, patient outcomes, system performance, and staff vitality.

Frontline dashboards can enable clinical microsystems to provide safe, timely, effective, efficient, equitable, and patient-centered care. Dashboards allow us to capture information that matters most about patients and organizational settings and to display this information in a manner that stimulates timely, responsive action. Clinical microsystems (such as primary care practices, emergency departments, neonatal intensive care units, inpatient care units, or spine centers) can build their own dashboards from combining the value compass and balanced scorecard frameworks.[16]

## Using the Cascades Metaphor to Measure at Different Levels of a System

Leaders of large and small health care organizations seek not only to transform care within the system, but also to measure this transformation in a manner that is both efficient and effective. Strategic and operating plans are linked to system-level *big dot* measures of success, such as quality, safety, value, innovation, core processes, customer satisfaction, and financial strength. This linking must occur at all levels of the organization and must include line-of-sight measures that *cascade* down from the top of the organization to frontline units where care is actually delivered and patients receive the benefits of treatment. Nolan summarizes the execution of cascading metrics in a 2007 white paper published by the Institute for Healthcare Improvement.[17]

Consider a macrosystem-level measure like health care costs per person or adverse events per 1,000 patients served, as shown in Figure 4.7. It is possible to disaggregate big dot measures at this organizational level to view performance at the meso and then the *little dot* microsystem levels that show the value of the measure at the level of the frontline clinical microsystem. We can envision cascading metrics that extend from the top of the organization downward and from the bottom of the organization upward. All these metrics capture the same priorities (indeed, the same performance) in vessels of different size and utility, depending on the needs of leadership, clinicians, and staff at different organizational levels. Macrosystem *big dot* metrics are pools formed by little dots produced in multiple contributing microsystems.

The aim of cascading metrics, when applied to clinical microsystems, is to connect these dots and to develop organizational alignment through common line-of-sight measures. (See Figure 4.8 for an example of how cascading metrics help connect the dots). These cascades are built through thoughtful identification of activities within the microsystem that contribute to frontline value and system-wide aims. Of course, such construction assumes micro and macrosystem participants have determined together which activities and outcomes count as valuable and what system features and products matter most to patients, families, clinicians and staff, macrosystem leaders, and external customers. The *Measure What Matters* worksheet, discussed next, offers an integration of the frameworks and metaphors we have previously reviewed and helps tie organizational and local priorities to specific cascading metrics.

**FIGURE 4.7    Cascading Metrics Using Adverse Event Rates as an Example.**

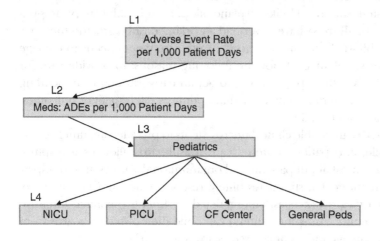

## FIGURE 4.8  Cascading Metrics.

| Microsystem |
|---|
| • Improve parent satisfaction above 80 percent in neonatal intensive care unit. |
| • Reduce staff turnover below 11 percent. |
| • Improve staff and physician satisfaction. |
| • Reduce neonatal intensive care unit hospital-acquired infections by 30 percent. |
| • Achieve NICU operating margin of 3 percent. |
| • Achieve labor expense per adjusted discharge at 40 percent. |
| • Increase infant deliveries. |

| Mesosystem |
|---|
| • Improve patient satisfaction to the 75th percentile. |
| • Improve employee and physician satisfaction. |
| • Reduce annual employee turnover. |
| • Reduce hospital-acquired infections in the Children's Hospital by 30 percent. |
| • Achieve supply expense per adjusted discharge at 40 percent. |
| • Achieve labor expense per adjusted discharge at 40 percent. |
| • Increase annual admissions. |

| Macrosystem |
|---|
| • Improve patient satisfaction to the 75 th percentile. |
| • Reduce employee turnover to 11 percent. |
| • Decrease mortality index to .8. |
| • Increase Inpatient admissions to 7 percent. |
| • Increase outpatient visits to 7 percent. |
| • Maintain supply and labor expense per adjusted discharges at 40 percent. |

### Measure What Matters Worksheet

The *Measure What Matters* worksheet (MWM) was designed by Godfrey and Nelson to identify key measures for managing and improving clinical unit performance, both in real time (now) and over time (future). The MWM, uses value compass and balanced scorecard methods to create unit-specific dashboards that relate to organization-wide measurement cascades. The MWM worksheet is available at www.clinicalmicrosystems. org. It provides a road map for creating a useful microsystem dashboard. We recommend the following steps for using the MWM worksheet:

1. Build a value compass for the microsystem or clinical unit to measure clinical status, functional status, risk status, satisfaction, and cost (see Chapter Four Action Guide).
2. Construct a balanced scorecard for the microsystem or clinical unit to measure strategic and operational progress on innovation and learning, key processes, customer satisfaction, finance, and growth (see Chapter Four Action Guide).
3. Determine the organization's strategic measures and illustrate how these cascade through the organization from the macro to the meso to the micro-level of the enterprise (see Chapter Four Action Guide).
4. Design a dashboard using selected and time-critical value compass and balanced scorecard measures to monitor progress and performance (see Chapter Four Action Guide).
5. Initiate use of the dashboard by plotting data points. Use run charts or control charts to demonstrate trends and illustrate key results in separate tables or figures.

To enhance the utility of this instrument and to support the development of rich information environments more generally, we also advise that users give special priority to *timeliness* and *attentiveness* of displayed data. To the extent that these displays represent *real-time* results, they will more effectively guide actions that are intelligent and timely. Similarly, when dashboards are highly visible in work stations and elsewhere, and when they are frequently referenced in brief huddles, in team meetings, in all-staff meetings and in annual retreats, they become an integral part of the microsystem and can more effectively influence the quality of frontline performance.

---

## CASE EXAMPLE: USING THE *MEASURE WHAT MATTERS* WORKSHEET IN NEONATAL INTENSIVE CARE UNITS

The Vermont Oxford Network collaborative (VON NIC/Q 2007) started with the bold aim of using measures embedded in the *Measure What Matters* (MWM)[18] worksheets to improve performance and enhance leadership. During an 18-month action-learning period, dozens of neonatal intensive care unit (NICU) teams learned how to adapt these ideas (about compasses, scorecards, dashboards, and cascades) to their own microsystems. In the final phase of this collaboration, the VON NIC/Q 2007 participants were introduced to the MWM and were shown an illustrative mock-up of the Measures for Improvement *data wall* shown in Figure 4.9. Participants were invited to use the instrument to integrate various domains of their prior work, which had heretofore been separated or neglected. For example, patient satisfaction feedback data, staff satisfaction feedback data, infection rate trends, and cost per discharge were often disconnected fragments of data that were never considered in context or over time or linked to improvement work at different levels of the system.

More than fifty NICUs met the challenge, constructed data walls, and shared them at the final session of the collaborative. There were many excellent examples of how different intensive care nurseries took these principles and methods, made them their own, and began using them to monitor, to manage, to evaluate, and to improve performance.

---

## CONCLUSION

We have reviewed cases, principles, and frameworks, which together demonstrate the value (and the feasibility) of constructing rich information environments in clinical microsystems. The purpose of measurement is not merely to score and tabulate performance retrospectively, but (much more importantly) to guide intelligent action prospectively.[19] High performing clinical microsystems embed data collection and interpretation into the work of patient care itself, and these data are used to support such diverse activities as monitoring, evaluating, managing, reporting, and improving core clinical and supporting processes.

Measuring what matters is a dynamic process because *what* matters will depend upon who requests, reviews, and responds to specific measures. Clinicians, support staff, administrative leaders, and patients and families are all empowered by information to identify emerging needs, to maintain successes, and to improve upon care processes that are not yet successful. Intelligent action depends upon intelligent design of information environments, and such design is essential for achieving the highest health care value.

FIGURE 4.9   Sample Layout: Measures for Improvement.

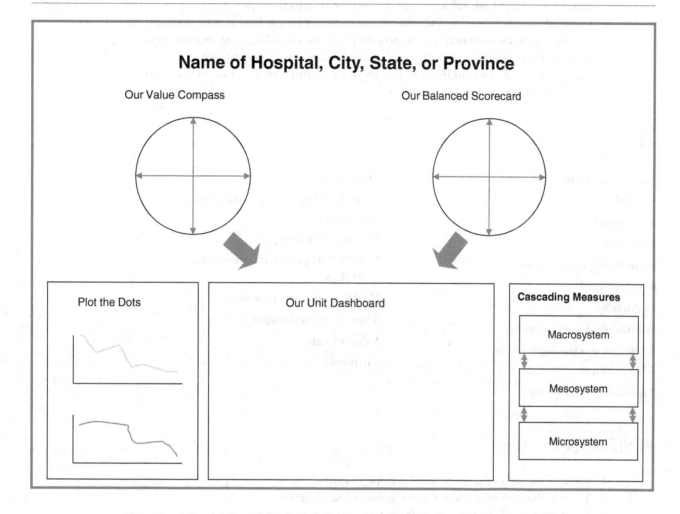

## SUMMARY

- In high functioning health care systems, the measurement-supported activities of monitoring, evaluating, improving, managing, and reporting are tightly linked and designed to cascade from one level of the organization to the next.
- Principles for using measures and building rich information environments include the following:
  - Design it—provide access to a rich information environment.
  - Connect with it—use information to connect patients to staff and staff to staff.
  - Measure it—develop performance goals and linked measures that reflect core values and core competencies.
  - Use it for betterment—measure processes and outcomes, collect feedback data, and redesign continuously based on data.
- Develop feed forward and feedback information flows to support doing the right thing in the right way at the right time and to provide a platform for evaluating, learning, improving, and innovating.

- Use value compass and balanced scorecard frameworks to help support the measured delivery of high value care and of efficient, effective operating performance.
- Use dashboards to enable the clinical microsystem to see how it is performing on key areas in as close to real time as possible, and use cascading measures to align the organization's strategic priorities at the micro, meso, and macro-levels.
- The purpose of measurement is not to score performance retrospectively but to guide intelligent action prospectively.

## KEY TERMS

Big dot measures

Cascade

Dashboard

Data wall

Generic value equation

Feed forward

Feedback

Information environment

Little dot microsystem levels

Measurement

Measuring what matters

Outcomes

Patient and customer satisfaction
  tracking

Patient value compass

Quality and productivity indicator
  tracking

Real-time process monitoring

Time to thrombolytics

Value of care

Virtuous cycle

## REVIEW QUESTIONS

1. What is the unit of analysis for the value compass?
2. What is the unit of analysis for the balanced scorecard?
3. What are four of the ten principles for designing rich information environments you could begin to implement?
4. What is the feedback and feed forward system for the Spine Center and the Overlook ED?

## DISCUSSION QUESTIONS

1. Think about the microsystem you are studying. What have you identified in data and information that can contribute to a rich information environment? What might you do to further enhance the information environment?
2. Have you found any evidence of feed forward–feedback systems in your clinical microsystem or between clinical microsystems? How might you start with a simple process to begin a feed forward-feedback system?
3. How might you approach microsystem leadership with the idea of enriching the microsystem data and information environment?
4. Discuss the *ideal* rich information environment for the microsystem you are studying. What might be the barriers? What aspects of the microsystem could advance the design and execution of the rich information environment?

# REFERENCES

1. Weinstein, J., Brown, P. W., Hanscom, B., Walsh, T., & Nelson, E. C. Designing an ambulatory clinical practice for outcomes improvement. *Quality Management in Health Care*, 2000, *8*(2), 1–20.

2. Nelson et al. Microsystems in health care: Part 1. Learning from high-performing front-line clinical units. *Joint Commission Journal on Quality Improvement*, 2002, *28*(9), 472–493.

3. Batalden, P., & Davidoff, F. What is quality improvement and how can it transform health care? *Quality and Safety in Health Care*, 2007, *16*, 2–3.

4. Rother, J., & Shook, J. *Learning to see.* Brookline, MA: Lean Enterprise Institute, 1998.

5. Splaine, M., Batalden, P., Nelson, E., Plume, S. K., & Wasson, J. H. Looking at care from the inside out: A conceptual approach to geriatric care. *Journal of Ambulatory Care Management*, 1998, *21*(3), 1–9.

6. Nelson, E. C., Batalden, P. B., & Ryer, J. C. *Clinical improvement action guide.* Oakbrook Terrace, IL: Joint Commission on Accreditation of Healthcare Organizations, 1998.

7. Nelson et al. Improving health care, part 1: The clinical value compass. *Joint Commission Journal on Quality Improvement*, 1996, *22*(4), 243–258.

8. Speroff, T., Miles, P., & Matthews, B. Improving health care: Part 5. Applying the Dartmouth clinical improvement model to community health. *Joint Commission Journal on Quality Improvement*, 1998, *24*(12), 679–703.

9. Griffith, J., Alexander, J. A., & Jelinek, R. C. Measuring comparative hospital performance. *Journal of Healthcare Management*, 2002, *47*(1), 41–57.

10. Kaplan, N., & David, P. *Strategy maps: Converting intangible assets into tangible outcomes.* Boston: Harvard Business Review, 2004.

11. Kaplan, R., & Norton, D. *The strategy focused organization.* Boston: Harvard Business School Press, 2001.

12. Kaplan, R. S., & Norton, D. P. The balanced scorecard—measures that drive performance. *Harvard Business Review*, 1992, January-February, 71–79.

13. Kaplan, R. S. & Norton, D. P. Putting the balanced scorecard to work. *Harvard Business Review*, 1993, September–October, 134–147.

14. Oliveira, J. The balanced scorecard: An integrative approach to performance evaluation. *Healthcare Financial Management*, 2001, *55*(5), 42–46.

15. Bossidy, L., & Charan, R. *Execution: The discipline of getting things done.* New York: Crown Business, 2002.

16. Nelson et al. Report cards or instrument panels: Who needs what? *Joint Commission Journal on Quality Improvement*, 1995, *21*(4), 155–166.

17. Nolan, T. *Execution of strategic improvement initiatives to produce system-level results. The innovation series white paper.* Cambridge, MA: Institute for Healthcare Improvement, 2007.

18. Horbar, J. D. The Vermont Oxford network: Evidence-based quality improvement for neonatology. *Pediatrics*, 1999, *103*(1 Supplement E), 350–359.

19. Wheeler, D. J. *Understanding variation: The key to managing chaos.* (2nd ed.) Knoxville, TN: SPC Press, 2000.

Chapter Four Action Guide provides tools and methods to design measurement and monitor microsystem performance to assess if desired goals and outcomes in patient care are being achieved for the patient or population being cared for and from the perspective of the overall performance of the clinical microsystem. In addition, a worksheet is included to help link performance measures from the clinical microsystem to the mesosystem and macrosystem to understand the connections of specific measures throughout the organization.

Tools that support measuring and monitoring, such as the patient value compass, the balanced scorecard sheet, the measure what matters worksheet, and data walls, are included in this chapter. As discussed within the chapter, a balanced approach that considers multiple aspects, measures, and stakeholders for the patient and population and for the microsystem and organization has high utility in measuring and monitoring performance.

## PATIENT VALUE COMPASS

The Patient Value Compass (PVC) (unit of analysis is the patient or population) is used to determine whether the microsystem is providing care and services that meet patient needs for high quality and high value. The PVC is designed to provide a balanced view of outcomes, which include health status, patient satisfaction, and patient care costs for an individual patient or for a defined population of patients.

Results of the interaction between patient, staff, and clinical and support processes produce patterns of critical results (such as biological status, functional status, risk status, patient perceptions of goodness of care, and costs associated with care) that combine to represent the value of care.

The PVC presents a balanced approach to measure and display value in health care. The worksheets that follow guide the process of creating a PVC for a patient or population of interest.

Figure AG4.1 (side A of the worksheet) provides guidance for completing the PVC steps starting with clearly identifying the selected population to study along with an aim of improvement for this selected population. Tips are listed on the left-hand column to help an interdisciplinary group work through identifying different measures and outcomes for the selected population. Figure AG4.2 (side B of the worksheet) provides space to define the operational definitions of the selected outcome measures on side

## FIGURE AG4.1   Clinical Value Compass Side A.

**Clinical Value Compass Worksheet, Side A**

OUTCOMES ➔ Select a population:_____
(specify patient population)

_____

AIM ➔ What's the general aim? Given our wish to limit or reduce the illness burden for this type of patient, what are the desired results?

_____

_____

TIPS: Path Forward ➔

Worksheet purpose: To identify measures of outcomes or costs that contribute most to the value of care.

1. Select a clinically significant population.
2. Assemble small interdisciplinary team.
3. Use brainstorming or nominal group technique to generate "long" list of measures.
4. Start with west (clinical) on the compass and go clockwise around the compass.
5. Use multi-voting to identify "short" list of four to twelve key measures of outcomes and costs.
6. Determine what data are needed versus what data can be obtained in real time at affordable cost.
7. Use Side B of worksheet to record names and definitions of selected measures of value.

**Functional**
- Physical function          _____
- Mental health              _____
- Social or role             _____
- Other (health risk)        _____
-                            _____

**Clinical**
_____ - Morbidity
_____ - Morbidity
_____ - Complications
_____ -
_____ -

**Satisfaction**
- Health Care Delivery       _____
- Perceived Health Benefit   _____
-                            _____
-                            _____

**Costs**
- Direct medical             _____
- Indirect                   _____
-                            _____
-                            _____

A. The importance of defining the conceptual and operational measures is listed on the left-hand side of the page.

## BALANCED SCORECARD

The Balanced Scorecard (unit of analysis is the microsystem/unit of care) provides measures to see if the system is meeting the members' needs while matching up with the strategic plan and larger organizational vision (see Figure AG4.3).

The four points of success measured include:

1. *Strategic learning and innovation.* To achieve our vision, how will we sustain our ability to change and improve as fast as times require? Are we learning and innovating in business critical areas?
2. *Key processes.* To satisfy customers, what key processes must we perfect? How are key processes performing?
3. *Customers' view of goodness.* To achieve our vision, how should we appear to our customers? How do we look in the eyes of our customers?

FIGURE AG4.2 Clinical Value Compass Side B.

| Clinical Value Compass Worksheet, Side B | | |
|---|---|---|

SPECIFIC OPERATIONAL DEFINITIONS ➜ for key outcome and cost measures

| TIPS: Writing Definitions ➜ | Variable name and brief conceptual definition | Source of data and operational definition |
|---|---|---|
| A *conceptual definition* is a brief statement describing a variable of interest. It should tell people **what** you want to measure and who "owns" it. | A.<br>Owner: _____ | |
| | B.<br>Owner: _____ | |
| | C.<br>Owner: _____ | |
| An *operational definition* is a clearly specified **method** for reliably sorting, classifying, or measuring a variable. It should be written as an instruction set, or protocol, that would enable two different people to measure the variable by using the same process; both people should produce the same result. The definition should explain to people **how** a variable should be measured. | D.<br>Owner: _____ | |
| | E.<br>Owner: _____ | |
| | F.<br>Owner: _____ | |
| | G.<br>Owner: _____ | |
| | H.<br>Owner: _____ | |

4. *Financial results.* To succeed financially, how should we appear to our shareholders and board? How are we doing at managing costs and making margins?

Additional examples of balanced scorecards can be found at www.clinicalmicrosystem .org.

## MEASURE WHAT MATTERS WORKSHEET

The *Measure What Matters* (MWM) worksheet provides a road map for creating your microsystem dashboard. Your measures will change over time so this dashboard is intended to be a dynamic display of current key measures at the macrosystem, meso-system, and microsystem level. The MWM worksheet demonstrates the connections between microsystem improvement and strategic enterprise-wide goals and targets. The idea is to identify a few current measures from the Value Compass and the Balanced Scorecard to track over time and to display measures of progress toward goals on the microsystem dashboard. Once measures are sustained at the goal level, new metrics can

FIGURE AG4.3   Strategic Performance Compass.

### Learning and Growth
How will we enhance our ability to change and improve?

| Objectives | Measures | Targets | Initiatives |
|---|---|---|---|
| 1. | | | |
| 2. | | | |
| 3. | | | |
| 4. | | | |

### Key Process
What key processes must we perfect?

| Objectives | Measures | Targets | Initiatives |
|---|---|---|---|
| 1. | | | |
| 2. | | | |
| 3. | | | |
| 4. | | | |

### Customers
How should we appear to our customers?

| Objectives | Measures | Targets | Initiatives |
|---|---|---|---|
| 1. | | | |
| 2. | | | |
| 3. | | | |
| 4. | | | |

### Financial
How should we appear to our board?

| Objectives | Measures | Targets | Initiatives |
|---|---|---|---|
| 1. | | | |
| 2. | | | |
| 3. | | | |
| 4. | | | |

be identified to track. Figure AG4.4 is the first page of the *Measure What Matters* worksheet and provides an overview of the process along with the path forward to begin to create a microsystem dashboard or instrument panel.

Creating a patient value compass of measures for the patient or population is the next step in the process to create a dashboard or instrument panel as seen in Figure AG4.5 (www.josseybass.com/go/nelson).

The next step is to create a balanced scorecard of measurement for the clinical microsystem performance (Figure AG4.6 www.josseybass.com/go/nelson).

When the AG4.5 and AG4.6 pages are laid side-by-side, you can see the space at the bottom of the pages to draft your dashboard or instrument panel taking key measures from the value compass and the balanced scorecard to begin to monitor performance over time.

The last page of the *Measure What Matters* worksheet is Cascading Measures: connecting performance measures from the microsystem to the mesosystem to the macrosystem (Figure AG4.7, www.josseybass.com/go/nelson). To determine what measures should be monitored, suggestions are offered to review organization annual reports, strategic plans, and senior leadership and board of directors' selected measures.

FIGURE AG4.4   Measure What Matters Page 1.

## Measure What Matters
### Clinical Value Compass
### Balanced Scorecards
### Microsystem Dashboards

**Unit Name:**_____ **Date:**_____

**Organization Name:**_____

**Aim**: Provide a clear path forward to identify key measures to track unit performance in real time *and* over time:

① Patient Outcomes (Clinical Value Compass)
② Microsystem Performance (Balanced Scorecard)
③ Microsystem Dashboard or Instrument Panel (① and ②)
④ Linkage to Organization Strategy (Cascading Measures)

**Background:**

Organized data displays provide feedback on system performance. Key measures that reflect the purpose and goals of the microsystem include population and/or subpopulation outcomes (clinical value compass) and system performance measures (balanced scorecard), both of which reflect microsystem results toward desired outcomes. The unit dashboard or instrument panel provides a method to monitor a blend of current indicators (clinical value compass and balanced scorecard) of a microsystem to provide real-time indications over time on how the unit is performing. It is important to remember the microsystem-level dashboard or instrument panel variables can change as improvements, priorities, and process measures change.

**Path Forward:**

① Create Clinical Value Compass
② Create Balanced Scorecard
③ Determine Organization's Strategic Measures
④ Create Microsystem Dashboard or Instrument Panel
⑤ Cascading Measures

## EXAMPLES OF DATA WALLS

A data wall is a clearly defined physical space where vital measures of performance can be posted. Data walls provide visual graphics of critical measures for the clinical microsystem to know if desired outcomes and performance are being achieved. The *Measure What Matters* worksheet aids clinical microsystems in building dashboards to post on data walls. The graphic displays can be handwritten and updated or produced from various electronic software programs.

Using a data wall requires the clinical microsystem members to identify who will maintain the data wall to ensure the measures are current and relevant. A data "captain" can oversee the data wall, remind staff to review it regularly, and alert staff to important changes in the data over time. Many clinical microsystems gather at the data wall monthly during all staff meetings to review performance and opportunities to continue to improve toward stated goals. Review of the data wall can provide a time to celebrate and acknowledge improvement efforts by all staff to achieve and maintain desired results while at the same time continuously reinforcing the need for improvement. Examples of *Measure What Matters* dashboards can be found at www.clinicalmicrosystem.org.

## REFERENCES

1. Kaplan, R. S., Norton, D. P. The Strategy-Focused Organization: How Balanced Scorecard Companies Thrive in the New Business Environment (Hardcover – Sep 2000).
2. Nelson, Batalden, Ryer, "Measuring Outcomes and Costs: "The Clinical Value Compass" Chapter Three, *Clinical Improvement Action Guide*, Joint Commission Resources 2001.
3. Kaplan, R. S., Norton, D. P. "Putting the Balanced Scorecard to Work" *Harvard Business Review*, September 1, 1993.
4. Kaplan, R. S., Norton, D. P. "The Balanced Scorecard: Translating Strategy into Action", Sep 1996
5. www.clinicalmicrosystem.org   Click on "tools on left hand menu, then streaming videos".
   - Measuring & Monitoring Video #2 – Value Compass Thinking
   - Measuring & Monitoring Video #3 – Balanced Scorecard Approach
   - *Both require Real Player*
6. Nelson, E. C., Edwards, W. H. Measure What Matters from NICQ 2007: Improvement in Action; Horbar, J D, Leahy, K, Handyside, J, editors. Vermont Oxford Network Burlington, VT, 2009. Published on-line at www.microsystem.org.

# STARTING THE PATIENT'S CARE IN CLINICAL MICROSYSTEMS

Marjorie M. Godfrey

Eugene C. Nelson

Paul B. Batalden

## LEARNING OBJECTIVES

- Describe and evaluate how patients enter a clinical microsystem, including the processes of gaining access in multiple ways.
- Identify and describe handoffs and transitions in care.
- Discuss the patient's orientation to the clinical microsystem and identify improvement opportunities.
- Observe the process of an initial health assessment and the consequent formation of a plan for care that matches the individual's needs, interests, and preferences.
- Explore mental models that limit or enhance relationships between clinical microsystems.

As patients enter into new relationships with clinical microsystems, several common *entry functions* serve as the foundation for subsequent and successful care. These functions are explored in detail in the present chapter. The microsystem must first assure safe and reliable access to all appropriate patients, either directly or via handoff from another clinical microsystem. Patients must then be effectively oriented to microsystem protocols, access pathways, and clinical resources, which facilitates informed partnership in brief or longer-term care. Finally, standardized assessment of patients' current health status and needs will facilitate design of a plan for care that is both patient-centered and problem-focused.

## THE ENTRY FUNCTIONS OF CLINICAL MICROSYSTEMS

Good beginnings. Every patient entry into a new clinical microsystem represents, for that person, both the *initiation* of an important healing relationship and a crucial *next step* in the lifelong journey of improving, restoring, or maintaining health. Individuals with specific health needs hope to benefit from appropriate information, advice, and treatment, and to do so in partnership with competent, compassionate, and caring health professionals. This partnership requires that patients and families are empowered to access, engage, and navigate the microsystem effectively.[1] It simultaneously requires that health professionals within that microsystem know the patient well, through reliable handoffs and sound assessments that permit design of appropriate care plans. In this context, the microsystem entry functions of patient access and transition, orientation, assessment, and care plan development are closely linked; we therefore consider them as a unit in this chapter. Together, these functions provide a necessary foundation to address specific care needs in preventive, acute, chronic, and palliative domains, topics we discuss in subsequent chapters (see also "Patient Entry and Plan of Care").

As Table 5.1 reveals, the process of patient entry into clinical microsystems involves several discrete (although overlapping) steps. Although every patient brings unique needs to the care relationship, and although every microsystem implements special processes to assess and to meet those needs, we can identify a number of common

Table 5.1 Critical Steps in the Health Care Journey

| Beginning Points | Ending Points |
|---|---|
| Patient enters the microsystem or is assigned to the microsystem. | Patient and clinicians have knowledge of each other's intent. |
| Patient is explicitly connected to a specific clinician, team, or associate. | Patient is able to meet health needs by using the following skills to leverage the microsystem:<br>• Scheduling visits, encounters, sessions<br>• Communicating with the clinician, team, or associate<br>• Reporting health status changes<br>• Obtaining needed medications and test results<br>• Exploring plan for care options |
| Patient arrives for the first visit, is admitted or is transferred to a new clinical microsystem. | Overall health risk and health status assessment completed and plan of care established to guide delivery of care to patient. |

process components. In general, clinical microsystems must assure optimal functioning in the following critical areas:

- Safe and reliable patient access to the microsystem, either directly or via handoff from another clinical microsystem
- Effective orientation of individuals to microsystem protocols, access pathways, and resources, so patients can function as informed and engaged partners
- Sound assessment of the patient's current health status, which lays the groundwork for developing an appropriate plan for care

In the present chapter we examine each of these entry functions in detail and explore essential principles, methodologies, and monitoring strategies to evaluate success.

## Access and Handoffs

In general, patients enter or gain access to a particular microsystem via one of two pathways. First, in ambulatory settings (such as doctor's office, cardiovascular rehabilitation program, or emergency department) the patient or someone acting on the patient's behalf (such as a family member or referring physician) makes contact by phone, e-mail, fax, or shows up unannounced. These are *direct* modes of entry into the microsystem to access services. Alternatively, in inpatient settings such as intensive care units, surgical suites, post-anesthesia care units, or inpatient medical units the patient is usually transferred from one setting to another by professional staff. This *transfer mode of entry*, or transition of care into the microsystem from one setting into the next, involves a handoff of information, of care responsibility, and often, quite literally, of the patient. Both *direct* and *transfer modes of access* present specific opportunities for quality improvement and safety design. Let us scrutinize these functions more closely.

### Access to Care and Services

An old aphorism suggests the good physician provides superior care by being accessible, affable, and able.[2] Indeed, good patient access is a precondition for high-quality care. As the Institute for Healthcare Improvement (IHI) has summarized in its Idealized Design of Clinical Office Practice initiative, patients depend upon clinical microsystems that "give me exactly what I want and need exactly when I want and need it."[3]

Good access not only meets the patient's need to receive desired services in a timely manner, it also promotes the following:

- *Effective care* by decreasing delays between recognition of clinical need and delivery of illness-reducing services
- *Efficient care* by improving flow of services and speed of transition from one source of care to the next, thus decreasing *backlogs* (patients waiting in queue), improving throughput, and increasing productivity
- *Improved satisfaction with care* by meeting or exceeding the expectations of patients, families, referring physicians, and third party payers
- *Improved staff morale* by enabling care providers to perform their own best work in a timely and effective manner

As we consider specific strategies to optimize access in clinical microsystems, we must recognize the increasingly diverse forms of interaction that may be appropriate for patients with diverse needs. While traditional approaches to improving access have focused largely on patient visits, modern forms of patient care must be considered more broadly as forms of patient contact. In many contexts, of course, face-to-face interaction, such as an office visit or an inpatient experience, remain essential. But in other contexts appropriate care (including information exchange, clinical assessment, and treatment) may be provided either in real time or asynchronously (with some agreed-upon time lag) via telephone, e-mail, text message, telemedicine, or any number of rapidly evolving electronic media.

### Systematically Improving Access to Care

Mark Murray and others have pioneered and popularized methods for improving access to care, with attention to system redesign.[4,5] Four fundamental activities drive this important work:

1. Shape demand
2. Match supply and demand
3. Redesign the system to increase supply
4. Do today's work today

As Murray demonstrates, access problems are delay problems, and delays result from system design features. Batalden reminds us, "Every system is perfectly designed to get the results it gets."[6] If the desired result is elimination of unwanted delays, then microsystems must commit themselves to intelligent change. This is achieved through careful self-assessment of current resources and through exploration of processes that use these resources to maximize capacity, to meet patient needs, and to avoid unnecessary costs. In general, this can be accomplished by taking the following actions:

- Analyze the current state of supply and demand for microsystem services
- Predict and manage patient demand and service supply on a daily, weekly, and monthly basis, based on review of real-time data
- Increase efficiency of operations and streamline patient flow within and between care settings

### Methods to Increase Access and Improve Flow

Figure 5.1, from *Advanced Clinic Access*,[7] a publication prepared for the Veterans Health Administration (VHA) by the Institute for Healthcare Improvement, summarizes concepts and methods that can effectively improve access to care for outpatient services. The methods reviewed in this *Access Improvement Bible* (as it is called among some health care leaders) have been successfully adapted throughout North America and Europe. The full booklet can be viewed at www.clinicalmicrosystem.org. Figure 5.1 summarizes core principles, related change concepts, and specific methods to improve access to care. Variants for primary care and specialty care are considered as well. Ten key change concepts are reviewed in the IHI and VHA report:

1. Work down the backlog
2. Reduce demand
3. Understand supply and demand
4. Reduce appointment types
5. Plan for contingencies
6. Manage the constraint

FIGURE 5.1   Change Concepts for Advanced Clinic Access.

## SHAPE DEMAND

### 1. Work Down the Backlog
➢ Gain immediate capacity.
➢ Temporarily add appointment slots.

### 2. Reduce Demand

PRIMARY CARE
➢ Maximize activity or appointments.
➢ Extend intervals for return appointments.
➢ Create alternatives to traditional face-to-face interactions.
➢ Optimize patient involvement in care.

SPECIALTY CARE
➢ Build service agreements between primary and specialty care.
➢ Extend intervals for return appointments.
➢ Reduce demand for physician visits by optimizing team roles.
➢ Discharge patients to primary care from specialty care.
➢ Create alternatives to traditional face-to-face interactions.

## MATCH SUPPLY AND DEMAND

### 3. Understand Supply and Demand

PRIMARY CARE
➢ Know your demand.
➢ Know your supply.
➢ Consider doing today's work today.
➢ Make panel size equitable based on clinical FTE.

SPECIALTY CARE
➢ Know your demand.
➢ Know your supply.
➢ Consider doing today's work today.
➢ Establish input equity for specialty clinics.

### 4. Reduce Appointment Types
➢ Use only a small number of appointment types.
➢ Standardize appointment lengths.

### 5. Plan for Contingencies
➢ Manage demand variation proactively.
➢ Develop flexible, multi-skilled staff.
➢ Anticipate unusual but expected events.

## REDESIGN THE SYSTEM TO INCREASE SUPPLY

### 6. Manage the Constraint
➢ Identify the constraint.
➢ Drive unnecessary work away from the constraint.

### 7. Optimize the Care Team
➢ Ensure all roles in practice are maximized to meet patient needs.
➢ Use standard protocols to optimize use of other providers.
➢ Separate responsibilities for phone triage, patient flow, and paper flow.

### 8. Synchronize Patient, Provider, and Information
➢ Start the first AM and PM appointments on time.
➢ Do patient registration by phone when confirming the patient appointment.
➢ Check the chart to make sure it is complete, accurate, and present at the appointment.
➢ Use health prompts to anticipate full potential of today's need.
➢ Make sure that rooming criteria include having the patient ready.

### 9. Predict and Anticipate Patient Needs at Time of Appointment
➢ Use regular "huddles" to anticipate and plan for contingencies.
➢ Communicate among care delivery team throughout the day.

### 10. Optimize Rooms and Equipment
➢ Use open rooming to maximize flexibility.
➢ Standardize supplies in exam rooms and keep stocked at all times.

7. Optimize the care team
8. Synchronize patient, provider, and information
9. Predict and anticipate patient needs at time of appointment
10. Optimize rooms and equipment

Although most published work on access improvement focuses upon ambulatory care, similar attention has been given to access issues in inpatient settings and to access across entire *episodes of care,* meaning the experience of receiving care for a health problem that requires care over time and in different locations. How, for example, can accessibility and flow be improved for patients across an entire illness experience from doctor's office, to emergency department, to surgical unit, to post-anesthesia care unit, to surgical inpatient unit, and to skilled nursing home after hospital discharge? The capability to *move* a patient from one inpatient microsystem to the next, based upon that patient's evolving health needs and clinical status requires open access in each of the next downstream units that participates in this episode of care. Substantial preplanning and coordination is required to assure seamless flow of both patient and patient information, and *complete access* includes timely presence of not only clinical staff but also whatever supporting services (diagnostic tests, consultations, and medications) may be required.

Most of the concepts and methods listed in Figure 5.1 for ambulatory care can also be adapted to inpatient care and to prolonged *episodes* of care across the larger meso-system.[8] Table 5.2 lists some specific methods used by hospitals and clinical mesosystems to improve access and flow. See also the discussion in Chapter Seven on access issues.

Reflection on these change concepts and methods reveals that specific attention to improved access can also support more comprehensive redesign of clinical microsystems and mesosystems. Readers will appreciate the general relevance and applicability of these ideas. Consider in particular the value of changing and optimizing roles, changing processes and work flows, changing the flow of information, enriching the information environment, continuously measuring and monitoring, and making adaptations based on tests of change (PDSA cycles) and learning (reflection on improvements and new information gained from the PDSA cycle).

### Evaluating Successful Access to Care

Access is an essential dimension of *measurable* system performance, and access metrics are commonly included in balanced scorecards, dashboards, and instrument panels. Some typical access metrics for outpatient and inpatient care are as follows:

### Outpatient

- Appointment slots open at beginning of day
- Over and under counts at end of day (that is, the number of appointment slots filled vis à vis the number of appointment slots available)
- Time to third available appointment
- Future appointment capacity (next month or quarter)
- Abandoned incoming phone calls from patients
- Time spent waiting on phone to talk to staff person
- Time spent waiting in office to see a provider
- Patient perceptions of access to care and waiting times
- Patient no-show rates

Table 5.2 Methods for Improving Access and Flow in Clinical Mesosystems

| Change Concept | Illustrative Method |
|---|---|
| Use service agreements to shape demand. | Establish clear agreements between clinical programs or units to indicate when patients should and should not be transferred and what information should accompany the transfer. Plan regular meeting times to provide feedback between microsystems regarding the transfer process. |
| Use standard order sets across the continuum of care. | Develop evidence-based standard orders for subpopulations of patients that provide a default plan of care for typical patients as their care episode progresses from microsystem to microsystem over time. |
| Precondition and pre-educate patients. | Make patients more fit for surgery or better prepared for inpatient care by offering pre-procedure physical conditioning, training, and education. |
| Establish and update plan of care. | Establish a plan of care and update it regularly; focus plan of care on actions needed to achieve clinical milestones that will enable progression to next downstream clinical microsystem. |
| Continuously monitor patient flows. | Establish a system (flow boards and daily organization bed/census meetings) to measure the capacity and the percentage of capacity filled for each clinical microsystem within the continuum (for example, within the ED, intensive care units, inpatient units, and surgical units) in real time |
| Use decision support. | Embed decision support into patient care flow to enrich the information environment by building in reminders, safety checks, and evidence-based care protocols. |
| Schedule early discharges. | Establish policies and processes to target discharges from a unit to be accomplished by a certain time. |
| Make and use contingency plans. | Establish policies and practices for making real-time adjustments in staffing and flow of patients based on unexpected increases in patient demand or on decreases in number of staff. |
| Enhance relationships between microsystems. | Establish regular daily meeting time between microsystems that are part of the mesosystem of care for patients to productively plan transfer of information, data, and plan of care in anticipation of the transition from one microsystem to another. Create conditions for memory of the patient and family across the continuum of care. Design processes for the receiving microsystem members (a nurse from a medical surgical unit, for example) to visit the sending microsystem (an intensive care unit, for example) to meet patient and family in advance of transfer to the medical surgical unit. |

## Inpatient

- Number of beds open at midnight
- Time from request to transfer to arrival at unit
- Time from *outside* request to transfer to admission
- Time from scheduled surgery to arrival at surgical unit
- Time to transfer patient out to *external* location
- Failed transfers resulting in patient return to previous microsystem
- Delayed transfers resulting in failure to admit new patients in a timely fashion
- Diversion of transferred patients resulting in lost customers and lost revenues

When planning methods for measurement of clinical access, inclusion of multiple metrics will enhance value. Real-time metrics on instrument panels or dashboards permit frontline microsystems to monitor and support rapid resource adjustments, enabling constant matching of supply and demand. Concurrent use of longitudinal

metrics                                                        on
run charts and control charts will identify vital trends over time, enabling clinical and administrative leaders to plan future resource allocations and program developments. These separate functions of measurement are discussed in greater detail in Chapter Four (see also *Measuring Access Improvement: Patient Focused Access Measures*[9] at www .clinicalmicrosystem.org.

## Transitions and Handoffs

It is the nature of systems that all parts are connected, but these connections may be direct or indirect, and they may be flawless or faulty. As a patient leaves home or community and enters the health care system, or as movement occurs from one microsystem to another, care may be delayed, hastened, coordinated, or fragmented. Just as we may improve access to care by designing and redesigning unique clinical microsystems, we can (and must) improve coordination of care across microsystems through similar attention to design. How do we optimize the safety and effectiveness of handoffs and other care transitions?

Imagine viewing a patient's entire clinical journey, over time, from being up on a *catwalk,* as industrial assembly line processes are sometimes viewed. Imagine (as in

**FIGURE 5.2   Patient Access to Care from the Catwalk.**

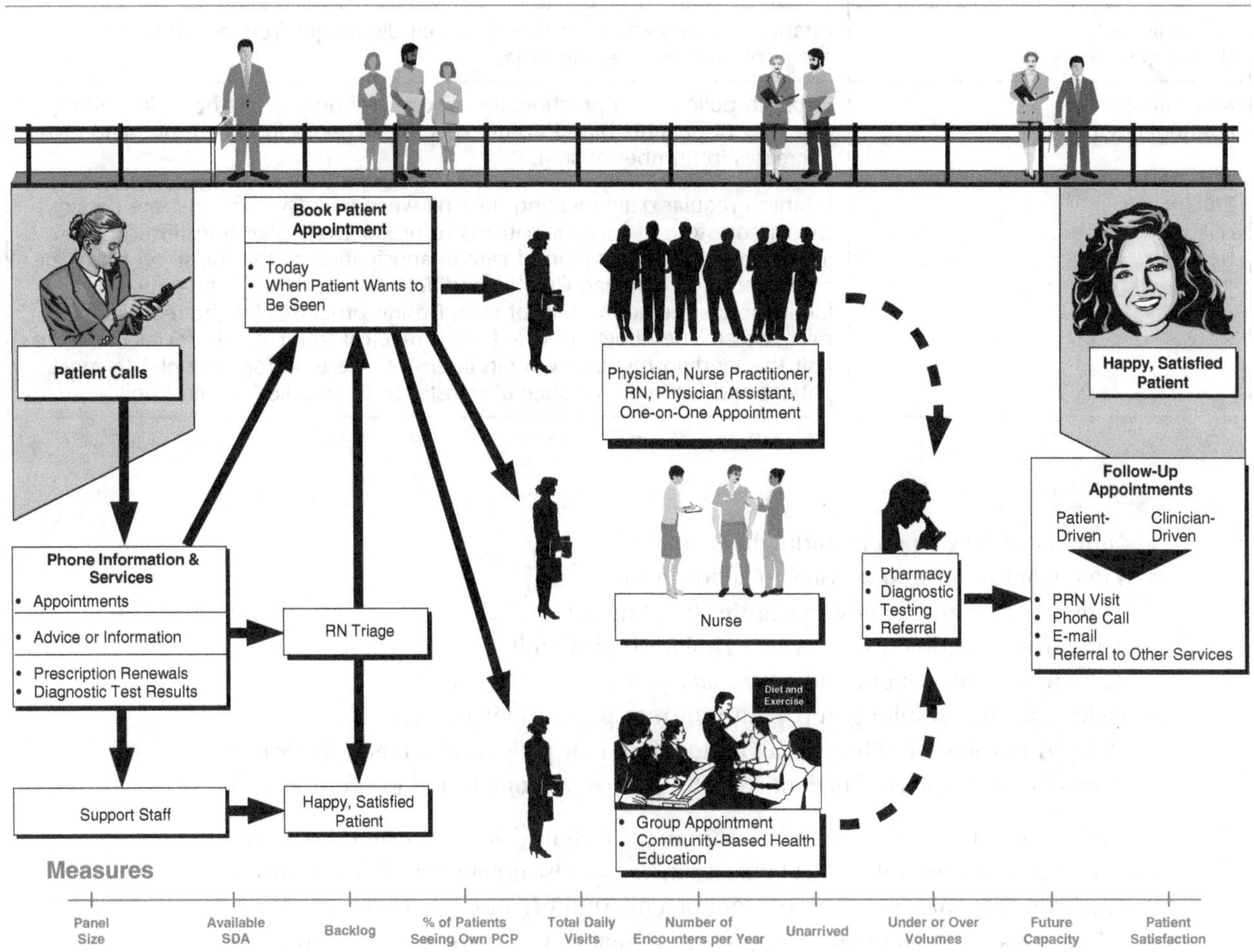

## MATCHING PATIENTS' NEEDS WITH THEIR PLAN OF CARE

Americans use a great deal of health care. They make more than 1.6 billion visits to doctors' offices, hospital outpatient departments, and emergency rooms,[1] and they receive more than 2.6 billion orders for prescribed medications.[2] In addition, each year Americans spend more than 220 million days in hospitals[3] and more than 1.2 billion days in nursing homes.[4] That adds up to a lot of care.

All of these visits, prescriptions, and stays in hospitals and nursing homes provide myriad opportunities for poor quality and waste in the form of overuse, underuse, and misuse of care and services. These types of waste have been well-documented by the Institute of Medicine[5] and the RAND Corporation.

If we step back to analyze this situation, we recognize that the process of *entering* into a clinical microsystem and of developing a plan of care are incredibly high-leverage, high-impact events. If the right patient gets to the right place at the right time, and if the clinical team can work with the patient to get the right assessment and a high-quality plan of care (that "increases the likelihood of desired health outcomes . . . consistent with current professional knowledge"[6]), then the need for care will match the need for service in the optimal way. This in turn can produce best value health care by matching the patient's needs for a health benefit with needed and appropriate treatments and services.

### References

1. National Center for Health Statistics. *Health, United States, 2006 with chartbook on trends in the health of Americans, Table 89.* Hyattsville, MD, 2006.
2. National Center for Health Statistics. *Health, United States, 2006 with chartbook on trends in the health of Americans, Table 92.* Hyattsville, MD, 2006.
3. National Center for Health Statistics. *Health, United States, 2006 with chartbook on trends in the health of Americans, Table 100.* Hyattsville, MD, 2006.
4. National Center for Health Statistics. *Health, United States, 2006 with chartbook on trends in the health of Americans, Table 102.* Hyattsville, MD, 2006.
5. Institute of Medicine. *Crossing the quality chasm: A new health system for the 21st century.* Washington, DC: Committee on Quality of Health Care, 2001.
6. Lohr, K. (Ed.). *Medicare: A strategy for quality assurance.* Washington, DC: National Academies Press, Committee to Design a Strategy for Quality Review and Assurance in Medicare, Division of Health Care Services, 1990.

Figures 5.2 and 5.3.) looking down on the flow of care and witnessing sequential hand-offs and transitions, as information, responsibility, and even the patient are transferred in space and time. This catwalk perspective will commonly reveal that a disproportionate number of quality and safety challenges arise at precisely these points of transition (see "Matching Patients' Needs with Their Plan of Care").

When we reflect on the properties of systems and the connections within and between systems and on the patient's journey over time and through different clinical microsystems, the following observations are pertinent:

- The health care system is a set of interdependent parts that work together to promote health and reduce the burden of illness.
- The performance of the health care system depends upon the quality of the parts and their interactions.

**FIGURE 5.3    The Catwalk of Post-Anesthesia Care.**

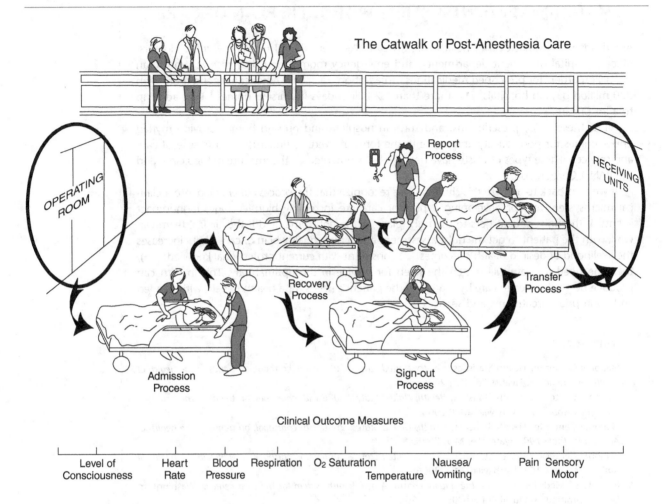

The Catwalk of Post-Anesthesia Care

OPERATING ROOM

RECEIVING UNITS

Report Process

Recovery Process

Transfer Process

Admission Process

Sign-out Process

Clinical Outcome Measures

Level of Consciousness — Heart Rate — Blood Pressure — Respiration — O₂ Saturation — Temperature — Nausea/Vomiting — Pain — Sensory Motor

- The interactions between the parts occurs in the *white spaces* separating individuals, units, and organizations; responsibility and accountability are unclear in the *between* microsystems space. White spaces exist throughout a patient's health care journey. When a patient is transferred between clinical microsystems within an organization or when a patient is transferred to another facility the white space exists where there is unclear accountability and responsibility for the patient.
- The white spaces may not be owned or claimed by anyone and are often ill-defined and unrecognized.
- An individual patient's care frequently involves a wide variety of interdependent professionals delivering care (or supporting the delivery of care) across multiple locations.
- Optimal care requires design of transitions and handoffs to provide coordination and continuity of care (between locations and between caregivers) so gaps in care occurring in the white spaces are eliminated.

Recognizing that many major and minor quality and safety problems are white space problems, the American Board of Internal Medicine (ABIM) asked a consortium of multiple professional societies in 2007 to address this issue and to develop some useful definitions on care transitions.[10] According to Greiner, coordination of care and transitions in care are functions that help "ensure that the patient's needs and preferences for health services and information sharing across people, functions and sites are met over time."[10] Freisen et al. describe handoffs in care as the "transfer of information (along with authority and responsibility) during transitions in care across the continuum for the purpose of ensuring continuity and safety of patient care.[11]

### Principles of Effective Transitions and Handoffs

Successful transitions and handoffs depend upon honoring the following essential principles:

*Staff responsibility:* Assign responsibility to professional staff to establish reliable methods for implementing care transitions and handoffs.

*Two-way communication:* Employ bidirectional and mutually confirming forms of communication between locations of care and between providers to inform evaluation, to secure appropriate follow-up, and to integrate all facets of care.

*Include patients:* Engage patients to the greatest extent possible in all transitions, but do not rely upon them to complete these functions.[10]

*Prepare patients:* Communicate effectively to establish cooperation, realistic expectations, follow-up, and contingency plans; check to ensure the patient understands all these components.

*Culture of cooperation:* Foster a culture of cooperation in the health care community to address patient needs, including those that require assistance from different organizations and disparate parts of the health care system.

### Methods

We recommend the following steps to improve transitions and handoffs.

1. Identify places in the process flow where transitions and handoffs occur and where breakdowns are likely, such as:
   - Transfer of patients into a hospital or nursing home or within a facility from one unit to another
   - Patient referrals for a consultation or for specialized care
   - Shift changes among nurses, MDs, respiratory therapists, social workers, and other professionals
   - Communication of critical diagnostic test results
   - Arrangements for an on-call clinician to provide assistance with changing patient needs and the transition process

   Chapter Five Action Guide provides simple instructions and examples to help you construct a flowchart of the processes to see what actually happens in daily work.

2. Establish shared expectations for all of the microsystems involved in the patient's care for transitions and handoffs; use standard processes for making transitions and handoffs across the mesosystem of care. A patient who has an acute myocardial infarction (AMI) receives care from the emergency department, the cardiac catheterization laboratory, cardiac care unit, and rehabilitation unit. These clinical microsystems would need to meet to establish clear aims for AMI patients including

expectations and processes to ensure safe transitions and handoffs across the different clinical microsystems.

3. Select a standard approach and develop a clear process map for accomplishing the transition or handoff (checklist, protocol).
4. Educate staff on the standard process (what, why, when, how) and practice under simulated and real conditions.
5. Monitor and measure the success of transitions and handoffs and discuss this topic within the mesosystem to facilitate ongoing improvements.
6. Engage leaders at the mesosystem level to create conditions for the linked microsystems to establish and review transition processes.

The Joint Commission's 2009 National Patient Safety Goals[12] require a standard approach to handoff communication, including an opportunity to ask and respond to questions. National Patient Safety Goals include the following:

- Allow opportunity for questioning between the giver and receiver of patient information.
- Communicate up-to-date information regarding patient care, treatment and services, condition, any recent unanticipated changes, and what to watch for in the next interval of care.
- Develop a process to verify the received information, including repeat back or read back as appropriate.
- The receiver of the handoff information reviews relevant patient historical data, which may include previous care, treatment, and services.
- Limit interruption during handoffs to minimize the possibility of information being altered or lost.

Various methods are now widely used to improve the efficiency and reliability of communication at transition points and handoffs.[13] A well-known tool is based on the acronym, *SBAR*:

- *Situation*: description of current issue
- *Background*: brief description of preceding events
- *Assessment*: key features of current state
- *Recommendation*: suggested action(s) to take next

*SBAR* is a mnemonic device for effective communication. Its value is directly linked to its reliable use at the front line when patient and information transfers take place.

Different adaptations of the SBAR method are illustrated in Figures 5.4, 5.5, and 5.6. Each of these adaptations maintain the SBAR framework and also reflect the unique cultures and settings of various clinical microsystems. Another mnemonic I PASS the BATON is presented in Figure 5.7. I PASS the BATON is understood as follows:

Introduction
Patient + Assessment + Situation + Safety concerns
Background + Actions + Timing + Ownership + Next

FIGURE 5.4 Handoff Communication Checklist for Surgery.

## HANDOFF COMMUNICATION

**S** — Complete on all patients going to surgery or procedure

Reason for Procedure: _____

- ☐ Cardiac Cath
- ☐ Dialysis
- ☐ Endoscopy
- ☐ Medical Imaging (Angio, CT, US, Nuc Med, MRI)
- ☐ Outpatient Treatment Center
- ☐ OV/CVOR
- ☐ Pediatric Outpatient Treatment Center
- ☐ Unit
- ☐ Other: _____

Date: _____  Unit Sending Patient: _____  Unit Patient to Return to Post Procedure: _____

Primary RN: _____  Name Patient Prefers to Be Called: _____

☐ Nursing Physical Assessment Completed

Level of Consciousness: ☐ oriented ☐ cooperative ☐ anxious ☐ uncooperative ☐ confused ☐ other: _____

Pain Assessment: Pain Level: _____  Scale Used: _____  Pain Goal: _____

Last dose of pain medication: _____

Medication Reconciliation Complete: ☐ yes ☐ no

Spouse/Significant Other with Patient: ☐ yes ☐ no  Name: _____  Location: _____

Vitals (to be done within the hour prior to leaving unit):

Time: _____  Temperature: _____  Pulse: _____  Respirations: _____  Blood Pressure: _____  O₂ Sat: _____  Room air/O₂ _____ l/mi

NPO Status: Time of last oral intake of clears: _____  Solids (including milk products): _____

Pre-Procedure Meds: Ordered: ☐ no ☐ yes  Given: ☐ no ☐ yes (see MAR)  Prep Complete: ☐ no ☐ yes

Recent Weight: _____ kg. ☐actual ☐ yes  Height: _____ cm

Consents signed: ☐ surgery/procedural ☐ anesthesia/sedation ☐ blood ☐ sterilization

**B**

| | Ordered | | | Results on Chart | | | | Ordered | | | Results on Chart | | |
|---|---|---|---|---|---|---|---|---|---|---|---|---|---|
| CBC | ☐ yes | ☐ no | ☐ NA | ☐ yes | ☐ no | | UA | ☐ yes | ☐ no | ☐ NA | ☐ yes | ☐ no | |
| CMP | ☐ yes | ☐ no | ☐ NA | ☐ yes | ☐ no | | 12-Lead EKG | ☐ yes | ☐ no | ☐ NA | ☐ yes | ☐ no | |
| PT/INR/PTTT | ☐ yes | ☐ no | ☐ NA | ☐ yes | ☐ no | | Chest X-Ray | ☐ yes | ☐ no | ☐ NA | ☐ yes | ☐ no | |
| Type & Cross | ☐ yes | ☐ no | ☐ NA | ☐ yes | ☐ no | | Blood Sugar: _____ | ☐ yes | ☐ no | ☐ NA | ☐ yes | ☐ no | |
| HCG | ☐ yes | ☐ no | ☐ NA | ☐ yes | ☐ no | | Other: _____ | ☐ yes | ☐ no | ☐ NA | ☐ yes | ☐ no | |

Abnormal results?: ☐ No ☐ Yes, If, Yes, Physician Notified: _____  Time Notified: _____  Notified by: _____

Orders received?: ☐ No ☐ Yes, If, Yes, See Orders

In Chart:
- ☐ History and Physical
- ☐ Pre-Operative Note
- ☐ Conditions of Admission
- ☐ RN Flowsheet/progress notes
- ☐ MAR
- ☐ Allergy Sheet
- ☐ PCMP
- ☐ MRI Checklist
- ☐ Contrast Form

For patients receiving bowel prep: Results Clear: ☐ Yes ☐ No

**** Also complete this section if going to surgery ****

| | | | | |
|---|---|---|---|---|
| Jewelry removed | ☐ Yes | ☐ No, if No, Secured | ☐ NA | |
| Prosthesis removed | ☐ Yes | ☐ No | ☐ NA | |
| Dentures removed | ☐ Yes | ☐ No | ☐ NA | |
| Contacts removed | ☐ Yes | ☐ No | ☐ NA | |
| Glasses removed | ☐ Yes | ☐ No | ☐ NA | |
| Skin prep done | ☐ Yes | ☐ No | ☐ NA | |

Denture cup labeled and sent to pre-op ☐ Yes ☐ No ☐ NA

Pneumatic/therapeutic hose on patient to pre-op ☐ Yes ☐ No ☐ NA

If ordered

Pre-operative incentive spirometer reading: _____

Time of Last Void: ☐ Diaper ☐ Foley ☐ Bedpan ☐ Bathroom Privileges ☐ Incontinent

**** Also complete for Cardiovascular Patients ****

1st Shower: _____  2nd Shower with clipping (less than 4 hours from OR time): _____

**A**
- ☐ Patient ready for transfer
- ☐ Patient transferring for intervention

Accompanied by: ☐ transporter ☐ nurse ☐ nurse & monitor  Transported via: ☐ cart ☐ wheelchair ☐ bed ☐ ambuatory

Report called to: _____ at: _____  Report faxed to: _____ to ext: _____

Please call: _____ at ext. _____  for any questions.

**R**

Signature(s) of staff Sending Patient: _____  Date: _____  Time: _____

Signature of Pre-op/Procedural Staff Receiving Patient: _____  Date: _____  Time: _____

Comments: _____

S: Situation    B: Background    A: Assessment    R: Recommendation

FIGURE 5.5  RN to RN Handoff Tool.

# RN to RN HANDOFF TOOL
(O.R. – PACU – CVICU)

Date: _____

## SITUATION (patient history)

Patient's Age and _____

Pre-Operative Diagnosis: _____

Pertinent Medical History: _____

Operative Procedure: _____

Allergies                    ☐ NKDA           ☐ Yes _____

Sensory Impairment           ☐ No             ☐ Yes _____

Family Present               ☐ ASU Waiting Room  ☐ 5th Floor – CVOR Waiting Room

Religious/Cultural Issues     ☐ No             ☐ Yes _____

Isolation Precautions         ☐ No             ☐ Yes _____

Interpreter Required          ☐ No             ☐ Yes _____

Valuables/Belongings (disposition) _____

## INTRAOPERATIVE BACKGROUND:

Meds given intraoperatively _____

Blood Given:        ☐ Yes    ☐ No    Transfused: _____ RBCs _____ Platelets _____ FFPS

Units Available: _____

Assessment of Skin Integrity: _____
(include pressure sites, positioning related to areas, and incision site)

Musculoskeletal Restrictions   ☐ No    ☐ Yes _____

Tubes/Drains/Catheters         ☐ N/A   ☐ Yes _____
(include size and location)

Dressings/Cast/Splint          ☐ No    ☐ Yes _____

Count Correct                  ☐ Yes   ☐ No    ☐ X-ray taken

Other: (labs, path, results) _____

Patient Transferred to    ☐ PACU    ☐ CVICU

Report Given To: _____ RN    Report Given By: _____, RN (relief only)

Report Given To: _____ RN    Report Given By: _____, RN (relief only)

Report Given To: _____ RN    Report Given By: _____, RN

FIGURE 5.6  SBAR Patient Report Guideline for Perioperative Services.

| | **SBAR** Patient Report Guidelines: Perioperative Services | |
|---|---|---|
| Report Given by: | Time: | Phone: |
| Report Received by: | | Phone: |
| **S** | **Situation:**<br>❑ Patient's Name<br>❑ Age, Gender<br>❑ Diagnosis/Procedure being performed | ❑ NPO Status (# of hours)<br>❑ Allergies<br>❑ Advanced Directive, Code Status |
| **B** | **Background:**<br>❑ History/Past hospitalization<br>❑ Infection control/Isolation<br>❑ Primary language<br>❑ Legal Status | ❑ Special Needs – spiritual, cultural, learning, communication<br>❑ Religious Needs – refuses blood transfusion<br>❑ Disposition of Patient Belongings |
| **A** | **Assessment:**<br>❑ Current Status – Preop or OR<br>➤ Planned surgical procedure<br>➤ Surgical procedure verified and marked<br>➤ Planned anesthesia type<br>➤ Allergies<br>➤ Mental status<br>➤ Language barriers<br>➤ Blood products/Consent<br>➤ Medications received in preop<br>➤ Antibiotics to be given<br>➤ Blood products available<br>➤ Significant medical history (elevated BP, cardiac, asthma)<br>➤ Equipment needs (SCD)<br>➤ Catheters, drains<br>➤ Musculoskeletal/Skin: breakdown, casts, wounds, dressings<br>➤ Surgeon has spoken with patient/family<br>➤ Family waiting/contact information?<br><br>❑ Current Status – OR to PACU/Critical Care<br>➤ Surgical procedure<br>➤ Allergies<br>➤ Blood products remaining<br>➤ Drains and catheters<br>➤ Motor activity (neuro)<br>➤ Peripheral circulation issue<br>➤ Positional issues<br>➤ Skin integrity<br>➤ Equipment needs<br>➤ Additional issues or concerns<br>❑ Communication with family regarding:<br>➤ Clinical condition<br>➤ Change in condition | ❑ Current Status – OR RN to OR RN<br>➤ Current stage of procedure<br>➤ Anesthesia type<br>➤ Position of patient/devices used<br>➤ Allergies<br>➤ Significant medical history<br>➤ Blood products/Consent<br>➤ Recent changes in condition<br>➤ Medications on the sterile field<br>➤ Irrigation fluids in use<br>➤ Instrumentation on/off field — needed<br>➤ Equipment device needs<br>➤ Implants needed available<br>➤ Vendor present — needed<br>➤ Specimens on and off field<br>➤ Drains and catheters<br>➤ Counts<br>    ○ Sponges<br>    ○ Needle/small items<br>    ○ Instruments<br>❑ Communication with family regarding:<br>➤ Clinical/Change in condition<br>❑ Current Status – OR Scrub to OR Scrub<br>➤ Current stage of procedure<br>➤ Anesthesia type<br>➤ Allergies<br>➤ Medications on the sterile field<br>➤ Irrigation fluids in use<br>➤ Location and count of all countable items currently in use<br>➤ Instrument trays in use and counts of all instruments<br>➤ Extra instruments available in room<br>➤ Implants on field/in room<br>➤ Number and location of specimens, on and off the field<br>➤ Any additional issues or concerns |
| **R** | **Recommendation:**<br>❑ Plan for continuing care interventions<br>❑ Nursing orders/Nursing plan of care<br>❑ *Additional Questions/Comments* | ❑ Abnormal results and related |

**FIGURE 5.7   I Pass the Baton Handoffs and Health Care Transitions.**

| | Handoffs and Healthcare Transitions with Opportunities to Ask QUESTIONS, CLARIFY, and CONFIRM | |
|---|---|---|
| **I** | **Introduction** | Introduce yourself and your role/job (include patient) |
| **P** | **Patient** | Name, identifiers, age, sex, location |
| **A** | **Assessment** | Presenting chief complaint, vital signs, and symptoms and diagnosis |
| **S** | **Situation** | Current status, medications, circumstances, including code status, level of (un)certainty, recent changes, response to treatment |
| **S** | **SAFETY Concerns** | Critical lab values, reports, socio-economic factors, allergies, alerts (falls, isolation, etc.) |
| **THE** | | |
| **B** | **Background** | Co-morbidities, previous episodes, past/home medications, family history |
| **A** | **Actions** | What actions were taken or are required AND provide brief rationale |
| **T** | **Timing** | Level of urgency and explicit timing, prioritization or actions |
| **O** | **Ownership** | Who is responsible (nurse/doctor/team) including patient/family responsibilities |
| **N** | **Next** | What will happen next? Anticipated changes? What is the **PLAN**? Contingency plans? |

Another acronym-based model is the TeamSTEPPS educational process, developed by the Agency for Healthcare Research and Quality (AHRQ).[14] TeamSTEPPS aims to improve patient safety through enhanced communication and teamwork skills among health care professionals. The process relies upon the following aims to increase team awareness:

- Role and responsibility clarification
- Conflict resolution
- Improved information sharing
- Optimized use of information, people, and resources to achieve the best clinical outcomes for patients

The reader is invited to explore further applications of handoffs and care transitions in Chapter Seven, where these functions are specifically considered in the context of acute care.

### Evaluating Successful Care Transitions

Care transitions, like initial access interventions, must be monitored to assure they remain both safe and effective. Pertinent information may be directly obtained via monitoring of transition metrics or may be indirectly inferred through assessment of *downstream* outcomes.

### Direct Assessment and Monitoring of Transition Metrics

- Observation of transitions and handoffs
- Reports and ratings by patients and families about handoffs and transitions that involve them directly
- Reports and ratings by staff who *receive* the patient, assessing the extent to which they felt adequately informed to take responsibility for care of the patient

### Indirect Assessment and Monitoring of Downstream Outcomes

- Rate of harm, including adverse drug events such as nosocomial infections, falls, and pressure ulcers
- Use of health resources, such as emergency department visits, avoidable hospital admissions, delays in discharges, readmissions within thirty days, and return to sending microsystem due to patient acuity and instability. Avoidable hospital admissions are often due to inadequate patient education at discharge from the hospital resulting in patient inability to identify and respond to changes in health status at home resulting in readmission to the hospital.

## Orienting Patients to Navigate Care

As an individual health care journey unfolds over time, patient and family will likely enter and exit many different clinical programs and clinical microsystems. Each new entry will require patients learning not only health-specific care strategies ("How do I lower my blood pressure?" "How do I prevent spread of my current infection?") but also microsystem-specific processes and structures ("How do I contact the inpatient nurse when I need more pain medication?" "How do I reach my doctor on weekends with an urgent concern?") This learning requirement is even more challenging when the patient must navigate multiple microsystems in quick succession, or even simultaneously.

Consider, for example, Bob Judd, who at the age of 55 experiences a myocardial infarction (heart attack), and must spend time sequentially in the emergency department, coronary catheterization unit, coronary care unit, inpatient step-down unit, cardiovascular rehabilitation program, and then outpatient follow-up with his family physician and a new cardiologist. As he endeavors to integrate important new clinical information, Bob must learn to navigate real-world health systems as well. The quality of his care depends not only on the skills of his several clinical teams, but also on his own learned capacity to make use of and to gain full value from the skills and the services available. Of course, Bob cannot be expected to secure this extensive knowledge on his own. It is the responsibility of clinical microsystems to anticipate the clinical *and* the systems knowledge patients will require and to design processes that effectively orient patients to both.

### *Principles for Orienting Patients to Microsystems*

Careful reflection is required to fully anticipate patient and family knowledge needs when entering a new system of care. In designing the orientation process that supports patients' acquisition of this knowledge, a number of key principles warrant consideration:

1. *Patient needs:* The aim of orientation is to establish reliable and helpful methods for patients to communicate needs, to navigate systems, to receive timely and appropriate services, and to anticipate clinical outcomes.
2. *Patient perspective:* What is the view of the microsystem from the perspective of patients and families who are totally new to this particular setting. What will they need to know so they can function as full partners in care?
3. *Must haves:* The following are common *must haves*.
   - *Safety:* What does the patient or family need to know to be safe and to protect the safety of other patients?

- *Team members:* Who is on the patient's or family's microsystem team, and what is their role?
- *Navigate:* What services and care is located where and how does the patient or family get there?
- *Access:* How can the patient or family make arrangements to get new or continuing services?
- *Decisions:* How can the patient or family learn what is needed to make a good decision in light of current health status, personal preferences, and potential treatment options?
- *Utilization:* How can the patient or family make wise use of self-care skills and professional health resources to retain or regain their health?

### Methods of Improving the Orientation Process

One way to improve the orientation process is to develop a practical patient and family-centered *user's manual,* meaning a guide on how to make use of a service, for the new patient and family. This can promote partnering with patients and can enhance the effectiveness and efficiency of the entire system. The user's manual may be brief (a fact sheet) or extensive (a notebook), and it may be delivered in paper, electronic, video, or other formats. A specific example of the orientation process for a neonatal intensive care unit is shown in Figure 5.8; this deployment flowchart specifies who does what and in what order. Table 5.3 describes ways to improve the orientation process.

### Evaluating Success of the Orientation Process

Periodic feedback from patients and families will help microsystems determine the goodness of the orientation process. A review of the process and tools to partner with patients that are discussed in Chapter Two may be worthwhile to design a process to obtain patient and family feedback. Survey instruments can be used, or individual patients and families (especially those who are new to the microsystem) can be interviewed in a formal or informal manner. The following questions (to patients and families) may be appropriate:

1. What services are offered by the (microsystem name), and where are these services located?
2. Who works in the (microsystem name), and what do they do for you?
3. How do you go about the following activities:
   - Making arrangements to receive services or to get help when needed
   - Making decisions about what treatments to choose
   - Knowing what to do to take care of yourself
   - Getting important questions answered
   - Knowing what to do in an emergency or if you have an urgent need for help
   - Knowing what you can do to be safe and to avoid harm
4. If a friend of yours were to receive care from (microsystem name) for the first time, what would you tell him (or her) so that he (or she) could obtain appropriate treatment and service?

## Initial Assessment and Plan of Care

Yogi Berra once famously stated, "If you don't know where you want to go, you might not get there."[15] Effective entry into clinical microsystems must include determination

**FIGURE 5.8   Orientation Process for Parents Whose Infant Has Been Transferred to a Neonatal Intensive Care Unit.**

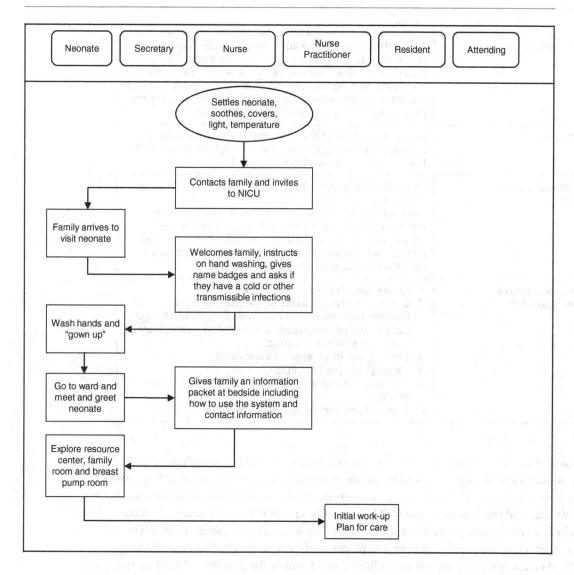

of where patients are, where they want (and need) to go, and how they may partner with care teams to get there. Initial assessment can richly characterize patients' needs, values, and resources, and can align these with a plan of care that fosters productive clinical relationships and generates best possible outcomes.

Consider the core clinical delivery process that is common to almost all microsystem work flows:

*Assess Time 1* → Diagnose → *Care Plan* → Treat → Outcomes → *Assess Time 2*

Note the bookend function of assessment at the beginning and end of all clinical episodes, and note the pivotal, central role of care plan formation. A correct and well-executed plan of care that is based upon initial assessment and that is intermittently modified based upon reassessments produces the best chance of optimal outcomes.

**Table 5.3 Steps and Methods for Analyzing and Improving
the Orientation Process**

| Steps | Methods |
|---|---|
| Assess current orientation process. | Assess the current orientation process: role play aspects of the orientation process (Through the Eyes of the Patient and Family worksheet in the Assess, Diagnose and Treat workbooks), use direct observation, or conduct individual or group interviews. Consider videotaping the process to share with members of the unit. |
| Identify benchmark exemplars. | Examine the best-of-the-best user manuals, orientation guides, and orientation programs to determine desirable features, functions, and delivery modes. |
| Consider alternative modes of communication. | Depending on patient needs and abilities, resources, and circumstances, consider alternative modes of communication for the orientation, such as fact sheet, brochure, notebook, video, web page, peer-to-peer orientation, group orientation, checklist (assisted), and face-to-face orientation by different microsystem team members as initial entry processes unfold. |
| Improve orientation process using Plan-Do-Study-Act. | 1. Create flowchart of current process. 2. Brainstorm change ideas: some may be done immediately and others may require tests of change such as the plan-do-study-act model to make changes using the scientific method. 3. Select a test of change to implement. 4. Develop the plan for PDSA. 5. Conduct the test and revise or implement the new process. 6. Seek patient, family, and staff feedback. |

Care plans have a hallowed place in the education of health professionals, in the daily work of clinical care itself, and in microsystem initiatives to continuously improve the quality of that care. Dr. Larry Weed's pioneering work on problem-oriented medical records featured the now-ubiquitous *SOAP note*. Using a SOAP note format, clinicians identify discrete health problems and for each problem develop plans of care based upon: *S*ubjective findings (reported symptoms and past history); *O*bjective findings (physical exam, lab work, and other studies); *A*ssessment of the problem (based on the findings and other information); and *P*lan on what actions should be taken to treat the problem.[16] Nurse educators have long emphasized the critical nature of a comprehensive, patient-centered, interdisciplinary plan of care.[17] More recently, innovators in medical education have promoted daily interdisciplinary bedside patient rounds, which engage the patient, the family, and the entire care team to improve the quality of care based on specific problem-focused plans.[18] These interdisciplinary rounds result in improved communication among patients, families, and interdisciplinary professionals; understanding by all of the care plan; and education of the care team to the patient's needs and care plan.

This model has gained traction in practice management and health policy discussions as well. The medical home movement, for example, makes the care plan a focal point for improving and coordinating health system performance.[19] *Medical homes* incorporate core primary care principles, relationship-centered patient care, new information technology, reimbursement reform, and plans of care derived from the Chronic Care

Model. This movement has garnered widespread support from all primary care specialty societies, including family practice, internal medicine, pediatrics, and osteopathic medicine. At the same time, diverse payers are making special arrangements to reimburse primary care practices for developing and implementing patient-specific plans of care.[20]

## Characteristics of Effective Care Plans

Care plans vary by setting and circumstance. The scope of the plan and the frequency of updates are tailored to the needs of patients in different clinical microsystems. Both assessment and care plan activities will vary, for example, in such diverse settings as a post-anesthesia care unit, an intensive care unit, a primary care practice, and a skilled nursing care facility. Therefore, although care plans will differ in meaningful ways across disparate clinical microsystems, some general principles are common across systems. Effective care plans frequently possess the following characteristics:

- *Patient-centered:* The care plan is based on the patient's current health status, preferences, and capabilities and is predicated on active engagement of patient and family.
- *Comprehensive:* The care plan takes into account clinical, psychological, social, environmental, and cultural factors that impact the patient's health and behavior.
- *Interdisciplinary:* The development and execution of an effective care plan often requires active engagement of different types of health professionals, who collaborate with each other and with the patient and family.
- *Adaptable:* Patients' health status, preferences, and capabilities change over time, so care plans must be designed to evolve in a continuous manner that aligns new clinical needs with appropriate clinical services.
- *Clear and accessible:* The care plan connects health problems with health goals, clarifies who is responsible for taking what actions, and is readily available to all care participants who have a stake in the patient's longitudinal health.

## The Wagner Care Model

Wagner has developed an influential model of planned care that can guide clinical microsystems in the design and implementation of patient-oriented and problem-specific planned services. Known most generally as the *Care Model*,[21,22] its specific realization in the *Chronic Care Model* is explored in detail in Chapter Eight. In the present chapter we consider the use of Wagner's model in the formation of plans of care.

As we depicted in Figure 2.4 on page 56, Wagner's model focuses attention upon productive interactions between an informed, empowered patient and a prepared, proactive clinician and interdisciplinary team. These interactions are supported by diverse resources within the microsystem, mesosystem, macrosystem, and larger community. As elaborated on in Chapter Eight, the model's successful execution hinges on careful planning and integration of: (1) patient self-management, (2) delivery system design, (3) decision support for patients and staff, and (4) clinical information system support. When these resources and structures are directed to specific clinical goals (as defined in negotiated plans of care), then productive patient-clinician interactions generate improved clinical outcomes.

The development of care plans and the delivery of effective planned care are seldom confined to a single office visit or to a specific hospital stay, nor are they limited to care provided by a single clinician or health professional. Planned care connects the present with the future, using knowledge from patients' past and present experiences to anticipate future needs and to optimize future outcomes.

Patient assessment, care plan development, and planned care delivery can be actualized in many forms. In the inpatient environment, methods to accomplish this may include the following:

- Full initial assessment to focus on admitting problem or health condition
- Daily interdisciplinary rounds engaging patient and family
- Use of a white board in the patient's room to show goals for the day and to identify the primary nurse and physician responsible for the patient's care and also invites patient and family involvement in care planning
- Hourly nursing rounds to check on patient's status and evolving needs
- Structured change-of-shift handoffs at the bedside to communicate essential information on patient status and specific care plan goals

In outpatient settings, microsystems may begin clinical assessment even prior to patients' arrival at the office. A paper or electronic health assessment survey can be sent to patients prior to initial workup and can be completed at home with results fed forward to the clinical site in advance of an actual visit.[23,24,25] Alternatively, CARE (Checking, Activating, Reinforcing, and Engineering) Vital Signs[26] are age-specific assessment tools that inform providers in advance of patients' unique needs and also offer patients need-specific educational materials. Chapter Five Action Guide provides more details about CARE Vital Signs. The structure of actual care plan documents will vary depending on conditions; such plans may be compact and focused or comprehensive and broad. The care plan for a critically ill ICU patient will differ substantially from one for a patient who seeks only preventive health services.

### Evaluating Care Plan Success

To improve the assessment and care planning process, it is wise to perform periodic audits or spot checks to answer questions such as the following:

- What proportion of patients have a care plan?
- Is the care plan current and up-to-date?
- Is the care plan based on an adequate assessment of the patient's health status?
- Are the patient and family active partners in care plan creation?
- Is the care plan accessible to those who need it?
- Is the care plan scope too limited or too expansive to be useful?
- How confident are patients, families, and staff in their ability to execute the care plan?
- What can be done to improve the care plan to achieve better outcomes?

## CONCLUSION

The first small step patients take into new clinical microsystems is in fact a very large step. In contexts that are associated with emerging (and sometimes urgent) health needs, patients and health professionals must find each other and learn about each other as a prerequisite to successfully *partnering* to achieve positive outcomes. The several *entry functions* of clinical microsystems parse the finding and learning into discrete and achievable tasks.

We have seen that thoughtful attention to microsystem design can optimize patients' access to care, and can facilitate safe and reliable transitions between microsystems when more extensive or integrated care is required. We have also observed that structured orientation and assessment will enrich patients' and caregivers' mutual understanding of each other and will provide a strong foundation for the development of targeted and shared care plans. As we focus attention on the clinical domains of preventive, acute, chronic, and palliative care in the next four chapters, we shall see that the *first step* of patient entry, when proactively supported by well-designed and well-tested microsystem care processes, establishes a clear path for the many important steps that follow.

## SUMMARY

This chapter explores the *entry functions* of clinical microsystems, with attention to transition points in the patient's health care journey between one microsystem and the next. The value of these transitions will be determined by the following variables:

- *Access:* the ease and timeliness of entry into each new microsystem
- *Transitions and handoffs:* the reliable conveyance of patient information to receiving clinical microsystems to afford continuity and correct care matched to needs
- *Orientation:* education of the patient on what one needs to know to gain maximum benefit and be engaged to the fullest extent possible
- *Assessment and plan of care:* the determination of what the patient wants and needs and how these needs can be met, based on available evidence and the patient's informed decisions

## KEY TERMS

Backlogs

CARE Vital Signs

Complete access

Direct modes of entry

Downstream outcomes

Entry functions

Episode of care

Handoff

I PASS the BATON

SBAR tool

SOAP notes

STAR Generative Relationship tool

TeamSTEPPS

Transition of care

User's manual

Wagner Care Model

White space

## REVIEW QUESTIONS

1. Define access to care and barriers to gaining timely access to a clinical microsystem.
2. What are the ten key change concepts to improve access?
3. Should all patient and family orientation materials be written materials? With deeper knowledge of patient populations, what other options might you consider?
4. What do transitions and handoffs refer to?
5. What process redesign steps create an improved transition or handoff process?

## DISCUSSION QUESTIONS

1. Consider the patient's journey and the flow of care in the microsystem you are studying.
   a. How do patients access care and how might you identify and measure delays in gaining access to care?
   b. Where are the transition points in patient flow?
   c. How could you assess the safety and reliability of the handoff process?
2. Think about your microsystem, mesosystem and macrosystem. What systems are currently in place to monitor access across the organization?
   a. What measures alert the system when patients have waits and delays?
   b. What measures alert the system of patients being turned away?

## REFERENCES

1. Nelson et al. The building blocks of health systems, part 1. *Joint Commission Journal on Quality and Patient Safety*, July 2008, *34*(7), 367–378.
2. Wild, J. *Quotes to live by*. Retrieved December 2, 2009, from www.cflconsulting.com/quotes.php
3. Berwick, D., & Kilo, C. Idealized design of clinical office practice: An interview with Donald Berwick and Charles Kilo of the Institute for Healthcare Improvement. *Managed Care Quarterly*, 1999, *7*(4), 62–69.
4. Murray, M., & Berwick, D. M. Advanced access: Reducing waiting and delays in primary care. *Journal of the American Medical Association*, 2003. *289*(8), 1035–1040.
5. Murray, M., Bodenheimer, T., Rittenhouse, D., & Grumbach, K. Improving timely access to primary care: Case studies of the advanced access model. *Journal of the American Medical Association*, 2003, *289*(8), 1042–1046.
6. Paul Batalden, personal communication to Eugene Nelson, DSc. Nashville, TN, HCA Corporate Headquarters, 1992.
7. Institute for Healthcare Improvement. Retrieved July 12, 2010 from www.ihi.org/IHI/Topics/OfficePractices/Access/ImprovementStories/MemberReportAdvancedClinicAccessInitiative.htm.
8. Proudlove, N., & Boaden, R. Using operational information and information systems to improve in-patient flow in hospitals. *Journal of Health Organization and Management*, 2005, *19*(6), 466–477.
9. Clinical Microsystem. *Measuring access improvement: Patient focused access measures*. Retrieved November 22, 2008, from www.clinicalmicrosystem.org
10. Greiner, A. *White space or black hole: What can we do to improve care transitions?* ABIM Foundation & SUTTP Alliance, 2007. Retrieved from www.abimfoundation.org/~/media/Files/Publications/F06–09–2007.ashx
11. Friesen, M., White, S. V., & Byers, J. F. *Handoffs: Implications for nurses*. Retrieved December 2, 2009, from www.ncbi.nlm.nih.gov/bookshelf/br.fcgi?book=nursehb&part=ch34 p. 1
12. Joint Commission Center for Transforming Healthcare. *National patient safety goals*. Retrieved December 2, 2009, from www.jointcommission.org/PatientSafety/NationalPatientSafetyGoals/09_hap_npsgs.htm
13. Haig, K., Sutton, S., & Whittington, J. SBAR: A shared mental model for improving communication between clinicians. *Joint Commission Journal on Quality and Patient Safety*, 2006, *32*(3), 167–175.

14. Agency for Healthcare Research and Quality. *TeamSTEPPS®: National implementation.* Retrieved December 1, 2009, from http://teamstepps.ahrq.gov

15. *Things people said: Yogi Berra quotes.* Retrieved December 2, 2009, from www.rinkworks.com/said/yogiberra.shtml

16. Weed, L. *Medical records, medical education and patient care.* Cleveland: Press of Case Western Reserve University, 1969.

17. Woody, M., & Mallison, M. The problem-oriented system for patient-centered care. *American Journal of Nursing,* 1973, *73*(7), 1168–1175.

18. Halm et al. Interdisciplinary rounds: Impact on patients, families, and staff. *Clinical Nurse Specialist,* 2003, *17*(3), 133–142.

19. Grumbach, K., & Bodenheimer, T. A primary care home for Americans: Putting the house in order. *Journal of the American Medical Association,* 2002, *288*(7), 889–893.

20. Starfield, B., & Shi, L. The medical home, access to care, and insurance: A review of evidence. *Pediatrics,* 2004, *113*(5 Suppl.), 1493–1498.

21. Bodenheimer, T., Wagner, E. H., & Grumbach, K. Improving primary care for patients with chronic illness: The chronic care model, part 2. *Journal of the American Medical Association,* 2002, *288*(15), 1909–1914.

22. Wagner, E. H., Austin, B. T., & Von Korff, M. Organizing care for patients with chronic illness. *Milbank Quarterly,* 1996, *74*(4), 511–544.

23. Hvitfeldt et al. Feed forward systems for patient participation and provider support: Adoption results from the original U.S. context to Sweden and beyond. *Quality Management in Health Care,* 2009, *18*(4), 247–256.

24. Nelson, E. Using outcomes measurement to improve quality and value. *New Directions for Mental Health Services,* 1996, *71*, 111–124.

25. Weinstein, J., Brown, P. W., Hanscom, B., Walsh, T., & Nelson, E. C. Designing an ambulatory clinical practice for outcomes improvement: From vision to reality—the Spine Center at Dartmouth-Hitchcock, year one. *Quality Management in Health Care,* 2000, *8*(2), 1–20.

26. How's your health. C.A.R.E. Vital signs. Retrieved December 2, 2009, from www.howsyourhealth.org/html/vital.pdf

# Chapter Five ACTION GUIDE

Chapter Five Action Guide focuses on tools to assess current processes including the value produced by the clinical microsystem, entry into a microsystem also known as *access*, and a tool to begin early assessment of patient needs.

## PROCESS MAPPING WITH FLOWCHARTS

Many types of flowcharts are used in health care improvement, including the following:

- High-level flowchart
- Detailed flowchart
- Deployment flowchart
- Value stream mapping (see Chapter Two Action Guide)

Process mapping creates a picture of the sequence of steps in a process, which helps identify the current state (of how the work of care and service delivery occurs in daily health care delivery) and helps plan improvement actions. The step-by-step pictures can illustrate waste, delays, and missteps in the process being studied. It is also helpful to use flowcharts to build consensus with an interdisciplinary group, to correct misunderstandings of the process, and to build common understanding. Different steps of the process are represented by boxes or other symbols on the flowchart.

An important reminder when starting improvement is to always flowchart the current process (not what one wishes or thinks it is). It is always wise to observe the process directly to match the conceptual flowchart made by an interdisciplinary group with the real process to identify inconsistencies. It is not uncommon to find in the process flowchart missing steps, extra steps, evidence of previously unknown work-arounds staff have created to deal with broken systems, disagreement amongst the interdisciplinary group on how the process works, and a tendency to draw the ideal version of the process flow. Observing the actual process after creation of the first draft process map is helpful to clarify the current process steps and then move to design the ideal process to test and measure to determine if the perceived ideal process creates better outcomes for patients and staff. Having members of the interdisciplinary group participate in the observation can often be enlightening for the individuals to gain further insights into the improvement process. Additionally, when creating a flowchart,

FIGURE AG5.1   High-Level Flowchart.

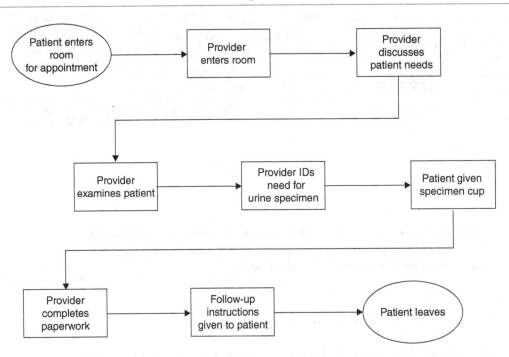

label it as a *draft* and post it for all staff to review and comment on, thereby engaging more staff in the improvement process, further identifying current state variation among interdisciplinary members, increasing awareness of the need to make improvements, and attracting more energy and interest to engage in improvement.

Processes of a clinical microsystem can be documented and studied as a high-level flowchart to provide an overview of the process (see Figure AG5.1).

High-level clinical microsystem process flowcharts can have additional detail added to the steps (or drill down in each high-level step) of high-level actions to result in a more detailed flowchart filled with important steps of the process (see Figure AG5.2).

The steps to create a flowchart include being very clear about the beginning and end of the process to be mapped. You must be able to state, "The process begins with _____" and "The process ends with _____." Remember this important aspect of the global aim statement in which you determined the aim of the improvement actions with a clear beginning and end of the process to be improved. To show all steps of the process, ask the following questions:

*What happens next?*
*And then what happens?*
*And then what happens?*

During this series of questions and responses by interdisciplinary members disagreements can occur on specific steps in the process. It is often helpful to document all versions being described by the members with the understanding the observation phase will help clarify what the current process is. The group may discover there are multiple versions of the current process during the observation phase. The variation that is discovered can be used to stimulate discussion about waste and unreliability that exists within the current process. A few examples of waste are:

FIGURE AG5.2    Drill Down Flowchart.

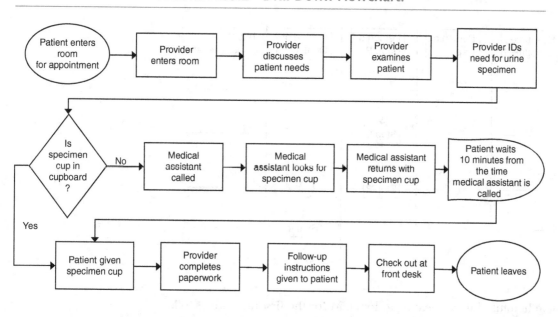

FIGURE AG5.3    Flowchart Symbol Key.

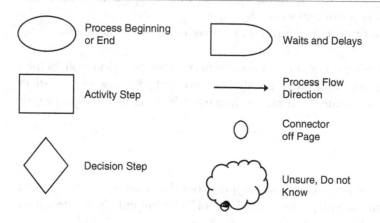

- Waiting for patients to arrive for an appointment
- Waiting for diagnostic test results
- Missing equipment and supplies
- Interruptions during a process resulting in rework or errors
- Hunting and gathering supplies and materials needed for patient care

The variation often leads to frustration among clinical microsystem members and unreliable outcomes of the process. Standardization of processes is the foundation for continuous improvement. When a process is carried out in the same way every time, new knowledge and insights to design an even better process can be discovered. Today's standardization leads to tomorrow's innovation.

Use the basic flowchart symbols depicted in Figure AG5.3 when constructing your flowchart.

**FIGURE AG5.4   Deployment Flow Diagram.**

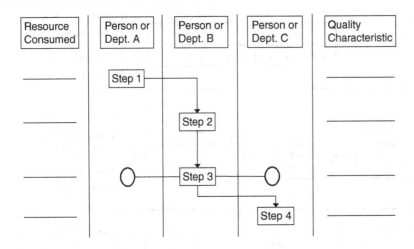

Some helpful hints in creating a flowchart for the first time are as follows:

- Determine the beginning and end of the process to be improved.
- Make a list of steps from start to finish by asking what happens first, then what happens, then what happens and so on.
- Turn the list of steps from start to finish into a flowchart using the symbols.

Some have found using sticky notes to document one step per sticky note helpful to then post on a flipchart; this makes it possible to move and add steps with the sticky notes. Others are able to create the flowchart immediately using the symbols directly on flipchart paper.

## Deployment Charts

Deployment charts are a type of process mapping tool that documents the process across roles or departments. This process mapping tool is very helpful when redesigning processes to optimize roles.

As shown in Figure AG5.4, the process of interest is drawn across roles or departments. If the action steps affect multiple people, the circle is drawn with a connector to show the multiple players for one step.

An example of a deployment flowchart (Figure AG5.5) shows each person's role and function during a patient's initial visit to a primary care physician's office.

# ACCESS MEASURES AND TOOLS

Access to a microsystem exactly when the patient wants it and needs it is a challenge in many health care settings. Timing and availability of services must be managed to ensure the right care is delivered at the right time by the right person, whether that care is delivered by a primary care provider, a medical specialist, or involves transfer from an intensive care unit to a medical unit bed.

## Initial Visit, Work-Up, and Plan of Care

**Aim**: To assess an individual patient's need and creating a plan for care
**Boundaries**: From the time an individual patient presents for the first visit to when the patient's symptoms
have been addressed and a care plan has been established

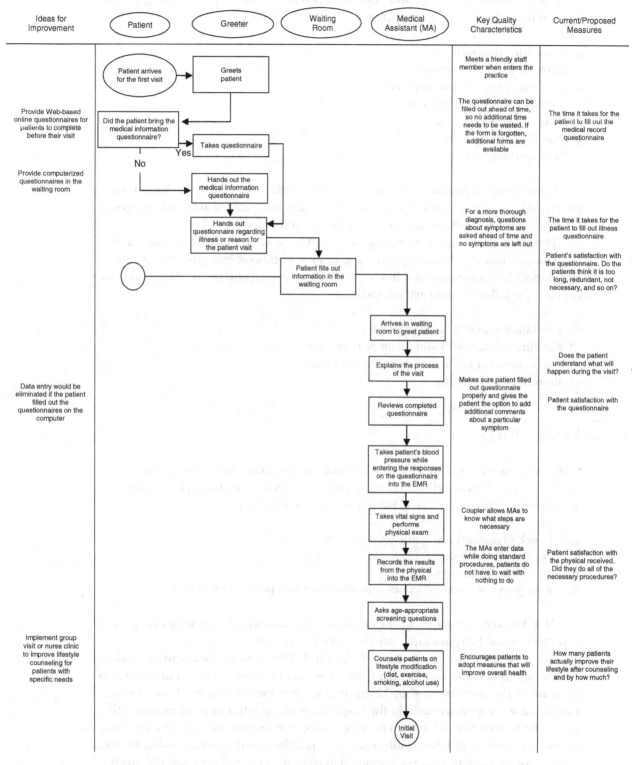

*Source:* Used with permission, Charlie Burger, MD, Norumbega Medical.
*Note:* EMR = electronic medical record.

Three helpful workbooks can be found at www.clinicalmicrosystem.org. The first two are *VHA Advanced Clinic Access* and *Improving Patient Access to Care*. These workbooks follow the Mark Murray and Catherine Tantau approach and offer many tools and worksheets to measure, assess, and improve access to care and services. The approach is based upon the following principles:

- Know your demand
- Know your practice capacity
- Shape and reduce your demand
- Increase your supply capacity
- Work down the backlog
- Plan for contingencies
- Redesign your system

In addition, the *Improving Patient Access to Care* workbook includes sections on measuring and monitoring access, tips for communication with patients and families, special considerations, leadership suggestions, and access resources.

The third workbook is *Measuring Access Improvement*. Mark Murray states in the introduction that the *Measuring Access Improvement* workbook gives the ship a rudder and shows what to measure and how to measure access improvement.[1] The workbook contains the following information and tools:

1. Introduction and general principles
2. Measures to start with and measure over time
3. Recommended maintenance and monitoring
4. Resources and reading

## CARE VITAL SIGNS

CARE Vital Signs is a manual worksheet tool for collecting useful information from patients and families that can be used to guide clinical actions and care planning during an office visit. The mnemonic CARE represents the following:

**C**    Check what matters to patients.
**A**    Act on the assessment.
**R**    Reinforce the actions.
**E**    reEngineer or build processes into staff roles and practice processes.

This low-tech method helps health care professionals gain insights into patient expectations and helps patients state their needs and expectations.[1]

Figure AG5.6 illustrates the front of the *CARE Vital Signs* worksheet where patient information is documented including what the patient wants to discuss or expects to be done at the ambulatory visit. Measures and questions you might find around a patient value compass are listed in the first column along with ranges of measures that should be further assessed and taken action on in the second column. The reinforce actions are listed as Web-based information or practice-based standing orders to plan the care for the patient. After considering staff roles and current processes, the practice processes could be re-engineered to build more standard practices and processes into

FIGURE AG5.6   CARE Vital Signs Page 1.

## CARE Vital Signs (For Adults Aged 19+)

Patient Name:_____   Date: _____   ID #: _____

What does patient want to discuss or expect to be done at this visit? _____
_____

| Measure or Question | Clinical Flag (Circle when noted) | Planned Care Standing Order | |
|---|---|---|---|
| | | Web-Based* | Practice-Based** |
| Height _____ BMI ____  Weight _____ | BMI 25 -30 → BMI 30+ → | *Exercise/Eating HYH* and diet evaluation | |
| BP ___/___ | >140/80 → <100/60 → | *Common Medical HYH* ------------- | |
| Pulse _____  RR _____ | <50; >100; irreg short of breath | ------------- ------------- | |
| Any of the following:  • Hypertension • Cardiac/Vascular Disease • Diabetes • Lung Problems/Asthma | Any concerns: _____ _____ _____ Or no previous use HYH Condition Form | Use www. howsyourhealth for condition management  *Common Medical HYH* | |
| Feeling Score (see reverse) | 4 or 5 → | *Feelings/emotion HYH* Evaluation | Phone follow-up for patients with emotion |
| Pain Score (see reverse) | 4 or 5 → | *Pain HYH* Evaluation | Phone follow-up for patients with pain |
| Pills making ill? (Yes, no, maybe, not taking) | yes or maybe | *Common Medical HYH* | |
| Not Good Health Habits (see reverse) | 4 or 5 → | *Health Habits HYH* | |
| Any other questions here** | | | |
| | | | |

**Patient Instructions:** Any checks or circles above? Go to the Web site before our next visit or phone contact.

Prevention: Circle if not completed.

| | 19-49 | 50-69 | 70+ |
|---|---|---|---|
| Female Only** | | | |
| Male Only** | | | |
| Both** | | | |

** Criteria to be completed by the office.

When instructed for the reasons listed above, OR for a general health check-up OR the HYH Chapters OR other special forms recommended by the office, go to **www.howsyourhealth.org** and type in _____ when you are asked for your passcode.

*Source:* Wasson, J., & Bartels, S. Care vital signs supports patient-centered, collaborative care. *Journal of Ambulatory Care Management,* 2009, *32*(1), 56–71.

| Height in Shoes | Weight Range "Normal"* | BMI 30+ Seriously Overweight |
|---|---|---|
| 4'10" | 91–119 | 145 |
| 4'11" | 94–124 | 150 |
| 5' | 97–128 | 156 |
| 5'1" | 101–132 | 162 |
| 5'2" | 104–137 | 167 |
| 5'3" | 107–141 | 173 |
| 5'4" | 111–146 | 179 |
| 5'5" | 114–150 | 184 |
| 5'6" | 118–155 | 190 |
| 5'7" | 121–160 | 195 |
| 5'8" | 125–164 | 200 |
| 5'9" | 129–169 | 206 |
| 5'10" | 132–174 | 212 |
| 5'11" | 136–179 | 217 |
| 6' | 140–184 | 223 |
| 6'1" | 144–189 | 229 |
| 6'2" | 148–195 | 234 |
| 6'3" | 152–200 | 240 |
| 6'4" | 156–205 | 245 |
| 6'5" | 160–211 | 250 |
| 6'6" | 164–216 | 255 |

*(BMI 25–29 "overweight" is between upper range of normal and BMI 30+ "seriously overweight")

## PAIN

During the past 4 weeks . . .
How much bodily pain have you generally had ?

| | | |
|---|---|---|
| No pain | | 1 |
| Very mild pain | | 2 |
| Mild pain | | 3 |
| Moderate pain | | 4 |
| Severe pain | | 5 |

COPYRIGHT © TRUSTEES OF DARTMOUTH COLLEGE/COOP PROJECT 1988
SUPPORT PROVIDED BY THE HENRY J. KAISER FAMILY FOUNDATION

## FEELINGS

During the past 4 weeks . . .
How much have you been bothered by emotional problems such as feeling anxious, depressed, irritable or downhearted and blue ?

| | | |
|---|---|---|
| Not at all | | 1 |
| Slightly | | 2 |
| Moderately | | 3 |
| Quite a bit | | 4 |
| Extremely | | 5 |

COPYRIGHT © TRUSTEES OF DARTMOUTH COLLEGE/COOP PROJECT 1988
SUPPORT PROVIDED BY THE HENRY J. KAISER FAMILY FOUNDATION

2

## HEALTH HABITS

During the past month, how often did you practice good health habits such as; using a seat belt, getting exercise, eating right, getting enough sleep or wearing safety helmets?

| | | |
|---|---|---|
| All of the time | | 1 |
| Most of the time | | 2 |
| Some of the time | | 3 |
| A little of the time | | 4 |
| None of the time | | 5 |

COPYRIGHT © TRUSTEES OF DARTMOUTH COLLEGE COOP PROJECT 1990
SUPPORT PROVIDED BY THE HENRY J. KAISER FAMILY FOUNDATION AND THE W.T. GRANT FOUNDATION

Source: Wasson, J., & Bartels, S. Care vital signs supports patient-centered, collaborative care. Journal of Ambulatory Care Management, 2009, 32(1), 56–71.

the care. The back of the *CARE Vital Signs* worksheet (Figure AG5.7) has helpful visual assessment tools to enable the patient to report on pain, feelings, and health habits.

Additionally, the CARE Vital Signs worksheet helps activate practice staff members when patient needs are identified. For example, protocols, self-management skills, and education can be initiated by frontline staff in real time as triggered by the screening worksheet. The screening categories include patient confidence in self-management, pain, medications, emotional issues, general health habits, and obesity. For additional information see, *CARE Vital Signs Supports Patient-Centered, Collaborative Care.*[1]

## REFERENCE

1. Godfrey, M., Patric, V. *Measuring Access Improvement.* Dartmouth College, Hanover, NH, 2002.
2. Wasson, J., & Bartels, S. Care vital signs supports patient-centered, collaborative care. *Journal of Ambulatory Care Management,* 2009, *32*(1), 56–71.

# CHAPTER 6

# DESIGNING PREVENTIVE CARE TO IMPROVE HEALTH

Joel S. Lazar

Paul B. Batalden

Marjorie M. Godfrey

Eugene C. Nelson

## LEARNING OBJECTIVES

- Define preventive care from the patient and microsystem perspective.
- Describe the four domains of care and how they are similar or different.
- Compare and contrast traditional prevention categories with action prevention domains.
- Describe the *Clinical Improvement Equation* and its implications for health care improvement.

Preventable illnesses account for half of our nation's deaths each year and for significantly more than half of our health care costs. The work of preventive care begins with thoughtful microsystem attention to patients' needs for proactive assessment and mitigation of health risks. Specific design strategies can then be used to plan, implement, and monitor the delivery of preventive services. In this chapter we first review an illustrative case study that reveals both the scope and the challenge of preventive care in frontline clinical microsystems. We next consider an action-based taxonomy of services to guide microsystems in planning appropriate care. Finally, we explore general and specific design principles that support successful implementation of preventive services and that generate lasting value through better health outcomes and lower health-related costs.

## THE WORK OF PREVENTIVE HEALTH CARE

When Iowa Senator Tom Harkin asserted in 2005 that "America's health care system is in crisis precisely because we systematically neglect wellness and prevention,"[1] he underscored the challenges and the opportunities of preventive health care. Approximately half the deaths in our country each year are due to preventable causes,[2] and far more than half of our nation's health care dollars are spent too late to manage injuries and chronic illnesses that earlier, anticipatory care could have prevented or mitigated.[3,4] These unfortunate data are all the more compelling because our collective deficiency is due not to lack of basic scientific knowledge (evidence in support of many specific preventive interventions is both broad and deep), but to inadequate systems to enable application of this knowledge. But here lies a great opportunity as well: as our knowledge and improvement of clinical microsystems grows, our ability to provide effective preventive care is likewise strengthened. In this chapter we draw attention to principles, planning, practices, and actual clinical experiences that support risk reduction at the front line of care. Through reflection on the daily work of clinical microsystems, the services Harkin identified as systematically neglected[1] can be effectively reprioritized.

*Preventive care* can be understood broadly as the full set of interventions and interactions that support proactive assessment and mitigation of health risks, before these risks progress to clinical illness or injury. *Preventive health interventions* are sometimes clustered intentionally in annual wellness exams (at which time, for example, scheduled immunizations may be administered or cancer screening exams performed). This care may also be incorporated opportunistically into clinical encounters whose original purpose was not specifically preventive (for example, when tobacco cessation counseling is offered to a smoker who presents with acute bronchitis). Prevention work occurs regularly in non-primary care settings as well (as when surgical teams complete pre-procedural checklists to assess and to mitigate risk of adverse surgical outcomes). Finally, many preventive behaviors of the microsystem are directed not toward patients at all, but toward the microsystem itself, through planned safety efforts that indirectly promote patient wellness by targeting health care-induced risk. For example, staff hand hygiene campaigns prevent patient infections in both inpatient and outpatient settings.

A list of preventive care activities appropriate to specific age-groups and to hospital and nursing home patients, is provided in Table 6.1. Note that preventive services in each age or population subgroup feature unique combinations of screening studies, behavioral counseling, and physical or pharmacologic interventions (for example, immunizations, prophylactic medications, and environmental changes). Later in this chapter, we consider these action domains in greater detail.

### Table 6.1    Sample List of Preventive Care Activities

**Infants and Children**
- Screen for congenital metabolic abnormalities (hemoglobinopathies, PKU).
- Vaccinate for preventable illnesses (DTaP, MMR, Polio, HiB).
- Screen for cardiac, growth, and cognitive-behavioral abnormalities.
- Assess feeding practices and counsel regarding breast-feeding and baby bottle tooth decay.
- Assess and counsel children regarding physical activity and healthy diets.
- Assess parent safety practices, including car seats, bicycle helmets, and poison control.

**Adolescents**
Review safety practices for infants and children. Focus also on the following preventive practices:
- Screen for tobacco use and provide tobacco cessation counseling.
- Screen for problem drinking and provide counseling.
- Screen for sexually transmitted diseases and provide counseling.
- Assess and counsel regarding exercise and healthy diets.
- Screen for obesity, glucose intolerance, and hypertension.

**Adults**
Assess and counsel for high-risk health behaviors (including tobacco, alcohol, and drug use) and review safety practices (including use of seatbelts and helmets and storage of firearms). Focus also on the following preventive practices:
- Screen women for cervical and breast cancer and also for osteoporosis (depending on age and risks).
- Screen men and women (age greater than 50) for colon cancer.
- Screen male smokers (age greater than 65) for aortic aneurysm.
- Vaccinate adults against influenza and (if age greater than 65) pneumococcal pneumonia.

**Hospitalized or Institutionalized Adults**
- Prophylax against deep vein thrombosis using heparin or compression stockings.
- Prophylax against gastritis or stress-induced gastrointestinal ulcer.
- Provide appropriate antibiotics prior to surgery.
- Routinely adjust position of bed-bound patients to minimize pressure-induced skin ulcers.
- Assess nutritional status and optimize nutrient balance.
- Implement staff hand hygiene practices for all staff.
- Review patient medication and allergy lists on a regular basis.
- Use pre-procedural checklists for all patients undergoing surgery.
- Standardize handoff protocols for blood products (transfusions).
- Standardize patient identification protocols to match individuals with interventions.

As these varied examples suggest, the microsystem's essential first function when planning for preventive health interventions, and when planning for frontline care improvements more generally, is to focus less on predefined specific *visit types* such as the annual health exam (although this may often be the setting for such care), *and more on the context-specific needs of patients and families themselves.* These needs are of course diverse, but can be broadly categorized, as shown in Table 6.2. This table provides not a provider-focused taxonomy of services already in place, but a patient-focused framework for development of new services. This framework provides a standard with which to judge success of continuous improvement work. By maintaining our focus on the needs of patients and on the actual work required to meet these needs, we validate the reality of clinical care as experienced by both patients and practitioners; we recognize that, in actual practice, the boundaries between *preventive, acute, chronic,* and *palliative care* domains are permeable to varying degrees. For example, screening a diabetic patient's retina could be classified as both preventive care *and* chronic care. We are empowered, in effect, to align microsystem resources with patients' expressed priorities.

Table 6.2    Overarching Care Needs of Patient and Family

| | |
|---|---|
| **Preventive care** | • Proactive assessment and mitigation of health risks |
| **Acute care** | • Timely attention to new or newly worsening disruption of health or function |
| **Chronic care** | • Longitudinal resiliency and support in self-management of ongoing disease |
| **Palliative care** | • Comfort and dignity in the context of underlying disease progression |

Thus, as Table 6.2 suggests, when the clinical team directs its attention to preventive care, its members are in fact asking the specific questions: "How do we meet the needs of patient and family for proactive assessment and mitigation of health risks?" "How do we anticipate and identify such risks, and how do we minimize their potential adverse impact on both individual patients and entire populations?" An illustrative case study follows to facilitate our exploration of these questions.

## CASE STUDY: THE SCOPE AND CHALLENGE OF PREVENTIVE CARE

Consider Peter Manson, a 64-year-old carpenter who rarely seeks medical attention. On one notable occasion, however, he does present to his primary care physician for assessment of fever and sore throat. At this visit his blood pressure is elevated to 160/90, as was also the case two years ago. His weight is significantly higher than the ideal range, and he continues to smoke one pack of cigarettes per day. He takes no regular medications, and he confirms (when questioned by the nurse during prescreening) that he has no allergies to medications. A throat swab is performed that confirms strep throat, and he is prescribed an appropriate dose of penicillin. Because his well-intended but very busy physician is running behind schedule on this day, no notice is made of last year's elevated serum cholesterol level in Peter's chart. (Elevated serum cholesterol levels, along with high blood pressure, obesity, and tobacco use, increase Peter's cardiovascular risk.) The physician also fails to note Peter's positive family history of colon cancer.

Now consider Peter's next encounter with the health care system, which unfortunately does not occur until two years later, when (even more unfortunately) he is admitted to the local hospital with acute myocardial infarction. He is given a baby aspirin at time of presentation, and other cardiac medications are prescribed prior to his eventual discharge. His hospitalization is prolonged, however, due to recurring chest pain, and he must spend a few days in the intensive care unit (ICU). The stress of this ICU stay provokes gastrointestinal bleeding due to a stress ulcer, and Peter requires a transfusion with two units of red blood cells to maintain his hemoglobin level. His situation stabilizes, and prior to hospital discharge he is visited by a nurse who initiates motivational interviewing to support tobacco cessation. Peter is scheduled for follow-up with his primary care clinician one week after discharge, to check on new symptoms, to monitor the new medications, and to pursue the discussion about quitting cigarettes.

The astute reader will recognize multiple opportunities in this case study for each clinical microsystem to proactively assess and perform preventive health interventions specific to the needs of *this* unique patient. Some of these opportunities were successfully realized and executed. For example, the nurse reviewed medication allergies prior to physician's penicillin prescription; cardiac medications were ordered in the emergency department and at time of hospital discharge; transfused blood was screened for blood-borne pathogens; and tobacco cessation counseling was initiated. Other opportunities were missed, such as the failed early correction of Peter's elevated blood pressure; the lack of anticipatory guidance (at time of his strep throat visit) regarding tobacco use and obesity; and the absence of prophylactic anti-acid therapy in a stressed ICU patient, where gastrointestinal bleeding occurs fairly commonly. Often, the same clinical microsystem will successfully anticipate and proactively respond to certain risks, although other risks are not adequately considered. The features that distinguish success from failure are often not practitioners' level of academic knowledge (in evidence-based guidelines), but the microsystem's capacity to perform risk assessment, to align planned interventions with the risks identified, and to actually implement frontline process improvements in the delivery of care.

These functions are important at the level of individual care and also at the level of entire populations. As mentioned in this chapter's introduction, approximately half of our nation's two million deaths each year are from preventable causes.[3] The majority of these deaths are due to high-risk behaviors such as tobacco abuse, poor diet, and inadequate exercise, problems that all respond to clinical (prevention-focused) intervention.[5] Also preventable, as reviewed in Chapter Three, are the nearly 100,000 annual deaths caused by medical errors and environmental hazards within the health care system itself.[6]

These are staggering statistics, especially when we consider the wealth of knowledge and resources already available to reduce the burden of collective disease. But this knowledge is imperfectly applied. In McGlynn's[7] 2003 large review of several thousand patients' medical records, the U.S. health care system provided only 55 percent of recommended preventive health interventions to eligible adults. Consider the impact of these missed opportunities for primary, secondary, and tertiary prevention.[3]

- *Primary prevention* (Prophylaxis before disease occurs): For example, we know that pneumococcal vaccine (Pneumovax) can save 10,000 lives per year, yet only 64 percent of eligible elders are offered this immunization.
- *Secondary prevention* (Screening before disease causes symptoms): For example, we know that colon cancer screening can prevent 9,600 deaths per year, yet only 38 percent of eligible persons are offered this screening study.
- *Tertiary prevention* (Treatment before disease causes more damage): For example, we know that aspirin administration after myocardial infarction (MI) reduces vascular deaths by 15 percent and recurrent infarction by 30 percent, yet only 61 percent of MI survivors receive this medication.

Of course, these missed opportunities are not perpetrated by uncaring or unskilled health professionals. Risk mitigation is a goal shared by all. But, as Batalden has succinctly expressed, "every system *is* perfectly designed to get the results it gets,"[8] and too often we have unwittingly designed health care (again, in Senator Harkin's words) to "systematically neglect" preventive care.[1] At the macrosystem level, short-term financial incentives remain aligned with high technology illness-based interventions, rather than with lower tech wellness-based services whose *return on investment*, although great, may be delayed by many years. Despite the collective health burden attributable to preventable illness and the substantial cost savings that can be realized by addressing health risks *prior to* development of actual illness, only 3 percent of U.S. health expenditures are allocated to preventive care.[9] Effective prevention is an essential priority for clinical systems if they are to deliver high value care.

## AN ACTION-BASED TAXONOMY OF PREVENTIVE HEALTH SERVICES

In the section titled "The Work of Preventive Health Care" we have introduced the traditional categories of primary, secondary, and tertiary prevention. This parsing has the advantage of broad understanding across multiple professional domains and points to a common language shared by clinicians, public health officials, and researchers. But there is also an arbitrary dimension to this taxonomy, which, in the end, is defined only in relative terms; it is unclear whether this traditional language actually facilitates microsystems' planning for frontline preventive care services. When, for example, does blood pressure control switch from a secondary to a tertiary prevention modality? Is dietary counseling a form of primary, secondary, or tertiary preventive care (or all of the above), and in which context? And do these distinctions add any real value from the patient's perspective?

Indeed, at the level of frontline care planning and systematic process improvement, categorical models prove valuable only insofar as they specify and support precise actions. Who on the interdisciplinary team does what? Are the processes standardized and known by all? If the goal of categorizing preventive services is to facilitate their planning and execution (regardless of primary, secondary, or tertiary status), then a more action-based taxonomy is required. We thus suggest that, at the broadest level, the work of preventive care may be divided into the following three *activity* domains:

1. *Screening* to identify silent risks before they produce clinical illness. Examples include: cholesterol testing to stratify cardiac risk; colonoscopy to identify cancerous or pre-cancerous colon tumors.
2. *Behavioral modifications* and *clinical interventions* to prevent risk development or to mitigate risk progression. Examples include: tobacco cessation counseling to reduce risk of lung disease or cancer; blood pressure medications to prevent future stroke or myocardial infarction; dynamic pressure redistribution mattresses to prevent skin ulcers in frail bedbound patients.
3. *System modifications* to anticipate and diminish iatrogenic (health care-imposed) risks. Examples include: hand hygiene protocols to minimize spread of infection; perioperative surgical checklists and protocols to assure proper patient identification and standardization of procedures.

Once these conceptual domains are recognized, many precise forms of clinical intervention fall naturally into each category. Thus, Table 6.3 provides a sample list of *screening activities* (history taking, laboratory, imaging), *clinical interventions* (counseling, immunizations, medications, environmental modifications), and *system safety modifications* (error-proofing, checklists, forcing functions that compel safety behaviors through physical design, and failure modes and effects analysis, discussed in Chapter Three). Clinical microsystems can use this list to effectively plan and implement in appropriate contexts, based on the anticipated risks of individuals and populations and on the resources of the microsystem itself. Moreover, as suggested in the chapter's opening paragraphs, this list also highlights the diversity of microsystem *settings* (both primary and specialty care, both medical and surgical practice, both outpatient and inpatient) where preventive care systems are prioritized and enacted.

Once we categorize preventive health services in this action-based manner, members of the clinical microsystem are poised to ask operational questions that drive implemen-

**Table 6.3    An Action-Based Taxonomy of Preventive Health Care**

| Preventive Health Action | | Primary Care | Medical and Surgical Specialty Care |
|---|---|---|---|
| Screening *to identify personal risk or asymptomatic disease* | History and exam | • Assess health risk behaviors<br>• Screen blood pressure | • Assess bleeding history prior to surgery |
| | Laboratory | • Monitor cholesterol<br>• Take PAP smears<br>• Screen for sexually transmitted disease | • Screen blood sample to identify hepatitis virus or HIV |
| | Imaging | • Mammography<br>• Colonoscopy | • Preoperative cardiac testing |
| Clinical interventions *to mitigate personal risk or to prevent disease progression* | Behavioral (counseling or coaching) | • Counseling on exercise, diet, and home safety<br>• Tobacco cessation | • Strengthening exercises prior to elective orthopedic surgery |
| | Immunizations | • Routine childhood and adult immunizations | • Special vaccinations for splenectomized patients or for those who will be traveling abroad |
| | Medications | • Baby aspirin, cholesterol-reducing medications to prevent cardiac disease | • Antibiotics prior to surgery<br>• Deep venous thrombosis (DVT) prophylaxis |
| | Surgical | • Excision of skin lesions with malignant potential | • Prophylactic mastectomy in women at very high risk of breast cancer |
| | Environmental | • Hazard reduction in the home to reduce fall risk | • Modification of the workplace to reduce needlestick injuries or exposure to toxic fumes |
| System safety features *to mitigate iatrogenic risk system safety features?* | Forcing functions | • Computer-prompted review of medication and allergy lists | • Patient-identifying wrist bracelets |
| | Checklists | • Age-specific screening checklists | • Perioperative surgical checklists |
| | Handoffs | • Tracking referrals to assure completion of referral process with patient being seen | • Blood product delivery from blood bank to bedside |

tation of actual caregiving processes and behaviors. As we asked above, who on the interdisciplinary team does what? Do all participants understand their roles? When patients' preventive needs have been translated into general and then into more specific *activities,* discrete tasks can be identified, owned, and executed by specific microsystem members. Do all members of the microsystem function at the highest possible level in their role, based on education, training, and licensure? Peter in our previous case study needs to stop his tobacco use, and multiple microsystem members can help him to achieve this goal: a medical assistant can implement routine screening to identify all patients in the practice who smoke (including Peter); a nurse educator can assess Peter's readiness for change and can counsel him on available options for cessation; and the physician can reiterate the value of tobacco cessation and can prescribe medications that support this important preventive goal.

## Principles for Designing and Improving Preventive Health Care in Clinical Microsystems

Having explored the breadth of opportunities and challenges in preventive care, and having considered a taxonomy of needs and services that corresponds to necessary actions at the front line of care, how *does* the well-functioning clinical microsystem meet the needs of patients and families for proactive assessment and mitigation of health risks? Given the diversity of patients' needs, and given the equal diversity of clinical settings in which such needs may arise (primary and specialty care, medical and surgical practice, outpatient and inpatient), what general principles may inform the planning and implementation of specific evidence-based preventive health interventions? What microsystem processes support optimal delivery of preventive care that is safe, timely, effective, efficient, equitable, and patient-centered?[10]

At a conceptual level, the essential prevention work of every clinical microsystem includes the following general tasks:

- Understanding populations
- Understanding individual patients
- Linking available information (of the patient, of the microsystem, and from the professional literature) with value-based actions
- Building reliability when screening for potential risks
- Building respect and positive relations when coordinating roles and responsibilities with interdisciplinary clinical colleagues and when coaching patients to make behavioral changes
- Assessing and designing local processes and systems to support role optimization, efficiency, and clinical vigilance

When planning for highest quality preventive care (as well as for acute, chronic, and palliative care), clinical microsystems must first understand the demographic, socioeconomic, and medical characteristics of the populations they serve. This essential information directs professional attention to local health risks and to appropriate risk reduction in both individuals and communities. Of course, *individual* and *community* are not one and the same. From a planning perspective, knowledge of *collective* risk is imperative, as this knowledge of risk guides resource allocation and informs care algorithm development. But in the end, as every good clinician is aware, full understanding of risk also incorporates awareness of the unique needs and preferences of this unique patient who is in the room, on the phone, or at the other end of an e-mail. It is here at the interface of general and specific knowledge that best care actually occurs.

This principle also applies when caregivers transition from gathering knowledge to making interventions. In order to link available information with value-based action, effective microsystems must have skill and capacity to perform both generalizable (replicable, algorithm-driven) and individualized interventions. When specific preventive care needs are simple or "merely complicated,"[11] to borrow Glouberman and

Zimmerman's term, then microsystems must prioritize *reliability* to maximize efficiency and effectiveness and to minimize errors of both omission and commission.[12] This is the case when monitoring for routine childhood immunizations; only rarely will such a recommendation be inappropriate, so standardized algorithms will promote consistent implementation. Another example of algorithmic preventive care occurs in the mammography microsystem as depicted in Chapter Six Action Guide.

But when preventive care tasks are more complex, as for example when counseling a heavy alcohol user to reduce consumption, then attention to respectful relationships may have greater clinical importance than procedural reliability. This notion of complexity is elaborated in Chapter Eight.

## The Clinical Improvement Equation

Attention to both generality and specificity and to both knowledge and intervention suggests a specific application of Batalden and Davidoff's *Clinical Improvement Equation*,[13,14] which integrates caregivers' knowledge of generalizable scientific evidence within the context of unique clinical practice environments and activities. Because this integration is so essential to the design and improvement of preventive care services, we shall briefly review the equation's essential features and then explore design implications and applications at the front line of care.

Consider the Clinical Improvement Equation's general form:

$$\text{Generalizable Scientific Knowledge} + \text{Particular Context} \rightarrow$$
$$\text{Measured Performance Improvement}$$

This construction appears at first glance to be naively simplistic, but closer inspection reveals it builds upon complex and interdependent systems of knowledge. Indeed, as Figures 6.1 and 6.2 suggest, not only the textual elements of this equation, but also

FIGURE 6.1   Clinical Improvement Equation.

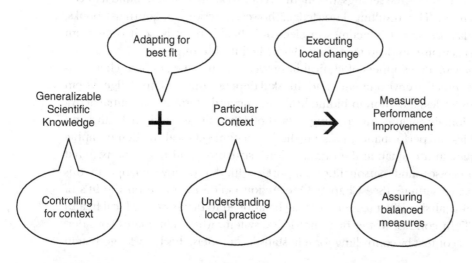

**Bringing Generalizable Scientific Evidence to Specific Contexts**

FIGURE 6.2    Knowledge Elements in Clinical Improvement.

| Generalizable Scientific Evidence | + | Particular Context | → | Measured Performance Improvement |
|---|---|---|---|---|
| Locating, acquiring, and evaluating new knowledge | Adapting evidence and redesigning practices | Characterizing practice environments | Executing changes | Measuring provider and system performance |
| Knowing how to: | Knowing how to: | Knowing how to: | Knowing how to: | Knowing how to: |
| ➤ Define well-formulated, answerable questions ➤ Identify or select good information sources, helpful reference librarians ➤ Critically appraise retrieved studies and summaries of evidence | ➤ Formulate clear improvement aims ➤ Identify alternative methods ➤ Assess benefit or compatibility ➤ Select the best fit | ➤ Evaluate individual patients and patient groups ➤ Assess current systems and processes ➤ Understand successful changes in the context ➤ Recognize local culture: what matters to people who work here | ➤ Identify and connect with what is strategically important for the future of the setting ➤ Discern the ways things work and regularly get done locally ➤ Attract and work interdependently with others in this setting ➤ Recognize and honor good work ➤ Foster the unlearning necessary to change | ➤ Design and interpret balanced measures of outcome ➤ Use self-assessment ➤ Measure and interpret performance over time, using statistical process control and graphic displays |

its syntactic connectors (the "+" and "→" signs) embed operational tasks and depend upon cognitive skills. A brief consideration of these separate functions will support our subsequent exploration of prevention-specific microsystem improvements.

The Clinical Improvement Equation can be further understood as follows:

- *Generalizable scientific knowledge.* The essential function here is locating, acquiring, and evaluating biomedical knowledge. Practitioners of clinical improvement must be skilled in forming answerable questions, retrieving and prioritizing information through Boolean searches, critically appraising retrieved studies, and interpreting the use of analytic techniques. Clinician-scientists navigate this system of knowledge with relative comfort, as it adapts the familiar methodologies of academic medicine and engages the traditional information base of biomedical literature. By testing hypotheses in context-free settings, the methods of this analytic system build a necessary foundation. The resulting knowledge, however, resides in journals, books, electronic databases, and sometimes in electronic health records, so it is far from sufficient to actualize improvement in real-world clinical settings.

- *Particular context.* Practitioners of clinical improvement must be adept at characterizing unique practice environments, and this skill depends upon a knowledge system that receives far less attention in biomedical training and literature. Essential activities in this domain include interpreting data (both quantitative and qualitative) on local priorities and performance, assessing the population's clinical and demographic characteristics, and evaluating the organization's structures and interactions. What patterns, processes, and personalities support or hinder positive change in this unique practice setting? (See Chapter One Action Guide for more on the 5Ps of microsystem analysis.) What techniques may be applied to diagnose the local health system itself? In contrast to the first knowledge system, which eliminates consideration of local context by controlling for it in statistical models, this knowledge system focuses sharply on the particular setting and all that contributes to its special identity.

- *The "+" sign.* The acquisition of generalizable scientific knowledge and particular context information does not assure that these separate forms of knowledge shall be successfully integrated. An additional bridging domain of knowledge supports adapting evidence and redesigning practices. Effective leaders of change know how to assess innovations for compatibility with the current system, design and sequence specific care algorithms to match locally available resources, and manage conflict and negotiation in the context of unique practice histories.

- *The "→" sign.* Once we bridge the general and the specific to identify strategies for local change that are grounded in scientific evidence, yet another domain of expertise is required to support executing changes. Masters of continuous quality improvement are skilled in effective communication, in articulating a vision that compels group coherence, in supporting staff during stressful transitions, and in sustaining and embedding strategies for long-term development. This knowledge system links strategic planning with human resource management to make things really happen in *this* particular place.

- *Measured performance improvement.* Successful improvement over time depends upon reliable and recurrent measuring of provider and system performance. This method of measurement preserves time as a variable and seeks direct insight into the quality of results as these vary over time. As discussed in Chapter Four, use of statistical process control charts, graphical displays, patient value compasses, and balanced scorecards ensure that all outcome perspectives are considered. Other clinical assessment tools provide not only feedback data on improvement trends, but also feed forward information to facilitate point-of-care improvement in real-time practice.

## Specific Questions to Support the Design and Improvement of Preventive Care

From the general principles suggested by the Clinical Improvement Equation, a more specific series of prevention-focused design questions can be derived. These questions and pertinent subquestions are depicted in Table 6.4. As the clinical microsystem reflects upon each of these items in turn, unique preventive care interventions are developed, or improvements are made, that integrate best evidence-based knowledge from the scientific literature with best localized knowledge from unique patients, populations, and the microsystem itself.

Interdisciplinary members of the clinical microsystem are encouraged to meet on a regular basis to discuss care and service delivery, safety, improvement, value, and outcomes of care and processes. Over a series of such meetings the group reflects upon its 5Ps (Purpose, Patients, Professionals, Processes, and Patterns), as detailed in Chapter One Action Guide. When comfortable with these building blocks of its own self-knowledge, the microsystem is prepared to ask itself the following prevention-focused questions:

1. In our microsystem, what diseases or hazards pose a risk to patients, and what evidence-based interventions can mitigate these risks?
2. What features of our microsystem support or impede risk reduction?
3. How do we maximize the likelihood that risk-reducing interventions are performed?
4. How do we monitor our performance?

**Table 6.4    Questions to Stimulate the Design and Improvement of Preventive Care**

| Question | Subquestions |
|---|---|
| 1. In our microsystem, what diseases or hazards pose a risk to patients, and what evidence-based interventions can mitigate these risks? | • Who are our patients?<br>• What are disease risks (based on age, gender, genetics, behaviors, health baseline, environment, and so on)?<br>• What iatrogenic (health care-imposed) hazards exist?<br>• What evidence supports specific preventive care? |
| 2. What features of our microsystem support or prohibit risk reduction? | • What available microsystem resources can facilitate risk reduction?<br>• What sources of unwanted process variation result in missed prevention opportunities?<br>• What are relevant features of patients and community that impact risk? |
| 3. How do we maximize the likelihood that risk-reducing interventions are performed? | • How are system changes planned, implemented, studied, and standardized?<br>• How do we engage all participants in the improvement process?<br>• How do we partner with patients and families? |
| 4. How do we monitor our performance? | • What indicators are tracked? How are they tracked?<br>• How are the data made available to frontline participants in the care process? |

*In Our Microsystem, What Diseases or Hazards Pose a Risk to Our Patients, and What Evidence-Based Interventions Can Mitigate These Risks?*

This question calls upon the clinical microsystem to first understand the demographic, socioeconomic, and medical characteristics of its own patient population (that is, in the language of the Clinical Improvement Equation, to expand knowledge of its own particular context), and then to explore in depth the generalizable scientific knowledge (another of the Improvement Equation's knowledge domains) that links specific health risks to specific demographic or clinical groups. In this stage of inquiry and planning, the microsystem reflects upon several important subquestions:

- *Who are our patients?* Review of administrative, clinical, and even community records can help answer this question. Pre-existing surveys and registries may identify discrete populations with well-defined health needs.
- *What are the disease risks?* The scientific literature directs clinicians to individual and population-specific health risks based on age, gender, genetics, behaviors, health baseline, and physical and social environment.
- *What iatrogenic (health care-imposed) hazards exist?* Members of the clinical microsystem must together walk through their daily administrative and caregiving activities. This review may proceed conceptually, with flowcharting in roundtable discussions, followed by observation of processes (see Chapter Five Action Guide), or literally, with physical re-enactments or simulations of entire clinical processes. Where in these processes are potential hazards identified? What essential information may be lost during which handoffs? What features of the physical environment may undermine safety for either patients or staff? (These questions are explored in greater detail in Chapter Three.)

- What evidence supports specific preventive care? Again, an extensive scientific literature provides abundant support for particular interventions that are tailored to specific clinical populations. But practitioners need not always review this primary data in exhaustive detail. Organizations such as the United States Preventive Services Task Force (USPSTF)[15] and the Cochrane Collaboration[16] have done much of the leg work, and subspecialty organizations (such as the American Diabetes Association and the American College of Cardiology) also publish systematic reviews of disease prevention. These findings, together with general and disease-specific recommendations, can be accessed online at reliable Web sites, and can guide frontline microsystems in preventive care planning and design.

The focus of practice-based and evidence-based investigation will of course depend on the needs of uniquely defined clinical populations. Depending on the context of care (primary versus specialist, medical versus surgical, outpatient versus inpatient), a broad array of evidence-based and locally pertinent preventive health interventions will be identified. Referring again to the practical taxonomy offered in Table 6.3, an evidence-based list might include the following:

- Screening to identify silent risks, such as mammography to detect hidden breast cancer; HIV testing in pregnant women to identify infection that may be transmitted to the newborn.
- Behavioral modifications and clinical interventions, such as gait training and hip protectors to prevent fall-induced hip fractures in frail elders; subcutaneous heparin (blood thinning injection) to prevent blood clots in immobile hospitalized patients.
- System modifications and standardizations to diminish iatrogenic risks, such as screening of blood products to prevent transmission of blood-borne illnesses at time of transfusion; hand hygiene protocols to minimize spread of infection.

### In Our Microsystem, What Patient and Practice Characteristics Support or Impede Risk Reduction?

With this question, the microsystem moves clearly from the Clinical Improvement Equation's first domain of generalizable scientific knowledge to its second domain of particular context. Demographic and patient-specific explorations from the first domain remain pertinent here, and new contextual features must be considered as well. The 5Ps microsystem analysis becomes especially salient, as self-exploration offers valuable insight into the Purpose, Patients, Professionals, Processes, and Patterns of the local system of care. What resources (personal, interpersonal, and technical) are available to the practice? How do staff interact with each other and with the patients and families they serve? How do leaders behave, and how are values and priorities communicated? What role do patient and family have in their own care?

As a result of such analysis, local risk factors are identified; these may be divided broadly into those factors that are attributable to the unique microsystem *practice* and those that are linked to patients and communities. Examples are as follows:

- *Practice features* include any system-specific characteristics that may impact the core principles of quality articulated by the Institute of Medicine (IOM) in 2001. (IOM principles of quality include thoroughness, safety, reliability, and accessibility of local care.[10]) For example, even if all professionals within the clinical microsystem are highly skilled, ineffective patterns of communication and nonstandardized patterns of practice can have profound deleterious effects on the quality of care delivered. In addition, the value of preventive services will be adversely affected by the unavailability of hand hygiene resources, by the absence of user-friendly data registry tools, or by prohibitive distances (for patients) to the nearest mammography center. These and other local features must be considered when planning for patients' total health risk burden.

- *Patient and community features* are inherent to specific populations, as well as to the environments in which the populations live and work and play. Are patients in *this* community financially and socially advantaged or disadvantaged? What level of education and literacy are typically attained? What sources of news and information exert local leverage? Are community resources in place to promote exercise and healthy food choices? Are local air and water quality compromised by industrial waste products from local factories? What other agencies and organizations touch the lives of patients in this microsystem, and how can these agencies be engaged to patients' advantage?

These considerations have obvious importance in planning local preventive care. Through reflective and intentional design of processes and systems, and through close examination of patient and community resources, variation in practice can be minimized and outcomes can be more reliably predicted. Best practices are identified and included in *playbooks* where collections of the microsystem's standardized best practices and processes are collected.[17]

### In Our Microsystem, How do We Maximize the Likelihood That Risk-Reducing Interventions Are Performed?

After exploring the generalizable scientific evidence that supports specific prevention priorities, and after reflecting upon local contextual features that make *this* community and *this* practice clinically unique, the microsystem enters next into the syntactic elements, the "+" and "→" of the Improvement Equation. How is knowledge of scientific evidence adapted to local context, and how are both coupled with meaningful action at the front line of care?

The microsystem's work in this syntactic domain is especially rewarding because it invites interdisciplinary members to collectively and creatively assess, diagnose, and treat the clinical microsystem itself. Participants work together to solve problems, to experiment, and to learn in real time through the PDSA cycle (that is, through iterative cycles of planning, doing, studying, and acting).[17] Much has been written on the specific processes that support frontline learning in service organizations, and growing literature adapts this general knowledge to the unique challenges and opportunities of the health care industry.

As editors of the present volume have described in two prior works, *Quality by Design*[17] and *Practice-Based Learning and Improvement*,[14] effective clinical microsystems build time for active and collaborative reflection in their daily work. This collective *processing time* is essential in the planning of preventive services. Microsystem members, including patients and families, share in defining global and specific preventive care aims that are supported by explorations of generalizable knowledge and local context. Members collaborate to: (1) map actual and ideal care processes; (2) reach consensus on cause and effect relationships internal to these processes; (3) identify benchmarks through formal or informal comparison with other organizations; (4) brainstorm new ideas in sessions enriched by varied perspectives; (5) adopt specific roles and test specific interventions for the patient's benefit; and (6) convene and reconvene to reflect on what has or has not worked, so each new cycle of care proves more successful.

The recurring theme in this work is interdisciplinary engagement. Specific preventive care processes (such as a new presurgical checklist or in a hand hygiene campaign, for example) grow robust in local settings not because these interventions are the best or the only way to solve a given problem, but because the microsystem has invested itself in their creation. The clinical literature offers many reports of prevention-focused tools and techniques, from automated clinician reminders and preprinted order sets to community alliances with churches and schools. Indeed, these interventions warrant attention for their potential positive impact. But in every case, the process by which interventions are developed and adapted will prove a stronger predictor of success than the content of the intervention itself. Batalden has repeatedly asserted that innovations and best practices cannot be simply installed or inserted into clinical care. Efforts to do so, in the absence of professional engagement and deep contextual knowledge, will result in short-lived execution and failed sustainability.

As explored in Chapter Two, mutual engagement in the work of preventive care extends most importantly to collaborating actively and repeatedly with patients and families. One of the most powerful design principles for improving the value of service is to turn the customer into the supplier. Because patients live the vast majority of their lives outside the walls of any clinical microsystem, and because patients are the ultimate stakeholder in decisions about preventive care, every effort must be made to prioritize and support strategies of *self*-care and to empower patients' enactment of these strategies. Thus, for example, patient self-management models developed by Kate Lorig and others[18,19] are ideally suited to the goals of preventive health care, and clinical microsystems can design local processes to support patients' participation in self-care programs. Similarly, formal incorporation of motivational interviewing techniques into frontline practice can leverage clinician-patient relationships in support of wellness-promoting patient behaviors, such as exercise, healthy diet, and tobacco cessation.[20] Not surprisingly, these same models of supported self-management also inform the design and delivery of *chronic illness* care, and in Chapter Eight we consider these models in greater detail.

### In Our Microsystem, How Do We Monitor Our Performance?

Having considered the adaptation of generalizable knowledge to local contexts, and having explored the design and implementation of appropriate preventive services based on this knowledge, our attention shifts in a deceptively linear manner to the right-hand side of the Clinical Improvement Equation (measured performance improvement). But this does not suggest that quantitative monitoring strategies are developed only *after* preventive services have been deployed. In the well-functioning clinical microsystem, measurement considerations must be considered earlier, and are built into the initial development of clinical services. By planning for measuring and monitoring performance, and by reflecting actively upon proposed measures, the microsystem gains clarity regarding what elements and outcomes of care it considers truly important. As explored in Chapter Four, microsystem participants ask themselves, "How will we know we are doing a good job?" (Are measures moving in the right direction?) and also, "What even *counts* as doing a good job?" (What is most important to measure?) Of great significance, when measurement planning also includes the patient and family, then the work of clinical improvement becomes focused sharply on outcomes that reflect patients' values and priorities.

Thus, in the context of available scientific knowledge, sound clinical judgment, and active patient engagement, the microsystem determines what indicators should be tracked, how these should be tracked, and for whose benefit. The *what* may combine process metrics (measures of microsystem function), such as percentage of encounters in which appropriate screening lab work is ordered, and *outcome* metrics (measures of reduced patient risk). These outcome metrics, in turn, may be categorized either as *surrogate markers* of risk reduction or as *direct indicators* of change in frequency or intensity of clinical events. Serum cholesterol level, for example, is a surrogate marker: it predicts future heart disease risk, but, in isolation, it is not a true clinical event like a myocardial infarction (which is a direct clinical outcome). Although direct measures of risk reduction are more robust, they are often more difficult to obtain in real-world settings than are surrogate markers; the latter are therefore more commonly used for continuous performance monitoring.

The *how* of measurement performance is sometimes neglected by frontline interdisciplinary teams who are committed to direct patient care, but who may fail to consider system requirements for continuous monitoring and improvement of that care. With intentional planning, the measurement of preventive care activities can be built into the provision of care itself in the following ways:

- Nursing staff may tabulate immunization counts each time they vaccinate a patient.
- Surgical technicians may tally preoperative checklists when these are completed and may enter aggregate data into electronic registries.
- Physicians may keep their own counts of specific preventive interventions performed and may document sequential successes or failures of performance that support continuous practice-based learning and improvement.

The process of role definition, which emerges through iterative discussion among interdisciplinary members of the clinical microsystem, enables individual participants to own specific steps in a clinical care pathway, and clarifies specific responsibilities in a *measurement* pathway.

Finally, if monitoring and measurement are to truly support the improvement of patient care (rather than simply to populate administrative records with lifeless data), then microsystems must consider for whose benefit each measurement is made and reported (see again Chapter Four). Who are the different stakeholders in preventive care, and how is pertinent performance information shared with each of them? Leaders of health care organizations, regulatory agencies, and (increasingly) insurers who incentivize preventive care through pay-for-performance fiscal models, will seek aggregate scorecards that summarize clinical care at the micro, meso, or macrosystem levels of service. Such summaries are important, but may be inadequate to stimulate performance change at the front line of care, where detailed individual dashboards or other forms of data display may more effectively guide local improvement efforts. In addition, patients who are active participants in their own preventive health care will also seek qualitative feedback on their personal efforts to achieve wellness. Many microsystems have thus developed customer friendly reports that enable patients to monitor their own progress over time toward desired health goals.

## CONCLUSION

As both the clinical and financial burden of preventable illness increasingly threaten the well-being of individuals and institutions (and ultimately the health of the nation), clinical microsystems are uniquely positioned to systematically embrace the work of preventive health that Senator Harkin suggests we have heretofore neglected. At the front line of care, professionals, staff, patients, and families are able to partner with each other to understand unique risks of both individuals and populations. They (we) are empowered to link this general understanding with specific knowledge of unique patient needs and practice resources, and to align this information with effective interventions that respect the concerns and requirements of all participants. These actions lead to measurable outcomes that are subject to monitoring over time. Patients and microsystems benefit when these outcomes are shared with all stakeholders. Regular feedback on achievement of specific targets and goals motivates individual patients to engage in wellness-promoting behaviors, and it also stimulates clinical microsystems to continuously improve the integrity and functioning of prevention-based care processes. In a very real sense, the health of our health care system depends upon this essential work.

## SUMMARY

- Preventive care can be understood broadly as the full set of interventions and interactions that support proactive assessment and mitigation of health risks, before these risks progress to clinical illness or injury.
- Effective planning for preventive care links caregivers' understanding of generalizable scientific knowledge with contextual information about unique clinical practice environments and activities.
- An action-based taxonomy of preventive care services includes screening activities, behavioral and biomedical interventions, and safety-focused modifications of the microsystem environment.
- In well-functioning clinical microsystems, proactive measurements are built into developing and implementing effective preventive care.

## KEY TERMS

Behavioral modifications

Clinical Improvement Equation

Clinical interventions

Collective risk

Disease risk

Generalizable scientific knowledge

Iatrogenic hazards

Measured performance improvement

Particular context

Preventive care

Preventive health interventions

Primary prevention

Processing time

Screening

Secondary prevention

Surrogate markers

Syntactic connectors (the + sign and the → sign)

System modifications

Tertiary prevention

# REVIEW QUESTIONS

1. What is the definition of preventive care? (Please include the four domains of care in your answer.)
2. How are the domains of care similar or different?
3. What are two examples of moving from traditional prevention categories (primary, secondary, tertiary) to action domains?
4. How can the Clinical Improvement Equation serve as a catalyst for embedding evidence-based care into daily practice?
5. What type of measurement tools display data over time to demonstrate a change has brought about an improvement?

# DISCUSSION QUESTIONS

1. Review the Clinical Improvement Equation and identify preventive activities that reside in your microsystem. Is there other generalizable scientific evidence on preventive activities that should be adapted to the microsystem? How might this equation help the process of standardizing and improving quality of care?
2. Think about your microsystem and identify pertinent processes that result in consistent delivery of preventive care. How are these processes measured and monitored?
3. Review the population of patients and the processes of care in your microsystem. What specific preventive processes occur during care delivery? Who does what?

# REFERENCES

1. Remarks by U.S. Senator Tom Harkin to the American College of Preventive Medicine. February 17, 2005. Retrieved February 10, 2010, from http://harkin.senate.gov/pr/p.cfm?i=232597
2. Mokdad, A., Marks, J. S., Stroup, D. F., & Gerberding, J. L. Actual causes of death in the United States, 2000. *Journal of the American Medical Association*, 2004, *291*, 1238–1245.
3. U.S. Department of Health and Human Services. *The power of prevention: Steps to a healthier U.S.* Report issued 2003. Retrieved August 10, 2010, from www.healthierus.gov/STEPS/summit/prevportfolio/power/index.html
4. Woolf, S. H. The power of prevention and what it requires. *Journal of the American Medical Association*, 2008, *290*, 2437–2439.
5. Kottke et al. The comparative effectiveness of heart disease prevention and treatment strategies. *American Journal of Preventive Medicine*, 2009, *36*(1), 82–88.
6. Institute of Medicine Committee on Quality Health Care in America. *To err is human: Building a safer health system.* Washington, DC: National Academy Press, 2000.
7. McGlynn et al. The quality of health care delivered to adults in the United States. *New England Journal of Medicine*, 2003, *348*(26), 2635–2645.
8. Paul Batalden, personal communication conversation with Eugene Nelson, CSc. Nashville, TN, HCA Corporate Headquarters, 1992.
9. Woolf, S. H. The big answer: Rediscovering prevention at a time of crisis in health care. *Harvard Health Policy Review*, 2006, *7*, 5–20.

10. Institute of Medicine Committee on Quality Health Care in America. *Crossing the quality chasm: A new health system for the 21st century.* Washington, DC: National Academy Press, 2001.

11. Glouberman, S., & Zimmerman, B. (2002). *Complicated and complex systems: What would successful reform of Medicare look like?* Ottawa: Commission on the Future of Health Care in Canada.

12. Liu, S., Homa, K., Butterly, J. R., Kirkland, K. B., & Batalden, P. B. Improving the simple, complicated and complex realities of community-acquired pneumonia. *Quality and Safety in Health Care,* 2009, *18*, 93–98.

13. Batalden, P., & Davidoff, F. What is quality improvement and how can it transform health care? *Quality and Safety in Health Care,* 2007, *16*, 2–3.

14. Nelson, G., Batalden, P. B., & Lazar, J. S. *Practice-based learning and improvement: A clinical improvement action guide.* (2nd ed.) Oak Brook, IL: Joint Commission Resources, 2007.

15. U.S. Department of Health and Human Services. Agency for Health Care Quality and Research. U.S. Preventive Services Task Force. Retrieved August 10, 2010, from www.ahrq.gov/clinic/USpstfix.htm

16. The Cochrane Collaboration. *Cochrane reviews.* Retrieved February 10, 2010, from www.cochrane.org/reviews

17. Nelson, E., Batalden, P. B., & Godfrey, M. M. *Quality by design.* San Francisco: Jossey-Bass, 2007.

18. Lorig, K., Sobel, D., Gonzalez, V., & Minor, M. *Living a healthy life with chronic conditions.* Boulder, CO: Bull Publishing, 2006.

19. Bodenheimer, T., Lorig, K., Holman, H., & Grumbach, K. Patient self-management of chronic disease in primary care. *Journal of the American Medical Association,* 2002, *288*, 2469–2475.

20. Miller, W., & Rolnick, S. *Motivational interviewing: Preparing people for change.* (2nd ed.) New York: Guilford Press, 2002.

Chapter Six Action Guide illustrates how preventive care like mammography occurs in radiology, a supporting microsystem and critical care. Every clinical and supportive microsystem has preventive processes embedded in daily operations but may not view the activities as preventive in nature. Many preventive behaviors of the microsystem are directed not toward patients at all but toward the microsystem itself through planned safety efforts that indirectly promote patient wellness by targeting health care–induced risk (so that staff hand hygiene campaigns, for example, prevent patient infections in both inpatient and outpatient settings).

## RADIOLOGY MICROSYSTEM PREVENTIVE ACTIVITY OF MAMMOGRAPHY AND VAP BUNDLES IN CRITICAL CARE

Preventive activities occur in all health care settings, not just in primary care. The mammography process in the radiology microsystem is illustrated using a deployment flowchart (see Figure AG6.1). It flows from the patient to referring physician, hospital microsystems, and individuals within radiology. Notice in this deployment flowchart that quality characteristics that increase value of the process from the patient perspective are listed for each step. Timeliness, organization, promptness, comfort, and accuracy of the process all contribute to a high-value process. Chapter Two Action Guide provides tools to learn from the patient what is important and valued in their care process. Building this customer knowledge into process redesign and then tracking and monitoring how well the key attributes exist in the processes using the potential measures can result in delighted patients and families.

Another example is intensive care; prevention occurs in the critical care setting specific to ventilator-acquired pneumonia (VAP) bundles for pneumonia prevention. The Institute for Healthcare Improvement www.ihi.org developed "bundles" to provide health care providers with evidence-based practices in a structured practice that has been documented to improve patient outcomes if carried out collectively and consistently. The key components of the ventilator bundle are:

FIGURE AG6.1 Radiology Flowchart.

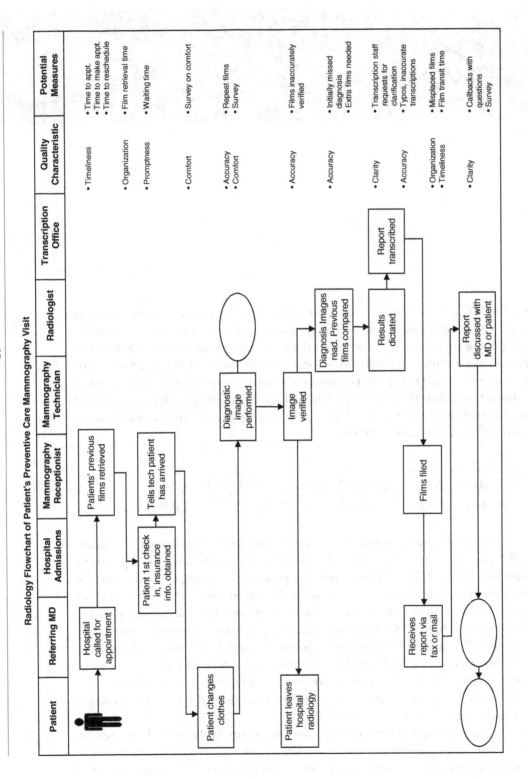

Radiology Flowchart of Patient's Preventive Care Mammography Visit

- Elevation of the head of the bed
- Daily "sedation vacations" and assessment of readiness to extubate
- Peptic ulcer disease prophylaxis
- Deep venous thrombosis prophylaxis
- Daily oral care with Chlorhexidine

# CHAPTER 7

# PLANNING FOR RESPONSIVE AND RELIABLE ACUTE CARE

Joel S. Lazar

Marjorie M. Godfrey

Eugene C. Nelson

Paul B. Batalden

## LEARNING OBJECTIVES

- Describe the role of clinical microsystems in acute care.
- Compare and contrast patient and microsystem perspectives on acute care.
- List five design requirements for acute care in clinical microsystems.
- Discuss the value and function of advanced access to health care.
- Describe how microsystems can optimize handoffs in patient care.

To effectively meet the acute care needs of patients and families, clinical microsystems must plan coordinated responses to foreseeable surprises. These responses are supported by evidence-based algorithms, structured decision-making processes, and well-defined (but flexible) roles for all participants. Acute care also demands timeliness, accessibility of service, and reliability of handoffs between sequential care providers. Specific design strategies can facilitate microsystems' delivery of care that meets these requirements and that is responsive to both predictable and unpredictable components of acute illness episodes.

## ANTICIPATING THE NEEDS OF ACUTELY ILL PATIENTS

The experience of acute illness is familiar to almost everyone, and invariably it entails not only the clinical distress of primary symptoms, but also greater or lesser degrees of emotional distress due to uncertainty about the *meaning* of primary symptoms. Patients are often overwhelmed by worries and questions, such as:

- Is this problem serious?
- Are therapies available to reverse my pain, fatigue, breathing trouble, and other symptoms?
- Once treated, will I return fully to my prior level of function?
- Can I even afford the treatment? And who will take care of my family while I'm sick?

Invariably, acute illness entails *disruption* not only to the patient and family but also to the clinical microsystem that provides care. Because such illness often emerges unexpectedly, clinical microsystems may not fully anticipate what resources (including personnel and material supplies) must be dedicated to acute concerns on a given day. Thus, the obvious disruption acuity brings to the lives of patients and families is matched, at least potentially, by disruption of usual processes within the microsystem.

In this context of urgency and unpredictability, where anxiety can easily extend from patient to caregiving microsystem, the Institute of Medicine's[1] prioritization of safety, timeliness, effectiveness, efficiency, equitability, and patient centeredness becomes especially salient. The role of clinical microsystems in acute care is thus to plan for the unexpected, to anticipate and to rehearse for foreseeable surprises, and to learn quickly from successes and failures. In this way, patient and microsystem disruption is contained, anxiety is reduced, and evidence-based care is applied in as timely a manner as possible.

In this chapter we explore needs of patients and families for acute care that is timely and accessible, that demonstrates tight coordination and effective handoffs, and that is equitable and efficient, evidence-based, and technically sound. We also examine features of clinical microsystems that are well-suited to meet these foreseeable needs.

## DEFINING ACUTE CARE NEEDS OF PATIENTS AND FAMILIES

As suggested in Chapter Six, and as reviewed again in Table 7.1, the clinical microsystem's essential first function when planning for acute care interventions, and when implementing frontline care improvements more generally, is to focus less on pre-defined specific visit types, such as the *urgent care visit* (although this may often be the

Table 7.1   Overarching Care Needs of Patient and Family

| | |
|---|---|
| **Preventive care** | • Proactive assessment and mitigation of health risks |
| **Acute care** | • Timely attention to new or newly worsening disruption of health or function |
| **Chronic care** | • Longitudinal resiliency and support in self-management of ongoing disease |
| **Palliative care** | • Comfort and dignity in the context of underlying disease progression |

context for acute care), and more upon the context-specific needs of *patients and families themselves.* Certain needs naturally cluster to contexts of acuity, and these needs suggest specific service and process design features (and microsystem planning activities that add clinical value), not only when applied in prespecified urgent care encounters, but also when incorporated into chronic or palliative contexts as foreseeable surprises arise.

For patients and families, the underlying need during times of acute illness is for timely attention to new or newly worsening disruption in health and function. The scope of acute care must therefore include the full set of microsystem interventions and interactions that address, in a timely manner, these new or newly worsening disruptions. As we have suggested, acute care needs may emerge from an otherwise healthy state (as when an otherwise healthy woman develops a new onset of deep vein thrombosis (blood clot in the lower leg), or may occur in the context of chronic or palliative care. A nine-year-old child with generally well-controlled asthma may experience a sudden flare-up of reactive airway symptoms (that require urgent modification of chronic therapy) at the time of a viral respiratory infection. A middle-aged man with stable congestive heart failure may experience acute exacerbation of his underlying cardiac disease, which prompts rapid medication change and even hospital admission. A frail, elderly nursing home resident, previously stable in palliative care, may fall and break her hip, necessitating prompt evaluation for pain control and possible surgery to optimize function.

Although these varied clinical settings imply diverse care strategies (and therefore diverse forms of preplanning) in all these acute care contexts, the microsystem is challenged to answer the same basic question: *How do we meet the needs of patient and family for timely attention to new or newly worsening disruption in health and function?* How, more precisely, do we prepare ourselves for these disruptions and rapidly respond in a proactive manner that reduces and hopefully reverses their adverse impact? How do we organize and apply our resources in anticipation of the unexpected?

## CASE STUDY: THE EXPERIENCE OF ACUITY

Joanne Wright describes herself as a healthy woman. In her mid-50s, she continues to exercise on a regular basis. Her diet is balanced, and she avoids cigarettes and excess alcohol. Although every few years she experiences an ear or sinus infection that requires antibiotics, these infections do not keep her down for long. This year, however, some three weeks prior to her scheduled preventive health exam, she develops cough and fever that feel out of the range of her past infections. In the first twenty-four hours of this ailment she applies home remedies (self-care that includes rest, fluids, and over-the-counter cough syrups) and experiences some subjective benefit. On day two of her illness she notes thicker, darker phlegm in her cough, and she feels winded with usual exertions. She explores health-related Internet sites that specify further self-care mea-

*(Continued)*

## CASE STUDY: THE EXPERIENCE OF ACUITY (Continued)

sures and that recommend physician contact if certain respiratory warning symptoms develop. By day three, feeling worse rather than better, she recognizes some of these symptoms herself: wheezing and shortness of breath, nausea and vomiting, ongoing fever and increasing fatigue. She phones the office of her primary care physician, Dr. Ben Daniels. Her subsequent journey is depicted graphically in the deployment flowchart of Figure 7.1.

Dr. Daniels' medical receptionist has been trained to use a *practice-specific triage protocol,* the details of which are specified in a standardized computer algorithm; patients with straightforward or non-urgent clinical concerns are scheduled automatically in upcoming appointment slots, whereas more urgent issues (including Joanne's call) trigger a phone handoff to the office registered nurse (RN). The office RN queries Joanne briefly and determines that a *same day* office appointment is required. Dr. Daniels has a tight schedule today, as do his practice partners, so some overbooking is required. Joanne may need to wait when she reaches the office, but she is reassured the doctor can see her this afternoon.

The pace of events begins to accelerate. Brought in to the office by her worried husband, Joanne continues to feel worse. She looks very unwell when the nurse escorts her to the exam room. Vital signs are checked using office protocols; extra parameters (also protocol-based and predetermined) are included in the nurse assessment, due to Joanne's poor appearance. She is wheezing and febrile, with elevated pulse and unexpectedly low blood pressure. Her doctor is still seeing another patient, but the nurse interrupts him, sharing her assessment and concern regarding Joanne's clinical appearance. Dr. Daniels thus excuses himself for a moment from his current patient, comes to Joanne's exam, and performs his own rapid assessment. She appears clinically toxic, and the lung exam suggests lobar pneumonia. Dr. Daniels orders stat oxygen therapy and medicated breathing treatment, which are administered by an office nursing assistant. He explains to Joanne and her husband that hospital admission is required, and he quickly obtains their consent to make preparations for transport.

Dr. Daniels asks his receptionist to phone for an ambulance and calls the local hospital emergency room to briefly review Joanne's status and reason for transfer with the on-call physician. Other patients in the office are kept waiting during this process, but they are informed (also per prerehearsed protocol) of the reason for this wait: "Dr. Daniels is attending an emergency situation, but he'll be with you shortly." These patients are given the option of rescheduling if they are unable to wait, and a secretary also checks to see if other team clinicians have capacity to accommodate a waiting patient. Meanwhile, the RN stays at Joanne's bedside until the ambulance team arrives. Essential information is exchanged, and the patient is transferred to gurney, to ambulance, and finally to the local hospital emergency room.

In the emergency room, further handoffs and protocol-based interventions are enacted. Oxygen is continued; intravenous fluids are administered to reverse Joanne's low blood pressure; a chest X-ray is ordered that reveals bilobar pneumonia. Evidence-based algorithms guide the choice of appropriate antibiotics, and a first dose is also intravenously administered within the first hour of Joanne's arrival. The hospital admission team is consulted, and, following further communication between clinicians and nurses, Joanne is transferred to the Intensive Care Unit, where additional prerehearsed activities follow. Oxygen levels remain low, and Joanne must be placed on a ventilator machine for forty-eight hours to support her respiratory function. A social worker checks in twice each day with Joanne's husband, whose worry for his wife has understandably heightened.

Thankfully, during the next few days the antibiotics prove effective. Joanne is weaned from her ventilator, and after a full eight days of hospital care she is well enough to be discharged home. A template-specified discharge summary is sent to Dr. Daniels so he will have full knowledge of her hospital care and of specialists' post-hospital recommendations when he meets her in a follow-up visit in the upcoming week. This appointment is scheduled before Joanne leaves the hospital. Additionally, several days before discharge at the daily interdisciplinary rounds that include both Joanne and her husband, the recommendation is made to activate home health services, which will provide care to Joanne in her weakened state and will support her continued recovery. In the aftermath of her ordeal, Joanne remains quite fatigued at her follow-up visit, but she is clearly, if gradually, on the mend. Dr. Daniels reassures her she can expect a full recovery to pre-illness level of function.

FIGURE 7.1   Pneumonia Deployment Flowchart.

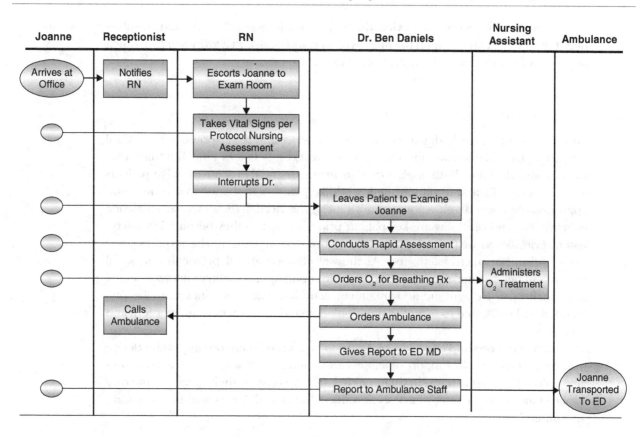

## AN OVERVIEW OF DESIGN REQUIREMENTS FOR ACUTE CARE

What experiential features of acuity are apparent in this case, and how do these determine the design features that a well-functioning microsystem must build into its provision of acute care? Clinical microsystems that support acute care rely on the following processes:

- Evidence-based algorithms
- Structured decision making and standard orders
- Advanced access
- Reliable handoffs
- Effective communication among microsystem members
- Rehearsal of coordinated actions

- Reflection and feedback after sentinel events
- Planning for the expected surprise

Medical professionals in these clinical microsystems demonstrate the following characteristics:

- Sensitivity to both timing and timeliness of care
- Well-defined (but flexible) roles
- Capacity to manage disruptions (both patient's and microsystem's)
- Active engagement of patients and families

In the present section, we review these elements in general terms, and in subsequent sections we expand upon the themes of *advanced access* and *effective handoffs,* which are essential components of any acute care delivery system.

### Time Is in the Foreground

Most notably, of course, both Joanne's illness experience and the response of her several interacting clinical microsystems unfold in a context compelled by time. But this is true in more ways than one. Both *timeliness* and *timing* are essential in acute care. For patients who are acutely ill, and for family members (like Joanne's husband) who acutely and appropriately worry about a loved one's illness, the need is *now*. Access, efficiency, effectiveness, and reliability are key patient priorities, and so they become key microsystem priorities as well. But Joanne needs more than timeliness; she requires good *timing* within her microsystem, too. As the well-choreographed protocols and serial handoffs in her case make clear, acute care builds upon tight coordination of sequential and synchronized diagnostic and treatment activities. These activities must be preplanned and well-timed to meet the situation's demands for urgency, agility, safety, and reliability.

Advanced access and effective care transitions (handoffs) are two important design features that specifically support timeliness and timing in clinical care. These features are explored in general terms in Chapter Five, and we consider their specific acute care applications in this chapter's later section titled "Advanced Access and Effective Care Transitions."

### Evidence-Based Algorithms and Structured Decision Making

Although Dr. Daniels and his colleagues cannot specifically predict *when* a given patient will call with some new and urgent disruption to health or function, they can predict more generally that such disruptions will occasionally occur. The 5Ps microsystem self-assessment model (see Chapter One Action Guide) provides insights into population needs, patterns, and local practice variations.[2] Microsystems can see the patterns of frequency and seasonal patterns of acute events and can plan accordingly with this new insight. Based upon such knowledge, well-functioning clinical microsystems anticipate the probability of acute presentations and preplan appropriate responses so real-time implementation is efficient and well-coordinated. The worst time to begin preparing for an emergency, of course, is at the time of that emergency. But microsystems often fail to prepare as broadly and as specifically as foreseeable situations require.

In broad terms, *evidence-based clinical algorithms* can be very beneficial. These algorithms embed knowledge from scientific studies within clinical care pathways, practice guidelines, and decision rules. What formal recommendations can guide frontline clinicians when Joanne presents with decompensated pneumonia? What evaluative measures (such as chest X-ray and sputum culture) can facilitate rapid diagnosis, and in what sequence should this evaluation occur? What antibiotics (directed toward which likely bacteria) does the literature suggest are appropriate? What supportive care measures (for example, oxygen and IV fluid hydration) are required? What clinical criteria support the decision to admit one patient to intensive care and to send another patient home?

Specific guidelines and algorithms, such as the pneumonia algorithm depicted in Figure 7.2, are developed by specialty and primary care medical societies and are easily accessible online or through professional publications. See, for example, www.icsi.org, the web site of the Institute for Clinical Systems Improvement, which serves as a clearinghouse for more than one hundred diagnostic and therapeutic care algorithms that are based on scientific evidence and expert reviews.[3] Individual microsystems can begin planning for the unexpected by considering potential urgencies that may arise in their practice setting (again, see the 5P model of microsystem self-assessment in Chapter One), and then by collecting and reviewing evidence-based recommendations that may be pertinent to these situations.

Readers will note at least three discrete, although overlapping, benefits of evidence-based algorithms. First, and perhaps most obviously, reliable third parties (professional organizations) have already done much of the legwork. Behind many formal algorithms stands a large body of primary research the guidelines summarize and synthesize. Second, these algorithms represent a *translation of knowledge into action*. Given the likelihood that Joanne has clinical pneumonia, what are specific members of her care team to do? What actions are justified by available evidence (or are at least reasonable in the current context, when good evidence is lacking)? How and when and by whom are discrete actions to be implemented? Finally, and nontrivially, well-designed algorithms generate action pathways that are relatively *simple* or are, at least, "merely complicated" (to borrow Glouberman and Zimmerman's[4] wonderful phrase), rather than overwhelmingly complex. Acute illness engenders anxiety, not only among patients, but also at times among providers and staff who must tend to this illness. The *if-then formulations of algorithm-based care*, although not appropriate to all clinical contexts, can in many acute settings provide welcome clarity and safety-promoting reliability (see Chapter Eight for further discussion).[5] *If* Joanne's chest X-ray shows W, *then* administer medication X; *if* her blood pressure is below Y, *then* treat with IV fluid Z. Experienced clinicians may modify such rules when the case at hand deviates from classic scenarios, but those rules do provide solid ground upon which to make decisions.

## Well-Defined (but Flexible) Roles Within the Clinical Microsystem

We have already suggested that clinical microsystems must prepare both broadly and specifically to manage potentially foreseeable acute patient needs. Clinical algorithms are directed to the breadth of this preparation. Careful role clarification and optimization based on education, licensure, formal training, and practical experience give the work specificity.

Many evidence-based algorithms falter in real-world clinical contexts because precise *actions* in a given pathway are not clearly linked to designated actors. It is one

## FIGURE 7.2   Pneumonia Care Algorithm.

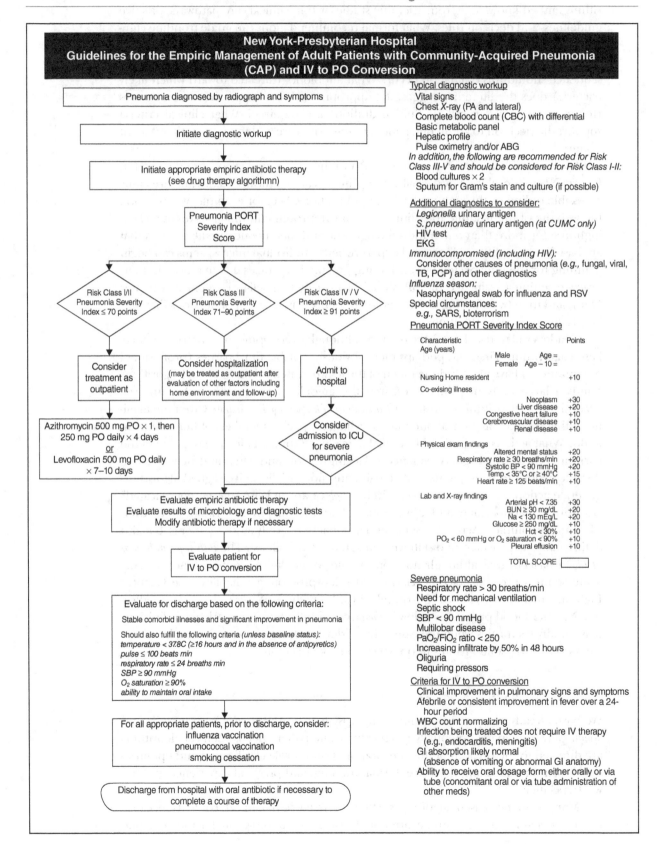

thing to record in flowchart boxes that patient is triaged, oxygen is administered, emergency room is called, and even other patients in the waiting room are notified of delay. But the well-functioning microsystem must customize and preassign ownership for each action. Thus, *receptionist* performs phone triage, *nurse* assistant administers oxygen, and *physician* calls emergency room. Again, in the heat of an acute event, and in less urgent contexts as well, individual team members may assume that someone else has performed that step. But without careful pre-assignment of roles, this someone may be no one. Deployment flowcharts facilitate role clarity and help ensure process reliability.

Of course, the relative rigidity of role assignments will vary with specific circumstances, and greater degrees of role flexibility will support greater adaptability of the microsystem overall. As Sarah Fraser and Trisha Greenhalgh have observed, "successful health services in the 21st century must aim not merely for change, improvement, and response, but for changeability, improvability, and responsiveness."[6] Novel situations arise with regularity in clinical care. By cross-training physicians, nurses, and other providers to adopt various roles as different scenarios require, and by building an open-endedness into the roles so these can be modified and expanded in the context of new learning, care participants can more fully use their skills in the service of patients and families with a common goal. The microsystem itself develops not merely *competence* (what individuals know and are able to do under normal conditions) but also, more critically, *capability,* which Fraser and Greenhalgh identify as "the extent to which individuals (and groups) can adapt to change, generate new knowledge, and continue to improve their performance."[6]

## Unique Role of Patient and Family

When considering the roles of each microsystem participant, we must not neglect the role of patient and family. In preventive, chronic, and palliative settings, the patients' behaviors and articulated priorities are perhaps more obviously a component of overall care. But even in acute care settings, where traditional descriptions of the *sick role*[7] assume the patient to have surrendered his authority and to have passively accepted whatever therapies the active health system administers, even here the role of patients and families is an active one.

At a most basic level, the individual with acute needs must first decide to access the health care system. This decision is by no means a foregone conclusion. As Figure 7.3 suggests, cross-sectional studies reveal that most persons who experience illness or injury do *not* seek attention in the mainstream health care system.[8,9] Individuals must first conclude that an experienced symptom, even if unpleasant, warrants specific intervention. Then, even when care is desired, further deliberation is required to clarify what form(s) of help to seek. Consider at right the internal monologue a person may perform all at once, or over the course of hours, days, weeks, or even months:

Is my new back pain an illness, or just a nuisance? Can I live with this discomfort, or should I do something about it? If I decide I should do something about it, then can I take care of this myself using knowledge I already have, or do I use one of several available resources at my disposal? Which of these resources is most appropriate, including family, friends, the Internet, a local physical therapist, alternative healers, my primary care provider, or the emergency room?

Only in the final phrases of the final sentence does the clinical microsystem appear, by which time a series of questions have been asked and a series of implicit or explicit decisions have been made. These sequential decisions are influenced not only by the intensity of experienced symptoms, but also by the

FIGURE 7.3    Who Seeks Care Where? Ecology of Medical Care 2001.

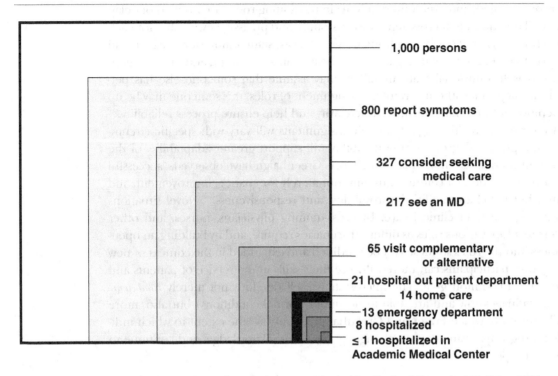

1,000 persons

800 report symptoms

327 consider seeking medical care

217 see an MD

65 visit complementary or alternative

21 hospital out patient department

14 home care

13 emergency department

8 hospitalized

≤ 1 hospitalized in Academic Medical Center

*Source:* L. A. Green et al. The ecology of medcal care revisited. *New England Journal of Medicine.* 2001, *344*, 2021–2025.

individual's personal beliefs and priorities, education and family background, social and financial resources, cultural expectations, and memory of past health care encounters.[10] This complex process requires active involvement by patients and families.

Acknowledging even this essential first role of patients in the initiation of their own care (not to mention later patient roles, which include negotiating treatment priorities, participating in shared decision making, and enacting therapeutic recommendations), the clinical microsystem can design effective acute care interventions that extend beyond the four walls of office or hospital settings. Langley's notion of *change concepts* permits us to think broadly about high-leverage process modifications within the microsystem that enhance quality and efficiency of care.[11] Figure 7.4 demonstrates that clinical microsystems can improve care by combining steps in a process, or by reordering or even eliminating steps. Care can also be improved by eliminating handoff failures between steps (see section titled "Advanced Access and Effective Care Transitions" in this chapter), or by replacing one step with an entirely new one of better value. Often neglected in such reflections is the possibility of *modifying the input* to a clinical process itself.[12] But here is precisely where in the process patient and family roles can be leveraged.

In particular, to support patients in the most effective use of available services, clinical microsystems can develop active education strategies that become decision-support resources for patients in need. The microsystem and patient together modify input to subsequent caregiving encounters through wellness strategies and acuity-modifying interventions that are outside the box of the health care setting. Children with chronic reactive airway disease, for example, are provided an *asthma action plan* that specifies self-care and system-care options based precisely on level of symptom acuity (see Figure

FIGURE 7.4   Change Concepts.

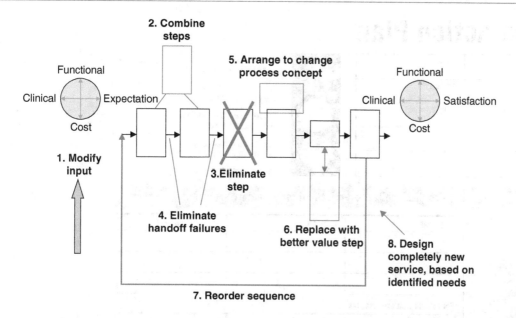

7.5). In this user-friendly model, symptoms in the upper go zone signify clinical stability and require no intervention. The middle caution zone symptoms trigger specific self-care actions that patient and family initiate at home. When such interventions are effective and the patient moves again to the upper go zone, an office or emergency room visit is appropriately avoided. Waste in the system is reduced, the self-empowered patient feels better, and system access is increased for the *next* patient, whose need for in-person care may persist. Only when the asthma patient experiences the lower danger zone symptoms must she contact the health care system directly, in which case the implementation of more aggressive therapy is very appropriate. Through a simple system-based modification of process inputs, the *entire* system more effectively directs the *right* level of care to the right patient at the right time.

## Planning for the Expected Surprise

As we have suggested, although clinical microsystems cannot precisely predict *when* a given patient will experience new and urgent disruption to health and function, they can predict more generally *that* such disruptions will occasionally occur. System resources and design elements that include evidence-based algorithms, decision-support structures, role optimizations, and input modifications can facilitate the microsystem's coordinated response to acute patient needs. Two further essential activities, which in effect integrate system resources and design elements, are thoughtful rehearsal of intervention strategies *before* true acuity arises, and careful reflection and debriefing upon microsystem responses *after* an acute event.

Fortified by evidence-based algorithms, clinical microsystems are well-positioned to pre-enact plausible urgent scenarios. Ideally this work involves realistic rehearsal of foreseeable events, as occurs in the mock codes administered by educators of advanced cardiac life support programs. Formal simulation centers have grown increasingly common and permit rehearsal of various acute scenarios in a safe environment. In these settings, unique role playing scenarios can be adapted to the special learning needs of

## FIGURE 7.5   Asthma Action Plan.

# Asthma Action Plan

| Name | Date |
|---|---|
| Doctor | Medical Record # |
| Doctor's Office Phone #: Day | Night/Weekend |
| Emergency Contact | |
| Doctor's Signature | |

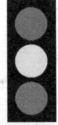

The colors of a traffic light will help you use your asthma medicines.

**Green** means **Go Zone!**
Use preventive medicine.

**Yellow** Means **Caution Zone!**
Add quick-relief medicine.

**Red** means **Danger Zone!**
Get help from a doctor.

Personal Best Peak Flow _____

### GO

You have _all_ of these:
- Breathing is good
- No cough or wheeze
- Sleep through the night
- Can work and play

Peak flow from ___ to ___

### CAUTION

You have _any_ of these:
- First signs of a cold
- Exposure to known trigger
- Cough   • Mild wheeze
- Tight chest   • Coughing at night

Peak flow from ___ to ___

### DANGER

Your asthma is getting worse fast:
- Medicine is not helping
- Breathing is hard and fast
- Nose opens wide
- Ribs show
- Can't talk well

Peak flow reading below ___

**Use these daily preventive anti-inflammatory medicines:**

| MEDICINE | HOW MUCH | HOW OFTEN/WHEN |
|---|---|---|
| | | |
| | | |
| | | |

For asthma with exercise, take:

| | | |
|---|---|---|

**Continue with green zone medicine and add:**

| MEDICINE | HOW MUCH | HOW OFTEN/WHEN |
|---|---|---|
| | | |
| | | |

**CALL YOUR PRIMARY CARE PROVIDER.**

**Take these medicines and call your doctor now.**

| MEDICINE | HOW MUCH | HOW OFTEN/WHEN |
|---|---|---|
| | | |
| | | |

**GET HELP FROM A DOCTOR NOW!** Do not be afraid of causing a fuss. Your doctor will want to see you right away. It's important! If you cannot contact your doctor, go directly to the emergency room. **DO NOT WAIT.**
Make an appointment with your primary care provider within two days of an ER visit or hospitalization.

 State of New York, George E. Pataki, Governor
Department of Health, Antonia C. Novello, M.D., M.P.H., Dr.P.H., Commissioner
COPY FOR PATIENT                                                   4850

_Source:_ Retrieved from www.health.state.ny.us/diseases/asthma/pdf/4850.pdf

participants. But even in the absence of special resources, microsystem participants can walk through essential steps of acute care processes. This may involve literal movements through a physical facility or handoffs rehearsed imaginatively around a conference table, with participants identifying potential gaps or pitfalls in simulated care (see Chapter Three Action Guide).

We have suggested the worst time to begin preparing for a clinical emergency is at the time of the emergency. Similarly, the worst aftermath of such an emergency (apart, of course, from any adverse patient outcome) is a failure to learn retrospectively from the event. Effective microsystems routinely build time for active reflection into the daily, weekly, or monthly activities of regular clinical operations. Formal morbidity and mortality conferences sometimes serve this function, as do prescheduled staff meetings. But these events may be remote in time from the actual provision of acute care, and opportunities for learning may be lost. Thus we recommend clinical microsystems engage in routine *huddles* to process the experience and to learn with all staff. Huddles can occur at either the start or the end of each clinical session or shift, and immediately after acute events. These checkouts may involve thorough debriefing of events, or may focus upon just three basic questions: "What did we do well in today's patient care?" "What might we have done better?" "What specific changes can we institute, based upon today's experience, to improve tomorrow's work?" When clinical acuity is associated with exceptional emotional intensity, as in the case of Joanne, who nearly died from her bacterial pneumonia, exploration of team members' feelings is also appropriate. Although technical algorithms and evidence-based guidelines help maintain objectivity and reliability in high-stake clinical contexts, personal reactions are inevitable in such settings. Leaders of clinical microsystems can create an emotional space in debriefing sessions that supports the safety of patients and also of caregiving professionals. In the end, effective and supportive processing of professionals' reactions builds trust and resiliency within the microsystem and strengthens team members' ability to provide highest quality care.

## ADVANCED ACCESS AND EFFECTIVE CARE TRANSITIONS

As we have suggested, timely access to care is an essential need of patients and families, especially in the acute context of new or newly worsening disruptions of health and function. But meeting this need in a consistent manner can be challenging for frontline microsystems. These microsystems typically plan their allocation of resources (including human resources) based upon extrapolations from past experience. How do we use this experience when planning for *tomorrow's* needs, which, of course, may vary in unforeseen ways from yesterday's and today's? How do we build just the right amount of clinical capacity, neither too much (which will engender waste) nor too little? Again, how do we organize and apply our resources in anticipation of the unexpected?

Murray and Tantau[13] have observed that health care organizations' traditional approach to the access problem presumes an insatiable demand for health care, so barriers must be constructed (such as complex scheduling models, multiple appointment types, and elaborate triage algorithms) to protect the system from being overwhelmed. But, in fact, such faulty solutions often diminish timely access rather than improve it. This is especially problematic, of course, when patients' needs are acute. Barriers to access in this context are also barriers to efficiency and effectiveness; satisfaction is reduced, and patient safety may be jeopardized.

As described in Chapter Five, optimal access requires that we reconceptualize clinical demand as a multifaceted design challenge where we actively balance supply and demand and match clinical resources with clinical needs.[14] In modern advanced access models, the goal is not to stave off existing demand into orderly (but time-wasting) queues, but to remove those queues to eliminate delays that detract from quality and value. Murray and Berwick[15] offer six elements of advanced access redesign that promote patient flow and build clinical capacity while dismantling long-established barriers to timely care. These elements are as follows:

- Balance supply and demand, which first requires understanding local supply and demand via the 5Ps microsystem self-assessment.
- Reduce backlog by working down cues of patients waiting for appointments, and by creating alternatives to traditional face-to-face interactions.
- Reduce the variety of appointment types and standardize appointment lengths.
- Develop contingency plans for unusual circumstances through development of flexible, multiskilled staff.
- Work to adjust demand profiles by maximizing activity at appointments and optimizing patient involvement in care.
- Increase the availability of bottleneck resources by managing constraints and optimizing care team efficiencies.

We can recognize in this recommendation to optimize care team efficiencies the obvious link between improving access specifically and improving microsystem efficiency more generally. The new model thus becomes familiar. Designing for advance access is, after all, about optimizing roles, standardizing protocols, implementing huddles, anticipating demand and supply, and reducing barriers to efficient workflow.

## Effective Care Transitions

Once we have reframed the challenge of building access as an invitation to actively manage (through system redesign) the balance between supply of clinical resources and demand for those resources, we are ready to embrace an even broader view that includes clinical handoffs and care transitions as special forms of advanced access. Recall the acute care requirements of Joanne, who suffers from progressing lobar pneumonia. Her journey requires smooth and timely access not only into her *receiving* microsystem (the office of her primary care practitioner), but also into *a series of subsequent microsystems* (the ambulance team, the emergency department, the inpatient intensive care unit), each of which must prepare itself to receive Joanne and her clinical information in a highly reliable manner.

The design of clinical handoffs thus becomes, in this view, a special subset of advanced access design. This is true in both outpatient and inpatient settings. Each clinical microsystem relies upon a next clinical microsystem downstream to receive the patient at a precise time, through precise transitional protocols, and with precise new needs to be met.[16,17] During her acute illness, Joanne travels through several clinical microsystems, each of which depends on the clinical microsystems both before (for appropriate information) and after (for safe and effective patient flow and for efficient management of resources). The *Transition and Handoff* worksheet in the Chapter Seven Action Guide provides a helpful tool to evaluate the volume and types of transitions into the clinical microsystem and the volume and types of handoffs to other clinical microsystems. In addition, the review of the transitions and handoffs allows deeper assessment of the processes in the transitions and handoffs to identify improvement opportunities to ensure safe and reliable patient flow. The special handoff protocols described in Chapter Five (including such mnemonics as "SBAR" and "I PASS the BATON") are in fact formalized tools to optimize access and communication within and between clinical microsytems.[18,19] Effective communication at these care transitions specifically links the *accessibility* priority with other quality emphases on safety, efficiency, and effectiveness.[13]

## CONCLUSION

We have observed that acute illness engenders unique feelings of urgency, anxiety, uncertainty, and disruption in patients and families, and that these feelings may be mirrored, to a greater or lesser extent, in members of the clinical microsystem. Such strong reactions coexist with the more technical challenges of acute care, which include the expectation of clinical excellence grounded in scientific evidence, the demand for rapid access, the need for reliable handoffs and coordination, and the requirement for responsive timeliness of care.

These challenges are met through careful preplanning of clinical services, through specific attention to patient and provider roles, through rehearsal of evidence-based algorithms, and through design and implementation of advanced access strategies and effective handoffs. These acute care features are subject to continuous improvement by using real-time reflection on specific value-added clinical processes. Indeed, although preventive, chronic, and palliative interventions may be similarly parsed into discrete process components (and these parsings are considered in Chapters Six, Eight, and Nine), acute interactions may be especially well-suited to process analysis. More so than in preventive, chronic, or palliative settings, the patient's experience of acute illness (and thus the microsystem's acute response to that illness) has well-demarcated beginnings and endings. The care is often inherently algorithmic, and thus its contours can be readily mapped. This mapping in turn facilitates application of specific change concepts to specifically improvable components of clinical care.

Consider again the idealized flowchart of Figure 7.4 and imagine that its separate boxes represent discrete steps in a particular acute care intervention. Several of Langley's change concepts are likewise depicted in this figure, and we can immediately appreciate their relevance to the design and improvement of specific microsystem care processes.[11,12] We have suggested already that the concept of modifying the input (in the form of pre-visit patient instructions and care plans) can enhance clinical care by directing the right intensity of care to the right patient at the right time. We have similarly seen that arranging to change a process concept from traditional to advanced access adds immediate value not only to the individual patient in need (whose urgent symptoms receive more rapid attention), but also to the overall system, whose resources and capacity are more effectively organized and distributed. Again, by eliminating handoff failures between steps, through predefined care transition algorithms, both patients and providers enjoy greater system safety and efficiency.

We can easily envision further microsystem improvements stimulated by change concept applications at discrete steps in the algorithm. What value might be added to patient triage, for example, if a clinical microsystem applied Langley's change concepts of combining and eliminating steps? What if participants explored the reordering or even reconceptualizing of entire sequences, thus creating a new sequence and indeed an entirely new service (telemedicine and Internet care, for example, instead of office care) to meet the same acute need? The possibilities are numerous, even as the reflective process that supports testing changes is reassuringly stable.

That process should by now feel familiar to students of clinical improvement. Clinical microsystem members collectively analyze the present pattern of care and then apply change concepts to identify discrete interventions that might improve the process in various ways. One such intervention is chosen for pilot testing; specific roles are defined, and a small test of change is implemented. Sufficient data are collected to demonstrate success (or not) of the given intervention, and clinical care is continually refined in large or small ways, based upon collective learning of all participants. Close attention to this process directly supports the planning for the unexpected that is crucial in acute care. The clinical microsystem is capable of linking inherently unpredictable health events with coordinated clinical services that set patients on a more predictable (timely, effective, reliable, and high-value) clinical journey.

## SUMMARY

- The urgency and unpredictability of acute illness requires that clinical microsystems anticipate patients' needs and rehearse tightly coordinated clinical responses.
- Reliability in acute contexts depends upon timely and accessible service, effective handoffs between providers, and care that is evidence-based and technically sound.
- Specific design features, including algorithm-based care, structured decision-making processes, and well-defined (but flexible) roles, will facilitate microsystems' delivery of the highest value acute care.

## KEY TERMS

Action plan

Acute illness

Capability

Change concepts

Clinical acuity

Competence

Evidence-based clinical algorithms

Huddle

If-then formulations of
    algorithm-based care

Practice-specific triage protocol

## REVIEW QUESTIONS

1. What is the role of clinical microsystems in acute care? Consider the microsystem staff and patient and family perspectives.
2. What are the fundamental design requirements for acute care in the clinical microsystem?
3. How does patient access to health care impact acute care and clinical microsystem processes?
4. What essential elements are necessary for ideal handoffs between microsystems?

## DISCUSSION QUESTIONS

1. Think about the clinical microsystem you are studying. Describe how the microsystem plans and prepares for acute care from both the patient and the microsystem staff perspective.

2. How easy is it for patients and families to access your microsystem for acute needs? What are some of the various access needs, such as access to appointments, to an inpatient bed, to information, to test results, and to prescription refills?

3. Think about the design requirements for acute care to answer the following questions:

   a. What are the specific timing needs within your microsystem from the perspective of both the patient (for example, rapid service) and the team members (for example, carefully orchestrated sequencing of process steps)?

   b. How are evidence-based practices, algorithms, and protocols embedded in the clinical microsystem? Describe how they are standardized and completed correctly by the right person at the right time every time.

   c. What opportunities exist to optimize interdisciplinary roles to achieve joy in work and to ensure the right person is doing the right thing at the right time, and that flexibility exists to meet changing needs?

   d. How are patients and families engaged in the work of your microsystem? Are there opportunities for patients and families to participate in design and innovation of care? Provide examples.

4. Discuss how your microsystem currently plans for the unexpected. What might you do to design improved acute processes that result in predictable responses and actions?

## REFERENCES

1. Institute of Medicine Committee on Quality Health Care in America. *Crossing the quality chasm: A new health system for the 21st century.* Washington, DC: National Academies Press, 2001.

2. Godfrey, M., Nelson, E. C., Wasson, J. H., Johnson, J. K., & Batalden, P. B. Planning patient-centered services. In E. Nelson, P. B. Batalden, & M. M. Godfrey (Eds.), *Quality by design: A clinical microsystems approach.* San Francisco: Jossey-Bass, 2007.

3. Institute for Clinical Systems Improvement. Retrieved February 10, 2010, from www.icsi.org/guidelines_and_more

4. Glouberman, S., & Zimmerman, B. *Complicated and complex systems: What would successful reform of Medicare look like?* Ottawa: Commission on the Future of Health Care in Canada, 2002.

5. Liu, S., Homa, K., Butterly, J. R., Kirkland, K. B., & Batalden, P. B. Improving the simple, complicated and complex realities of community-acquired pneumonia. *Quality and Safety in Health Care,* 2009, *18,* 93–98.

6. Fraser, S., & Greenhalgh, T. Coping with complexity: Educating for capability. *British Medical Journal,* 2001, *323,* p. 799.

7. Parsons, T. *The social system.* Glencoe, IL: The Free Press, 1951.

8. Green, L., Fryer Jr., G. E., Yawn, B. P., Lanier, D., & Dovey, S. M. The ecology of medical care revisited. *New England Journal of Medicine,* 2001, *344,* 2021–2025.

9. White, K., Williams, T. F., & Greenberg, B. G. The ecology of medical care. *New England Journal of Medicine,* 1961, *265,* 885–892.

10. O'Connor, B. *Healing traditions: Alternative medicine and the health professions.* Philadelphia: University of Pennsylvania Press, 1995.

11. Langley et al. *The improvement guide: A practical approach to enhancing organizational performance.* San Francisco: Jossey-Bass, 1996.

12. Batalden, P., Johnson, J. K., Nelson, E. C., Plume, S. K., & Lazar, J. S. (2007). Building on change: Concepts for improving any clinical process. In E. Nelson, P. B. Batalden, & J. L. Lazar (Eds.), *Practice-based learning and improvement: A clinical improvement action guide.* Oakbrook, IL: Joint Commission Resources.

13. *Advanced clinic access:* prepared for VHA by the Institute for Healthcare Improvement, Boston 2001.

14. Murray, M., Bodenheimer, T., Rittenhouse, D., & Grumbach, K. Improving timely access to primary care: Case studies of the advanced access model. *Journal of the American Medical Association,* 2003, *289*(8), 1042–1046.

15. Murray, M., & Berwick, D. M. Advanced access: Reducing waiting and delays in primary care. *Journal of the American Medical Association,* 2003, *289*(8), 1035–1040.

16. Friesen, M., White, S. V., & Byers, J. F. *Handoffs: Implications for nurses.* Retrieved December 2, 2009, from www.ncbi.nlm.nih.gov/bookshelf/br.fcgi?book=nursehb &part=ch34

17. Greiner, A. *White space or black hole: What can we do to improve care transitions?* Philadelphia: ABIM Foundation and SUTTP Alliance, 2007.

18. Agency for Healthcare Research and Quality. *TeamSTEPPS: National implementation.* Retrieved December 1, 2009, from http://teamstepps.ahrq.gov

19. Haig, K., Sutton, S., & Whittington, J. SBAR: A shared mental model for improving communication between clinicians. *Joint Commission Journal on Quality and Patient Safety,* 2006, *32*(3), 167–175.

As noted in Chapter Seven, acute care has many handoffs and transitions in the patient's course of care. In these white spaces the patient is at risk for transfer of incomplete, inaccurate, or absent information specific to the patient's unique needs and plan of care. Transition from ambulatory care to emergency medical systems such as an ambulance with trained staff and then to emergency departments requires exquisite communication and advance planning of the handoff processes.

Chapter Five offers standardized tools to support communication and handoffs between units including "SBAR" and "I PASS the BATON."

Figure AG7.1 is designed to help clinical microsystems reflect on the numbers and types of handoffs the microsystem participates in actively or passively. With an interdisciplinary group representing all roles in the clinical microsystem, include an agenda item in a meeting to discuss patient transitions and handoffs.

The group should answer the following questions:

- How many handoffs occur in the clinical microsystem each day?
- Do volumes vary by shift, day of the week, or seasonally?
- How many different clinical microsystems hand off patients to your clinical microsystem? How many times per day or week? Do you have all the information and data about the patients to smoothly assume responsibility for care and services?
- How many different clinical microsystems does your unit hand off to? Are there patterns in the handoffs? Do you know if the receiving microsystems have all the information they need to assume care for your patients?
- What is the process of communication and transition? How can it be improved?
- Have you discussed the handoff process with either sending or receiving clinical microsystems to determine each others' needs to provide safe and reliable care for the patient during the transition?

Once you have collected current data regarding volumes and patterns of handoffs in and out of your clinical microsystem, select a high volume, high frequency handoff. Invite the sending clinical microsystem to meet with your microsystem to assess the current transfer process to identify improvement opportunities.

FIGURE AG7.1   Microsystem Transitions and Handoffs.

Microsystem Name:_____          Date:_____

| Received | | |
|---|---|---|
| Location | Method | Frequency in 24 Hours |
| | | |
| | | |
| | | |
| | | |
| | | |
| | | |
| | | |
| | | |
| | | |
| | | |
| | | |
| | | |
| | | |

→ Microsystem →

| Sent | | |
|---|---|---|
| Location | Method | Frequency in 24 Hours |
| | | |
| | | |
| | | |
| | | |
| | | |
| | | |
| | | |
| | | |
| | | |
| | | |
| | | |
| | | |

| Most Frequent | |
|---|---|
| Received | |
| Sent | |
| Improvement Opportunities | |

# ENGAGING COMPLEXITY IN CHRONIC ILLNESS CARE

Joel S. Lazar

Paul B. Batalden

Eugene C. Nelson

Marjorie M. Godfrey

## LEARNING OBJECTIVES

- Explore the essential features of chronic illness care experienced over time and describe how these features require special considerations for the clinical microsystem, patients, and families.
- Identify the three essential goals of chronic illness care and how these interface with activities in preventive, acute, and palliative care.
- Discuss the framework of simple, complicated, and complex as it relates to chronic illness care.
- Examine the chronic care model, and explore its actualization in the clinical microsystem's design, delivery, and improvement of specific chronic care services.

Nearly half of all Americans live with chronic illness, and the impact is tremendous upon individuals and families, upon health systems, and upon our larger society. To effectively meet the needs of patients with chronic illness, clinical microsystems must align specific interventions with care needs that are simple, complicated, and complex in nature. Longitudinality, uncertainty, and relationship-dependence are especially salient features of chronic illness care that compel the clinical microsystem to engage principles of complexity in creative but still rigorous ways. The *chronic care model* provides a framework for partnering with patients, for coordinating resources, and for designing meaningful interventions that optimize clinical value. In the present chapter we explore this model, and we link it to specific applications of complexity theory in the frontline care of chronically ill patients.

## AN INVITATION TO COMPLEXITY

The design, delivery, and improvement of chronic illness care offer unique challenges and opportunities to members of the clinical microsystem, and to patients and families who partner in the management of their own health. The burden of chronic illness is tremendous in our health care system and in our society. Indeed, two-thirds of us will die of chronic illness, and half of us *live* (functionally or otherwise) with at least one chronic disease.[1,2] The majority of clinical encounters in America are focused upon longitudinal rather than acute illness care, as is 75 cents of every health care dollar.[3,4] But despite this abundant need, despite the resources expended, and despite the talents and best intentions of well-trained clinicians, nurses, technicians, and administrative staff, most patients with chronic illness receive care that falls demonstrably short of evidence-based quality goals.[5] Why have such goals been so difficult to achieve? Have we properly conceptualized the needs and experiences of chronically ill people? Have we appropriately framed the clinical and design questions that require attention? In the final analysis, how can clinical microsystems enhance the value of care delivered?

Neither these questions nor their solutions are simple, nor are they even (to borrow a pointed phrase from Glouberman and Zimmerman) "merely complicated."[6] Indeed, as we shall explore in the present chapter, we have entered a domain of problems that are *truly complex*, and it is the very recognition of this complexity that suggests new answers to our difficult questions. As we consider the unique demands chronic illness care places upon patients, families, and clinical microsystems, we quickly recognize that new conceptual paradigms and new forms of intervention are required. Chronic illness is not simply an expanded and extended form of acute illness. The differences between acute and chronic are qualitative (not quantitative), and these differences are enlightening.

Consider the comparison in Table 8.1 of acute and chronic disease, adapted and expanded from the work of Zimmerman and Plsek.[7] Note that *acute disease* most often begins abruptly and progresses (in the context of well-defined and often effective therapies) to a well-defined end point, typically with full and predictable restoration of a patient's normal health. *Chronic disease*, in contrast, begins gradually and is experienced continuously (in the context of therapies that may control but usually cannot cure the disease itself); there is no specified end point, but instead an expectation that *flare-ups* will manifest intermittently, unpredictably, and over a lifetime. The management of acute disease is most commonly office- or hospital-based, with the interprofessional team functioning as the authoritative center of knowledge and action. Chronic disease management, in contrast, may be *office-linked*, but is enacted predominantly in the home

### Table 8.1   A Comparison of Acute and Chronic Disease

|  | Acute Disease | Chronic Disease |
|---|---|---|
| Onset | • Usually abrupt | • Gradual over time |
| Course | • Well-defined endpoint, with a return to normal health | • Continuous, with flare-ups of instability |
| Specific therapy, technologic interventions | • Often available and effective | • No cure; indecisive technologies; therapies with adverse effects |
| Predictability | • Often high | • Often low |
| Autonomy, control, and knowledge | • Professional has more knowledge than patient | • Reciprocally knowledgeable participants in care |
| Site of care | • Office- or hospital-based | • Office-linked |
| Overarching need | • Reliability, timeliness | • Resiliency, relationship |

*Source:* Adapted and extended from Zimmerman, B., & Plsek, P. *Microsystems as complex adaptive systems: Ideas for improvement.* Retrieved February 10, 2010, from www.clinicalmicrosystem.org

and community by patients, families, and support systems, based on reciprocal knowledge and authority that includes all participants in active partnership. We may observe more generally that, and acute disease entails care that is reliably delivered *in* time, chronic disease requires care to be resilient and relationship-centered *over* time.

It is precisely this longitudinality, this care over time, and this interdependence of people and their support systems that underscores the challenge and the opportunity of designing and delivering chronic illness care. As we have already suggested, although most Americans will *die of* chronic disease, we also, for years and decades before, *live with* chronic disease. This illness, like the life of which it becomes a part, is no mere static event, but a necessarily (and continuously) changing experience. Its management requires dynamic and repeated negotiations over time. These negotiations are internal to the individual who is ill and also involve clinical systems that support the individual's self-care across years or decades of life. Predictability and unilateral authority are exchanged for adaptability and for a resilient and productive relationship. Simple aspects of chronic illness care may still be served by well-rehearsed triage strategies, and complicated components may still benefit from standardized clinical algorithms (such as those described in the acute care circumstances of Chapter Seven), but these strategies are no longer wholly sufficient. The overall caregiving environment is more complex, and the clinical microsystem must build into itself the capacity to engage this complexity.

The chronic illness experience thus invites us to explore and to expand both the content of clinical microsystem care and the process by which this care is designed and delivered. We shall observe that *care over time* implies a new role for the clinical microsystem, in response to newly emerging needs and capacities of patients and families. As outcomes become less predictable, as decision-making authority is necessarily shifted and shared, as the boundary between a patient's illness and his overall life becomes increasingly more permeable, we recognize the essential importance of partnership and relationship to achieve shared clinical goals.[8,9] As depicted in Table 8.2, the new need of patients and families is for longitudinal resiliency and support in self-management of ongoing disease. The clinical microsystem's realization of this need does not require abandoning technical rigor and formal process analysis. Rather it requires expanding these core qualities while engaging the new complexity implied in longitudinal relationship-centered care.

Table 8.2   Overarching Care Needs of Patient and Family

| | |
|---|---|
| Preventive care | • Proactive assessment and mitigation of health risks |
| Acute care | • Timely attention to new or newly worsening disruption of health or function |
| Chronic care | • Longitudinal resiliency and support in self-management of ongoing disease |
| Palliative care | • Comfort and dignity in the context of underlying disease progression |

In this chapter we first explore chronic illness care from the patient's perspective. We seek an intimate understanding that fully anticipates the needs of those the microsystem serves. Although each chronic disease presents unique challenges, we observe that common experiential themes emerge across varied diagnoses.[10] This commonality informs the patient's and the clinical microsystem's engagement in chronic illness. In this context we examine essential management goals and specific team-based strategies to realize them. In particular, we review the powerful *chronic care model* developed by Wagner and colleagues,[11,12,13,14] which provides both a conceptual framework and an operational blueprint for the planning, delivery, and improvement of frontline chronic illness care. Finally, we devote significant attention to the *interface* of patient and caregiving perspectives, for it is here in the partnership, in microsystem coordination and patient self-management strategies, that *care over time* is enacted. At this interface of patient and caregiving perspectives, we shall also further explore the principles of complexity science, which inform the microsystem's approach to the design and improvement of chronic care.

## THE EXPERIENCE OF CHRONIC ILLNESS

Chronic disease is ubiquitous and, as Table 8.3 suggests, can arise from dysfunction in literally any organ system of the body. Although the pathophysiologic origins of biomedical disease (in heart, lung, or intestine) may specify unique organ-based features, the final common pathway of all illness is a whole-person experience and one that is deeply embedded in familial, cultural, occupational, and financial contexts. Effective design and delivery of chronic illness care begins with a rich understanding of this whole-person experience and of these contexts, because microsystem interventions must have their effect on real patients and their lives.

Let us therefore consider one person's actual experience of chronic illness. We shall see in the following case study how medical, psychological, social, and economic issues all interact to create a clinical whole that is more complex and more challenging to manage than the sum of its discrete parts.

## CASE STUDY: THE EXPERIENCE OF CHRONIC ILLNESS

Carl Davis is a sixty-six-year-old high school teacher, grandfather, and amateur jazz guitarist. Although in the past he has found much joy in his work, his music, and especially in his time with his grandson, in recent years he has taken increasingly less pleasure in these and other activities. Distracting and fatiguing him now are several chronic diseases that individually, and in combination, draw on his time, energy, and emotional and financial resources.

Most important from his own perspective, Carl has lived these past ten years with type 2 diabetes mellitus. At his doctor's suggestion, he has tried to lose weight to bring this condition under better control, but he has experienced no meaningful success. Instead, persistent blood sugar elevations have necessitated initiation of one, then two, blood sugar-lowering medications. The second of these causes abdominal bloating and intermittent diarrhea, which have led to social embarrassment on more than one occasion. But Carl endeavors to comply with instructions for fear that stopping his medications will make matters even worse. Indeed, Carl's hemoglobin A1c level is persistently elevated to 9.0 (normal is less than 6.0), a value that suggests substantial chronic elevation of serum blood sugar levels and that indicates ongoing risk of eye and kidney disease (due to gradually accruing toxicity from the excess sugar). On one occasion he has been hospitalized for acute foot infection due to diabetes-induced neurovascular changes, also secondary to high sugars. The infection resolved, but his risk of future infections remains high. He now monitors the sugar level via fingerstick measurements he can perform at home, although he does so less frequently than his doctor has advised. He is frustrated by consistently poor sugar readings, which he experiences as daily reminders of his failure to improve and as a reminder of his own mortality. Because he is frustrated, he finds reasons to avoid the self-monitoring; sometimes he genuinely forgets due to his absorption in other life obligations, which include the need to tend to other chronic health conditions.

Like a substantial number of older Americans, Carl lives with not one chronic illness but several. Most notably he suffers from hypertension and elevated cholesterol, which (in combination with his diabetes) substantially increase his risk of dying prematurely from heart disease or stroke. Carl is uncomfortably aware of these risks. He takes daily medications to bring these conditions under control, and he also receives treatment for asthma and osteoarthritis, diseases that diminish his capacity to exercise and to improve his own health.

When clinicians and even family members ask how he is feeling, Carl typically responds, "I am fine." He is no complainer, and he feels shame regarding his several health conditions. He therefore downplays sensations and emotions that recur commonly in his life. Almost daily he experiences general fatigue and focal pain; he has difficulties at work due to poor concentration (and to frequently missed work days for clinic appointments). He worries about his finances because co-payments for office visits and expensive medications consume an increasing proportion of his monthly income. His wife observes him to be irritable at home and fears this is due to reactive depression the health care team has failed to diagnose.

After living ten years with his diabetes (and even longer with some of his other conditions), after adding a ninth chronic disease medication (with further side effects) to his growing list, after losing a few pounds but then regaining them, after setting aside his jazz guitar and reducing time with his grandson, Carl feels frustrated, sad, and generally disempowered. Simple and complicated elements of his care (such as blood sugar testing and algorithmic adjustment of medications) remain important, but these are insufficient to address the more complex reality of his situation. Even when he can focus successfully on one or two problems at a time, he cannot sustain the effort because other neglected problems become apparent. "There's just so much, doctor," he complained recently to his endocrinologist. "So much to take care of. . . ."

## THE BURDEN OF CHRONIC ILLNESS

As Carl's story suggests, there is indeed "so much to take care of" in the management of chronic illness. This is true for individual patients, for frontline clinical microsystems, and for the nation's health care system in its entirety. As we have already suggested, two of every three Americans will die of chronic disease. The top killers include heart

Table 8.3    Common Chronic Diseases in the United States

| | |
|---|---|
| **Cardiac (Heart)**<br>Coronary artery disease<br>Heart failure<br>Hypertension | **Blood**<br>Chronic anemia<br>Sickle cell disease |
| **Neuro (Brain)**<br>Cerebrovascular disease, stroke<br>Epilepsy<br>Alzheimer's disease<br>Parkinson's disease | **Gastrointestinal**<br>Chronic hepatitis<br>Cirrhosis<br>Inflammatory bowel disease (Crohn's,<br>    ulcerative colitis)<br>Irritable bowel syndrome |
| **Endocrine**<br>Diabetes mellitus<br>Thyroid diseases | **Chronic pain syndromes**<br>Degenerative joint disease (osteoarthritis)<br>Fibromyalgia |
| **Cancer**<br>Lung, breast, colon, prostate, ovary,<br>    uterus, leukemia, lymphoma | **Bone**<br>Osteoporosis |
| **Lungs**<br>COPD (emphysema, chronic bronchitis)<br>Asthma | **Inflammatory**<br>Rheumatoid arthritis<br>Lupus |
| **Skin**<br>Psoriasis<br>Eczema<br>Acne | **Mental and Behavioral**<br>Depression<br>Anxiety<br>Attention deficit disorder<br>Substance abuse |

disease, cancer, stroke, emphysema, diabetes, and Alzheimer's disease.[15] In addition, almost half of us, 125 million Americans, *live* with chronic illness, and millions more are diagnosed each year. Among people older than 65 years old (the highest growing segment of our population), 80 percent live with at least one chronic disease; 63 percent in this age group live with more than one chronic disease, and 25 percent (including Carl in our case study) live with four or more chronic conditions.[13]

Recognition of not only death rates but also of *life rates* has astounding implications. Although stroke is the third leading killer of adult Americans, a larger number of stroke victims survive their acute event and are left to live with small or potentially very large degrees of functional impairment and chronic clinical need. Stroke has left 1 million Americans alive with disabling conditions. A much smaller (although growing) number of people die each year from asthma, yet this condition accounts for 400,000 to 500,000 hospitalizations per year, 14 million missed school days, and 100 million days of restricted activity per year. Arthritis, by comparison, is only rarely a killer and rarely results in hospitalization (apart from surgical admissions for joint replacement), but it affects one in three adults and is the number one cause of disability in our nation.[2]

Of course, to the same extent that chronic illness impacts the personal lives of so many patients, it also impacts the professional lives of clinicians, nurses, technicians, administrators, and other interdisciplinary members of the clinical microsystem. These professionals appreciate that most of their work time is committed, directly or indirectly, to the care of people with chronic illness. This is true in primary care settings where the majority of patient visits are dedicated to such conditions as diabetes, hypertension, heart disease, and depression,[16] and in subspecialty medicine where entire fields like rheumatology, cardiology, pulmonology, and oncology have evolved to address clinical illnesses that are predominantly chronic in nature. Less obviously, but just as importantly, most inpatient admissions also represent flare-ups or decompensations of previously stable chronic conditions such as heart failure or chronic obstructive pulmonary disease, or adverse consequences of medications used in treatment. Surgical teams are similarly impacted. Rigorous consideration of and planning for chronic medications, disabilities, and disease-induced vulnerabilities is essential to assure best outcomes in operative care.

In the face of intense resource utilization, it is no surprise that such a huge proportion of our nation's health care costs are attributable to chronic illness. The United States' total health care expenditure in 2001 was $1.4 trillion, which represented an average cost of more than $5,000 for each American. Approximately 75 percent of this cost, or *one trillion dollars*, was spent on management of chronic disease. This economic burden particularly affects the older community and also the Medicare system that financially supports their care. As Table 8.4 reveals, more than half of all persons older than 65 have more than one chronic illness, and their care accounts for 95 percent of all Medicare expenditures. A full two-thirds of Medicare dollars are consumed by the one in four elders who live with four or more chronic conditions.[13]

And these are only the direct costs. Because chronic illness is experienced *over time*, substantial indirect costs also accrue from disability and diminished productivity. One in ten Americans experience major limitations in activity due to their chronic condition(s), and for many conditions the dollars due to lost productivity rival or exceed those spent on direct medical care. In 2003, cardiovascular disease, cancer, and stroke accounted for one-quarter of a trillion dollars of lost productivity. And ill people are not the only ones impacted; family members experience lost productivity as well. When children with asthma miss fourteen million school days per year, many care-providing parents will likely miss workdays as well.[2]

Chronic illnesses make up the majority of patients' articulated needs, occupy the majority of clinical microsystems' work time, and consume the majority of our nation's health care dollars. But even so we have not yet succeeded in meeting this great

Table 8.4    Number of Chronic Conditions per Medicare Beneficiary

| Number of Conditions | Percent of Beneficiaries | Percent of Expenditures |
| --- | --- | --- |
| 0 | 18 | 1 |
| 1 | 19 | 4 |
| 2 | 21 | 11 |
| 3 | 18 | 18 |
| 4 | 12 | 21 |
| 5 | 7 | 18 |
| 6 | 3 | 13 |
| 7+ | 2 | 14 |

*Source:* Improving chronic illness care. *Chronic care model.* Retrieved February 28, 2010, from www .improvingchroniccare.org/index.php?p=The_Chronic_Care_Model&s=2

challenge with the level of quality it deserves and requires. Large-scale surveys confirm that individuals receive only half of recommended interventions for chronic care needs.[5] This shortfall is apparent in both general reviews and disease-specific assessments. In community settings and academic centers, for example, fewer than 50 percent of diabetic patients (including Carl in our own case study) currently achieve target levels of control for blood sugar, blood pressure, or cholesterol,[17,18] and no more than 10 percent meet all three of these basic quality targets.[19]

There is, as Carl complained, "so much to take care of" in chronic illness care, and not only he, but also the several clinical microsystems with whom he interacts, can feel overwhelmed by the challenges. Let us therefore seek a broader perspective that helps us meet patients' needs more effectively and efficiently. In this chapter's remaining sections we first articulate the general and specific goals of chronic illness care in terms that reveal realistic pathways for partnership and intervention. We then explore conceptual models that frame these interventions more precisely, giving special attention to Glouberman and Zimmerman's *paradigm of complexity* and Wagner's chronic care model. We conclude by examining specific implications and applications of these models in frontline clinical microsystems, where design, delivery, and improvement of chronic care processes must finally occur.

## THE GOALS OF CHRONIC ILLNESS CARE

We have suggested in Chapters Six and Seven that the boundaries between conceptual domains of preventive, acute, chronic, and palliative care are in fact permeable. Classifying care in these domains permits powerful assessment and planning of discrete care components, which is a major strength of the entire clinical microsystem model. Even so, we must maintain our awareness that such classification may sometimes reflect the health care system's organization of services more than patients' actual experience of health and illness. In some microsystems, patients bring multiple needs simultaneously, and these may leap across the domains of preventive, acute, chronic, and palliative care.

When we consider chronic illness care in particular, the other elements of preventive, acute, and palliative care do not merely overlap; they are essential dimensions of chronic illness management. Because chronic diseases are experienced longitudinally, with many ups and downs, the illness will have many fluctuating manifestations *between* patients and even *within* the life of a given patient. Preventive concerns are an essential component of the chronic illness experience. Acute flare-ups and palliative needs must be similarly addressed. A patient-centered model of chronic illness care must anticipate such needs and must specify strategies for interdisciplinary members of the clinical microsystem to partner with patients in meeting them.

As proposed in this chapter's opening section (and depicted in Table 8.2), the underlying clinical need in chronic illness is for longitudinal resiliency and support in the self-management of ongoing disease. How does this *chronic* need manifest itself in the interconnected domains of preventive, acute, palliative, and chronic care? Careful reflection upon this question leads us to identify what are in fact the three essential goals of chronic illness care (see Table 8.5).

1. In the *preventive care* domain, patients with chronic illness need clinical microsystem support to reduce (through prevention) the morbidity and mortality associated

**Table 8.5  Three Essential Goals of Chronic Illness Care**

| Essential Goal | Interface with Other Domains | Examples, Comments |
|---|---|---|
| 1. Reduction of morbidity and mortality associated with late disease-related sequelae | Preventive care | • Amputations<br>• Renal failure<br>• Myocardial infarction (in patients with diabetes) |
| 2. Minimization of impact of short-term symptomatic flare-ups | Acute care | • Asthma exacerbation<br>• Heart failure readmissions<br>• Pain flare-ups in arthritis<br>• Diabetic ketoacidosis |
| 3. Optimization of quality of life, function, relationships, empowerment, and joy | Palliative care | • Not just a means to goals 1 and 2, but an end in itself |

with late disease-related sequelae. Thus, for example, proactive counseling, screening, and therapeutic interventions (of the kind discussed in Chapter Six) can help reduce a diabetic patient's future risk of renal failure, myocardial infarction, and amputation.

2. In the *acute care* domain, patients with chronic illness need clinical microsystem support to minimize the impact of short-term symptomatic flare-ups. Common manifestations of acuity in chronic illness (as suggested in Chapter Seven) include emergency department visits for exacerbations of asthma, hospital admissions for congestive heart failure, and presentations of life-threatening ketoacidosis in people with diabetes mellitus.

3. At the interface of chronic and *palliative* domains (as explored in Chapter Nine), patients with chronic illness need clinical microsystem support to optimize quality of life, function, relationships, empowerment, and joy. This attention to qualitative well-being is not simply a means to achieve the more quantitative goals 1 and 2 (*reduction of morbidity and mortality* and *minimization of impact of short-term symptomatic flare-ups, respectively*); rather it is an end in itself. Most people will live with chronic illness until they die, and *care over time* implies rigorous attention to the qualitative value of lived experience, including the optimization of longitudinal function and subjective well-being.

Although certain disease-specific manifestations are associated with one chronic illness or the next (such as the wheezing of asthma or emphysema, or the metabolic disregulation of diabetes), many experiential features of chronic illness are shared across different diseases and form a common and even predictable set of functional challenges that can respond to microsystem planning and intervention.[10] Carl, in our case study, has experienced ongoing pain and fatigue that require attention even apart from his blood sugar and cholesterol control. The following list shows the shared features of those of living with chronic illness:

• Fatigue
• Exertional intolerance
• Pain

- Sexual dysfunction
- Sleep dysfunction
- Occupational dysfunction and financial hardship
- Medication side-effects and management of polypharmacy
- Depression, isolation, challenges to self-efficacy

Critically, another shared symptom in so many chronic conditions is clinical or subclinical depression. As Carl has experienced in our case study, the very nature of chronic disease threatens loss of autonomy, triggers shame and isolation, and often diminishes real or perceived self-efficacy. These experiences are negative in their own right and can also perpetuate a vicious cycle of disengagement, self-neglect, and worsened clinical disease. As we shall soon discuss, an essential role of the clinical microsystem in chronic care is to actively promote patients' self-efficacy and self-management.[9] This emphasis not only facilitates improvement in quantitative biomedical outcomes, but also protects against (or helps to reverse) the sense of helplessness that can manifest as clinical depression. Achievement of mastery becomes its own reward.

## CLINICAL COMPLEXITY IN CHRONIC ILLNESS CARE

We have seen that although some characteristics of chronic illness are disease-specific, many experiential features are shared across numerous conditions. We have observed that these needs are broad and deep, encompassing clinical priorities that are both quantitative and qualitative in nature. As we turn our attention now to the clinical microsystem charged with addressing these needs, we observe that here, too, many system challenges, and many successful design features to meet these challenges, reappear across multiple illnesses. Most important, these design features must address not only discrete problems but also the whole person who presents for care. Clinical microsystems must therefore embrace a rich diversity of interventions that match the breadth and depth of patients' diverse and changing needs. Parchman observed, for example, that during an average seventeen-minute office visit for patients with diabetes mellitus, a full seventeen topics, questions, or symptoms were addressed.[20] How can the clinical microsystem begin to organize its resources (both human and technical) to meet such varied and numerous chronic needs?

A formal model of clinical complexity will help us meet this great challenge. Glouberman and Zimmerman,[6] and later Zimmerman and Plsek,[7] have proposed a framework of *simple, complicated, and complex problems* that may guide the microsystem's design and improvement of clinical care. These authors observe that problems of all sorts (not only clinical) may be categorized generally as simple, complicated, or complex in nature. These categories have practical consequences and, as we shall show, specific implications for the design of clinical services.

As depicted in Table 8.6, *simple problems* involve high degrees of predictability in contexts that are highly replicable. Glouberman and Zimmerman suggest that following a recipe is a quintessentially simple problem. All ingredients are known and stable, and no special expertise is required to accomplish the task (although cooking expertise may increase success rate). Recipes are designed to produce standardized products, and the best recipes give good results every time because variation is kept to a minimum.

Table 8.6    Three Types of Activities: Simple, Complicated, and Complex

| Simple | Complicated | Complex |
|---|---|---|
| *Following a recipe* | *Building a rocket* | *Raising a child* |
| No expertise required | Expertise required in specialized fields | Expertise helps, but is not sufficient to meet all challenges |
| Recipe tested to assure replicability of later efforts | Sending one rocket increases chance the next will be successful | Raising one child gives no assurance of success with next child |
| Parts and quantities are clearly defined | Parts are separated, and then coordinated | Parts cannot be separated from the whole |
| Outcomes are highly certain | Outcomes are certain with application of technical expertise | Outcomes are inherently uncertain |

*Source:* Adapted from Glouberman, S., & Zimmerman, B. *Complicated and complex systems: What would successful reform of Medicare look like?* Ottawa: Commission on the Future of Health Care in Canada, 2002.

*Complicated problems* depend similarly on stable and ultimately predictable components, but high levels of technical expertise are required to coordinate these components as a meaningful whole. Consider the task of *sending a rocket to the moon*. Technical formulae, rather than simple recipes, are required to solve such a problem. The full set of elements may not be immediately known, but such elements are inherently *knowable* to specialists who possess proper training. These elements remain stable in themselves and in relation to each other; an engine booster, for example, does not aspire to become a heating coil. As a result, and *because* such challenges can be approached technically, there is a high degree of certainty about outcomes. Rockets are similar to each other in essential ways, and although it is not easy to send one rocket to the moon, succeeding on one occasion substantially increases the likelihood of success on subsequent attempts.

But let us contrast the simple and the *merely complicated* (Glouberman and Zimmerman's term) with truly *complex problems*. Both stability of components and predictability of outcomes are diminished here, and this uncertainty arises not because more complicated technology must be applied, but because the full nature of inputs and outputs (and of the relationships between inputs and outputs) is *inherently* unknowable in a technical sense.

*Raising a child* is an iconic complex problem. Unlike recipe ingredients and rocket components, every child is unique and must be understood irreducibly as an individual. Formulae have little application, and indeed may be detrimental to achieving good solutions. The child changes over time in ways a rocket does not, and the parents engaged in child raising change as well (in part because of their interactions *with* that child). Raising one child successfully may provide experience but does not assure success with the next child; technical expertise is neither necessary nor sufficient to meet the most meaningful challenges. Complex problems thus differ from the complicated in a manner that is qualitative rather than quantitative. Like chronic illness compared with acute, the former is not merely like the latter, only more so; the two categories are fundamentally distinct.

# DESIGNING FOR COMPLEXITY THROUGH ALIGNMENT OF PROBLEMS AND PRACTICE SOLUTIONS

In clinical contexts, it is an oversimplification to suggest that all acute care problems are merely complicated and that all chronic care problems are complex. We shall see immediately below that chronic care in particular poses various challenges that are often simple, complicated, *and* complex in nature. But certainly, as Zimmerman and Plsek suggest,[7] the complicated-complex distinction provides valuable insight into different problems and practices in acute versus chronic care. Review again the distinctions between these clinical domains, as depicted in Table 8.1. Note in particular, in chronic disease management, the recurring suggestions of complexity (in the sense that Glouberman and Zimmerman use this term): predictability is low, technologies are indecisive, therapeutic benefits must be balanced with long-term adverse effects, and autonomy is shared rather than centralized. We have entered a new and potentially uncomfortable realm, and at least some subset of chronic disease interventions must address this complexity directly.

Why do these labels matter? However intellectually engaging this exercise may be, what functional value is gained by parsing problems as simple, complicated, or complex? We suggest the clinical microsystem's thoughtful categorizing of problems in this manner permits alignment with practice solutions of a similar (simple, complicated, or complex) nature.[21] Well-designed and well-implemented clinical interventions are characterized by a matching of challenge and response and by a proactive aligning of categorical levels of clinical problem and practice solution. If alignment is absent, then quality predictably suffers. These relationships are depicted in Figure 8.1.

As we shall discuss, simple problems respond best to simple solutions, whereas complex problems call for solutions that are likewise complex. Consider the specific consequences of *mis*alignment: one simple problem in chronic illness care is monitoring for and administering annual influenza immunization (in high risk patients, such as those with diabetes, asthma, or emphysema). This problem may be solved with a similarly simple practice. A licensed practical nurse (LPN) reviews the pre-populated immunization list in the patient's chart at time of office visit and automatically (via standard orders) administers the vaccine, assuming patient consent has been given. Alternatively, and less appropriately, the same simple problem might be mismanaged via practices that are complicated or even complex. The physician herself, during busy office hours, reviews the details of a disorganized medical record to discover the latest immunization date, then searches the hall for available staff, and then negotiates with two available nurses to determine who is more available to administer that same shot.

FIGURE 8.1   Aligning Levels of Problem and Practice Complexity.

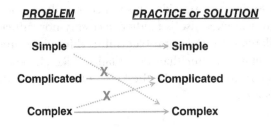

Table 8.7  Aligning Simple, Complicated, and Complex Activities with Appropriate Solutions

|  | Simple | Complicated | Complex |
|---|---|---|---|
| **Sample Problem** | Following a recipe | Building a rocket | Raising a child |
| **Prototype Solution** | Embedding yes or no functionality | Using if-then algorithms | Leveraging relationships |
| **Sample Solutions in Clinical Practice** | • Automating tasks<br>• Routinizing safety (check lists, forcing functions)<br>• Monitoring control | • Implementing care algorithms<br>• Adjusting therapies incrementally<br>• Standardizing education and treatment | • Building relationships<br>• Negotiating goals<br>• Managing uncertainty<br>• Evoking change |
| **Overarching Goal** | Ensuring reliability | Ensuring reliability | Ensuring resiliency |

In this scenario, the consequence of misalignment is at best an unnecessary waste of professionals' and patient's time, and at worst a failure to complete an important clinical task and evidence-based practice.

Or imagine the common but potentially more dangerous occurrence of complex problems that are met with merely complicated solutions. Our patient Carl grows more depressed due to his medical problems, functional limitations, and psychosocial concerns; he therefore neglects his medications, and his blood sugars further worsen, perpetuating a vicious cycle. His doctor responds to this sugar elevation with sequential increases in medication (a high tech solution) and with generic admonitions to improve diet and lose weight. Because Carl's true (and truly complex) problem of depression is not addressed in this battery of merely complicated solutions, diabetic therapy remains ineffective.

How then do clinical microsystems properly align levels of problem and practice complexity? Table 8.7 provides a template that links specific forms of clinical challenge (in chronic illness care) to therapeutic interventions of comparable complexity. Note that simple, complicated, and complex domains are all represented. The microsystem's task, when designing appropriate interventions, is to recognize what level of challenge is expressed in each clinical context and to match this problem to a practice solution of similar complexity.

Thus, as suggested in Table 8.7, *simple problems* in health care (the clinical equivalent of following a recipe) most commonly respond to solutions entailing *yes or no* functionality. For example, when a patient with emphysema develops clinical pneumonia, always check the oxygen saturation level (see Liu et al. for a sample application of this approach[21]). More generally, *simple practice solutions* in chronic care include automating tasks, monitoring control, and embedding safety via forcing function and checklists. In all these cases, the microsystem analyzes processes and empowers patients and professionals with well-specified tasks in well-defined roles. The expected outcome of such orchestration is increased service *reliability*.

*Complicated problems* call for reliability as well, but here the functionality is contingent or if-then in nature. Such problems benefit from sequential and well-designed decision nodes, also known as algorithms. When building a rocket or its clinical equivalent, such decision nodes are prominent and are derived from scientific evidence and technical expertise. For example, if Carl's blood pressure remains high (a complicated problem) after a trial of exercise and healthy diet, then add a medication of the ACE-inhibitor class. If his pressure remains high after two months, then double the dose. Complicated practice solutions in chronic illness care (and there are many) include implementing care algorithms, adjusting therapies incrementally, and standardizing patient education based on evidence from the scientific literature.

As suggested in our earlier discussion, complex problems are especially common in chronic illness care, and the functionality of solutions is no longer algorithmic but *relational*. When engaged in the clinical analogue of raising a child, absolute reliability is not possible. A more appropriate and achievable outcome is *resiliency* of relationship, the nurtured capacity of patients and health teams (together in partnership) to ride the waves of care over time. Essential values in this domain include autonomy, empowerment, and collaboration. Complex problem solutions entail building relationships, negotiating goals, managing uncertainty, and evoking behavioral changes in the patient.

This final list of complex problem solutions has taken us some distance from the familiar landscape of checklists and care algorithms. Building relationships and managing uncertainty sound at first glance more magical than practical, but in fact these behaviors are linked with skill sets and microsystem design features as grounded and specific as those that characterize simple and merely complicated interventions. Can we describe these features in terms that underscore their practical and functional nature? The answer is a resounding yes, and we shall devote this chapter's remaining sections to this task. But one further perspective on complexity is required to establish the context of that discussion.

## THE NATURE OF COMPLEX ADAPTIVE SYSTEMS

Our conception of complexity relies upon a rich history of research in such diverse fields as molecular biology, ecology, evolutionary theory, organizational psychology, economics, and systems theory.[22,23,24,25,26,27,28] From such conversations over the past few decades, the new field of complexity science has emerged, and it is this framework that provides the intellectual and practical foundations of our present discussion. *Complexity science*, as defined by Zimmerman and colleagues,[28] is the interdisciplinary study of complex adaptive systems (CAS), which in turn are collections of individual agents with "freedom to act in ways that are not always predictable, and whose actions are interconnected so that one agent's actions change the context for other agents."[29] Such systems are notable for their distributed rather than centralized control, for their nonlinearity and nonsingularity of relationship between cause and effect, and for their capacity to learn and adapt based on continuous feedback in a spontaneously self-organizing manner.[28]

These dynamics should now sound familiar. Although early writings on complexity theory identified such classic CAS examples as immune systems, insect colonies, financial markets, and business organizations,[29] the reader will immediately recognize that individual patients who live with chronic illness, these patients' families and communities, and the clinical microsystems that serve patients all represent adaptive systems that are equally, if not more, complex.

We may therefore frame our further discussion of chronic illness care as an exploration of complex adaptive systems. As we seek to understand truly complex dimensions of clinical microsystem planning, design, and implementation in chronic care settings, what specific features of complex adaptive systems can ground us in our study? Table

Table 8.8   Features of Complex Adaptive Systems, Design
Implications, and Examples

| Properties of Complex Systems | Implications for Design of Chronic Illness Care | Examples |
|---|---|---|
| Observed outcomes arise from multiple and mutually interdependent causes. | Design systems with explicit planning of multiple interacting inputs. | Chronic care model |
| Each agent's actions change the context for action by other agents in the same system. | Attend closely to handoffs, transitions, and care coordination. | Care coordination work |
| Agents are free to act in ways that are not totally predictable. | Design interventions that feature autonomy as an asset rather than as an obstacle in clinical care. | Self-management support |
| Boundaries are fuzzy rather than rigid. | Think broadly about influencing factors, unexpected resources, and community assets. | Link to community resources |
| Precise outcomes do not always follow from precise interventions. | Build good principles of interpersonal communication into every interaction. | Effective team communication |

8.8 provides a partial list of such features, together with specific implications and applications in chronic care. The reader is invited to consider this list carefully as we now examine specific design features in clinical microsystems at the (complex adaptive) interface of patients and care-providing teams.

## THE CHRONIC CARE MODEL

As suggested in Table 8.8, an essential property of complex adaptive systems is that observed outcomes arise from multiple and mutually interdependent causes. For clinical microsystems to effectively support complex patients with complex chronic illness, interdisciplinary team members must design care systems with explicit planning of multiple interacting inputs. The multidimensionality of clinical need must be matched with the multidimensionality of practice solutions. The chronic care model, developed by Wagner and introduced in Chapter Two, offers a powerful framework for designing and implementing such solutions.[12,14,30]

Although the chronic care model is complex in its structure and interrelationships, its conceptual foundation (as visually depicted in Figure 8.2) is beautifully simple. Improved functional and clinical outcomes are achieved through what Wagner calls *productive interactions* between patients and practice teams, each of which has been primed (informed, activated, prepared) for this partnering by a series of supportive resources and planning activities at the level of both micro and macrosystem. Of course, this straightforward and almost intuitive framework is challenging to implement. We now focus on its separate components to deepen our understanding of the design implications for clinical microsystems engaged in frontline care.

## FIGURE 8.2    Chronic Care Model.

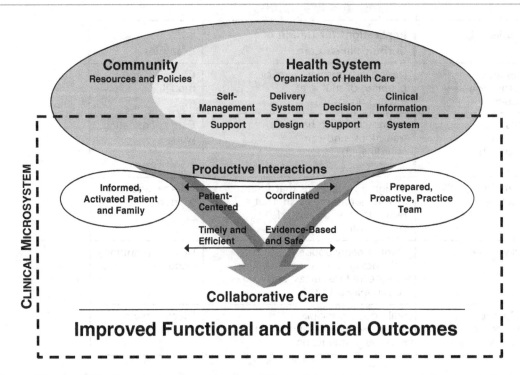

*Source:* Wagner, E. H. Chronic disease management: What will it take to improve care for chronic illness? *Effective Clinical Practice,* August 1998, *1*(1), 22–24.

Beginning at the final step and then working backward in the chronic care model's pathway, we appreciate that the ultimate goal in chronic illness care is improved outcomes. As we have already discussed, the expectation in chronic illness is usually not eradication or cure of disease, but optimal living in the context of ongoing disease. This optimal living includes reduction of disease-related morbidity and mortality, minimization of short-term symptomatic flare-ups, and achievement of full function in work and relationships. Table 8.5 summarizes these essential goals of chronic illness care in greater detail.

Readers familiar with the clinical value compass model (see Figure 8.3) will recognize a direct link between that tool's quality domains and the essential goals of chronic illness we have described. For Nelson and colleagues, *value* means improvement in clinical status, functional and risk status, and patient and family satisfaction against patient need, all in the context of reduced direct and indirect costs (Value = Quality/ Costs).[31] These are the same priorities we recognize in our present discussion of chronic illness goals and in Wagner's understanding of improved outcomes.

As the chronic care model suggests, these outcomes are necessarily achieved through productive interactions between an *informed, activated patient* and a *prepared, proactive practice team.* Activated patients have the motivation, information, skills, and confidence necessary to effectively make decisions about their health and to manage it.[13,30] Prepared and proactive practice teams, in turn, are enriched by patient information, decision support, and skilled staff, which help them deliver high-quality care. This chapter's subsequent sections will explore several forms of preparation and implementation that empower patients and practice teams (or clinical microsystems) to form effective partnerships.

FIGURE 8.3 Clinical Value Compass.

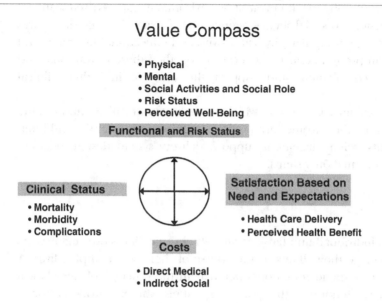

FIGURE 8.4 Embedded Systems.

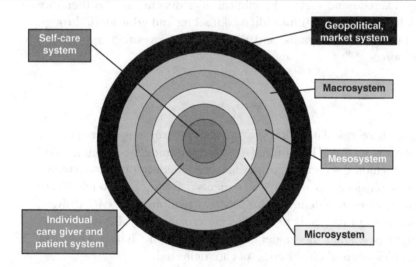

Specific resources facilitate both the activation of patients and the preparation of staff. Just as chronic illness is experienced in nested contexts of individual and family, local microsystem, larger macrosystem, and greater community (see Figure 8.4), so too do empowering resources cohere at levels from individual self-management and microsystem design to macrosytem organization and community policy. Although our attention in this chapter is focused on the clinical microsystem, we briefly acknowledge here the important role of macrosystem and community contributions. *Health care organizations (macrosystems)* provide leadership, vision, and material resources that support quality improvements at the front line of microsystem care. (For example, the prioritization of clinical quality may be articulated by organizational leaders, and decision support resources and clinical information systems may be appropriately integrated.) *Proactive communities* offer health-promoting environments, access to educational resources, and connections to social service agencies. (For example, accessible parks enable residents to engage in regular physical activity, and educational programs and community services can promote effective self-care.) Together, these institutional and community resources complement and support the work of individual clinical microsystems.

At the level of clinical microsystems, to which we dedicate our full attention in the remainder of this chapter, the chronic care model recognizes four essential and interacting design elements: self-management support, delivery system design, decision support, and clinical information systems.

## Self-Management Support

As we have suggested, individuals and families *live with* chronic illness over many years and must learn to manage their illness in the course of their own complex lives. A typical, stable patient may spend four hours per year in the office(s) of her clinical provider(s); the other 8,756 hours of that year are spent elsewhere: at work, at home, in community activities, and so on. It is the patient (not her clinical providers) who, in the end, defines care priorities, monitors physiologic parameters such as home blood sugar and weight, administers and adjusts medications, and maintains a healthful lifestyle (through exercise and diet). The clinical microsystem's role is therefore to actively support self-efficacy through individual counseling and education, through professional or peer-led group programs, and through access to other appropriate self-management resources.[8,9,10]

## Delivery System Design

Ostbye and colleagues have calculated that greater than 10 working hours per day (every working day of the year) would be required to provide all guideline-recommended chronic disease care (including screening, counseling, and medication management) to a typical primary care physician's panel of 2,500 patients.[32] Traditional models of care are clearly inadequate to meet such demand. But proactive planning of service delivery, with attention to processes of care and to the specific capacities of all professionals within the microsystem (see again the model of 5Ps discussed in Chapter One) can greatly enhance the efficiency and effectiveness of care delivered.

Clinical microsystems can (and must) define specific roles for different participants, and planned care visits can specify the sequence and implementation of discrete interventions, which may occur in person or asynchronously, via telephone, secure e-mail, or the Internet. Thus, a practice secretary may use standard orders to schedule retinal screening exams on all diabetic patients; a nurse assistant may review patients' home blood pressure readings; an on-site nutritionist or behavioral health professional may counsel patients regarding lifestyle changes; a nurse practitioner or physician may adjust medications based on evidenced-based guidelines; and a registered nurse may phone the patient two weeks after office visits to assess response to latest interventions. Finally, when patients with complex longitudinal needs are determined to be at high risk due to psychosocial or other factors, a care manager or health coach may assist the patient, for example through personal behavioral counseling.

## Decision Support

Excellent chronic illness care requires deep knowledge of best scientific evidence. But as suggested in the Chapter Six review of Batalden and Davidoff's Clinical Improvement Equation,[33] knowledge of evidence-based guidelines, although necessary, is not sufficient to assure delivery of optimal care. Rather, scientific knowledge must be linked to reliable actions embedded in frontline practices of *this* clinical microsystem. Paper or electronic task lists linked to unique patients or to patient visits may facilitate this work and will enhance reliability of simple and complicated components of chronic illness care. Each task is informed by scientific evidence; its execution is assigned to a pre-specified member of the interdisciplinary care team who signs the form once the task is completed. Guidelines can be embedded in the workflow, and their use can be prompted with paper or electronic reminders.

## Clinical Information Systems

As described in Chapter Four, efficient and effective care requires access to good information about both individual patients and entire practice populations. This is especially true in chronic illness care, where so many measures of care require attention and where such monitoring has relevance not only *in time* (as with today's blood sugar level and blood pressure reading), but also *over time* (as with cholesterol changes from year to year and recommended date for the next retinal exam). Electronic or paper registries can facilitate individual care planning and can prompt patients and clinical teams to pursue specific evidence-based care. In addition, as discussed in Chapter Four, clinical information systems permit monitoring and feedback to care teams on recent performance. Such systems provide instant access to statistical information including, for example, how many patients with heart failure have been prescribed appropriate medications to preserve cardiac function, or how many emphysema patients have missed their annual flu immunization.[30]

The increasing availability and use of electronic health records (EHRs) will enhance chronic illness management in the years ahead, but we must remember that even the finest technical innovations do not guarantee improvement in clinical care. Crosson and colleagues assessed quality of diabetic management in fifty family medicine practices. Thirteen of these practices used EHRs, and the remainder did not. The authors found that overall quality of diabetic care (in terms of processes, treatments, and intermediate outcomes) was significantly *poorer* in the practices using EHRs.[34] There may be several reasons for this finding, but one likely contributing factor is the misalignment described earlier in this chapter between problem and solution levels of complexity. EHRs, however valuable, are *merely complicated* solutions to problems that may be truly complex in nature, whether these problems are specific to the chronically ill patient or to the interpersonal processes that necessarily inform how technology is integrated into practice.

As we rely increasingly on electronic resources to fortify the clinical microsystem, there are still necessary points of contact between computers and the humans who provide clinical care. Students and practitioners of quality improvement are advised that *wetware precedes software and hardware*. The human patterns and interpersonal processes at the front line of care (what we may call *wetware*) must be effectively coordinated before they can optimally leverage the technology (*software* and *hardware*) that supports such care. As Taiichi Ohno has written of a different, nonclinical but value-based organization, "In the Toyota production system, sequencing of work and work standardization come first. . . . If *equipment* improvement comes first, work processes will never be improved."[35]

### Is the Chronic Care Model Effective?

At levels of both the micro and macrosystem, there is compelling support for the model's efficacy to improve multiple quality indicators across diverse chronic conditions (including heart failure, asthma, diabetes, and depression). Notably, although each of the chronic care model's separate design components (self-management, delivery system redesign, decision support, and clinical information system) yields demonstrable benefit, there is an added effect when multiple interventions are combined.[13] In one review of thirty-nine studies that assessed improvement in diabetic care, thirty-two studies demonstrated benefits in processes or outcomes. In addition, the five studies of clinics that adhered to all four design components all showed positive results.[12] Perhaps not surprisingly, the component most consistently associated with care improvement was self-management support (refer to www.improvingchroniccare.org for illuminating resources and reviews of chronic illness care).

What does this model look like for individual patients? Let us recall Carl, whose several interacting chronic illnesses became "so much [indeed too much] to take care of." In his more recent care, several components of the chronic care model have been implemented with beneficial effects. He has learned in a series of group education sessions (*self-management support*) to more effectively modify his diet, to monitor his own blood sugars, and to self-adjust his insulin based upon sugar levels. A registered nurse care manager (*delivery system redesign*) phones him at specified intervals to assess progress and address potential problems. His primary care physician and endocrinologist (*decision support*) now co-manage his intense medication regimen during planned visits (more *delivery system redesign*) every three months. Finally, an electronic health record (*clinical information system*) provides care reminders and flags potentially hazardous medication cross-reactions. As a result of these varied interventions (and likely the result of all of them in combination), Carl's blood sugar and blood pressure readings have demonstrably improved during the past year. His adherence to medication regimens is more consistent, and he reports taking greater pleasure in daily activities. He and his clinical microsystem are together dealing with the complexity of chronic illness care and have benefited from this engagement.

## CARE COORDINATON AND TRANSITIONS

Referring again to Table 8.8, we note a second important property of complex adaptive systems: each agent's actions change the context for action by other agents in the same system. This is certainly true in chronic illness care and in the design and improvement of that care. To engage this element of clinical complexity, microsystems must attend closely to handoffs, transitions, and care coordination.

Such a requirement draws our attention again to the chronic care model and to its emphasis on delivery system design and context. Handoffs and care transitions are common in the management of chronic illness, but close reflection reveals these functions have a different form and meaning than they did in our Chapter Seven exploration of acute care. Recall that chapter's discussion of Joanne Wright, whose frightening experience with bilobar pneumonia is depicted in the deployment flowchart of Figure 7.1. The well-orchestrated handoffs in that case were linear and unidirectional, as is

FIGURE 8.5    Radial Handoffs and Transitions in Chronic Illness Care.

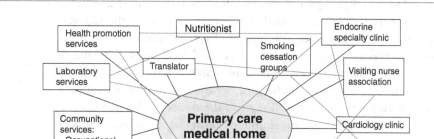

common in acute care. Joanne's journey took her sequentially from nurse to primary care physician, then to ambulance team, emergency department, and intensive care unit. Transitions were complicated, highly technical, and tightly coordinated, but they were not (in the sense that Glouberman and Zimmerman use the term) truly *complex.* Once the nature of acute microsystem disruption was established, formal algorithms for resuscitation, care transfer, and medication management brought reassuring predictability to the events.

Now consider the form of care transitions in chronic illness. As depicted in Figure 8.5, handoffs and communications are, for the most part, not linear but *radial* in nature. A central microsystem coordinates care, transferring both patient and patient information to various clinical microsystems that provide specified services and then return the patient (so to speak), along with now-modified information, to the central coordinating hub. Note that these handoffs are neither sequential nor unidirectional. A patient may interact with multiple microsystems simultaneously, and information is *exchanged* rather than simply passed down the line. Moreover, as Figure 8.5 suggests, the several clinical microsystems need not confine their own interactions to those with the central hub. As occurs commonly in complex systems, these semi-autonomous nodes are free to interact among themselves in a manner that may benefit or (if not carefully coordinated) harm the patient in question. An essential (complex) function of clinical microsystems in chronic illness care is therefore to coordinate the numerous and multidirectional handoffs of patient and patient information *over time* (as opposed to handoffs *in time* during acute care), so these efforts collectively serve the patient's best interests.

This coordinating function is frequently performed by a primary care medical home, but this is not always the case. The Dartmouth-Hitchcock Spine Center, for example, functions as a central hub for patients with chronic back pain who may require various combinations of surgical, medical, radiologic, anesthesia, physical therapy, and psychological service. Nephrology practices coordinate care for patients on dialysis with end-stage renal disease, and oncology teams similarly manage complex care transitions for cancer patients requiring numerous therapeutic and supportive interventions.

The common theme in these examples is *care coordination,* and the common function is management and transfer of information in a manner that supports the essential goals of chronic illness care. Informed by the 5Ps self-assessment discussed in Chapter

One, highly effective clinical microsystems attend to the processes and patterns of their own communication and to the roles of patients and professionals in sharing and securing that information. Delivery system design and redesign (to use again the chronic care model's terminology) facilitate proper assignment of coordination functions. In some settings a physician is the most appropriate conveyer and receiver of radial hand-offs, but in many contexts this role is well-served by a specially trained registered nurse or social worker. Clinical information systems (another chronic care model element) will certainly facilitate information transfer, although at their core such transfers are relational in nature and depend upon not only simple or *merely complicated* communication algorithms, but also upon complex negotiations and clarifications that cannot be entirely reduced to protocol. Chapter Eight Action Guide offers specific actions and a *STAR* generative tool to build stronger relationships between microsystems.

## PATIENT SELF-MANAGEMENT

One characteristic of complex adaptive systems has special relevance in the management of chronic illness. As we have discussed (and as Table 8.8 makes explicit), agents in complex systems are free to act in ways that are not totally predictable. This reality is often unsettling in clinical contexts, where health professionals (who are commonly trained to manage acuity rather than chronicity) often seek to maximize predictability and control to eradicate disease. But to engage the inherent uncertainty and complexity of chronic illness, clinical microsystems must design interventions that feature patient autonomy in clinical care as an asset rather than as an obstacle.

Indeed, patient autonomy and authority are the natural and necessary state of affairs in the experience of chronic illness. The patient, rather than her clinical team, will monitor physiological parameters such as blood pressure and weight at home. She will administer and adjust medications and will maintain a healthful lifestyle (that includes exercise, proper diet, and tobacco cessation). Ultimately, it is the patient who defines care priorities, and the clinical microsystem provides professional knowledge, training, and support so these priorities can be effectively addressed. As suggested in this chapter's opening section, predictability and unilateral authority give way in chronic illness care to adaptability and partnership and to resilient and productive relationships.

Successful implementation of the chronic care model depends upon an informed and activated patient who makes health decisions and performs self-care. This activation requires patients to possess knowledge, motivation, skills, and confidence. Numerous tools and techniques have been developed to stimulate *patient self-efficacy*, which extends beyond a patient's desire to modify behavior to achieve specific goals, and includes *confidence* in the skills required to make such goal-directed change. Self-efficacy has been linked to healthier behaviors and is an essential attribute of people living successfully with chronic illness.[9,10]

As we briefly review techniques that support self-efficacy (with attention to practice design and implementation), keep in mind that the goal of these interventions is both to *educate* patients about healthy behaviors and self-management and to *elicit* and refine self-knowledge and capacities that are already present. The role of counselors or health coaches is to help patients' discover their own expertise so patients can more fully align personal health priorities with actual health behaviors.[36]

Glasgow and colleagues[37,38] have described a broadly applicable model of collaborative self-management support called the *5As approach*. This model was initially

FIGURE 8.6    The 5As Cycle of Self-Management Support.

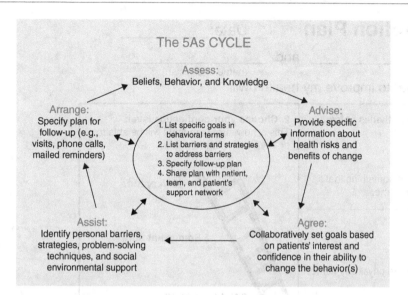

*Source:* World Health Organization. *Self-management support for chronic conditions using 5 As.* Geneva, Switzerland: World Health Organization, 2004, p. 4. Retrieved from www.who.int/diabetesactiononline/about/WHO%205A%20ppt.pdf.

developed to counsel patients in tobacco cessation, but more recently the U.S. Preventive Services Task Force has adopted it to provide a general framework for patient-centered coaching in various clinical contexts, including self-management in chronic illness. As depicted in Figure 8.6, Glasgow's 5As are *assess* (or *ask*), *advise, agree, assist,* and *arrange.* Appropriate to the complex (rather than merely complicated) nature of self-management problems and solutions, this series of interventions is in fact a sequence of *interactions.* As Westley and colleagues have observed, in complex systems, "our interventions are *always* interactions."[39]

In planned encounters that may be initiated by either clinician or staff (or even incorporated into pre-visit screening questionnaires), the clinical microsystem first assesses the patient's readiness to engage in health-promoting behaviors. For persons living with chronic illness, such behaviors may include renewed attention to exercise or diet, tobacco cessation, stress reduction, adherence to medications, or numerous other *patient-directed* possibilities. As illustrated in the action plan of Figure 8.7, clinical microsystems can (and should) use specific tools to identify and stimulate specific health behaviors, but the actual choice of behavior is always the patient's. (This information is also available online at www.familymedicine.medschool.ucsf.edu/research/research_programs/actionPlan.aspx.)

*Readiness to change* is a complex state that varies over time. Researchers and practitioners of *motivational interviewing* (an especially powerful interactive technique to effect health-promoting change) have observed that this readiness is influenced by both *motivation to change* ("On a scale of 1 to 10, how important is it to you to reduce the sugar in your diet?") and *confidence* that change is possible ("On that same scale of 1 to 10, how confident are you that you could make a dietary change in the upcoming week?")[36] These separate dimensions must each be assessed, as the nature of counseling will vary depending on which factor (motivation or confidence) presents the greater

FIGURE 8.7　My Action Plan.

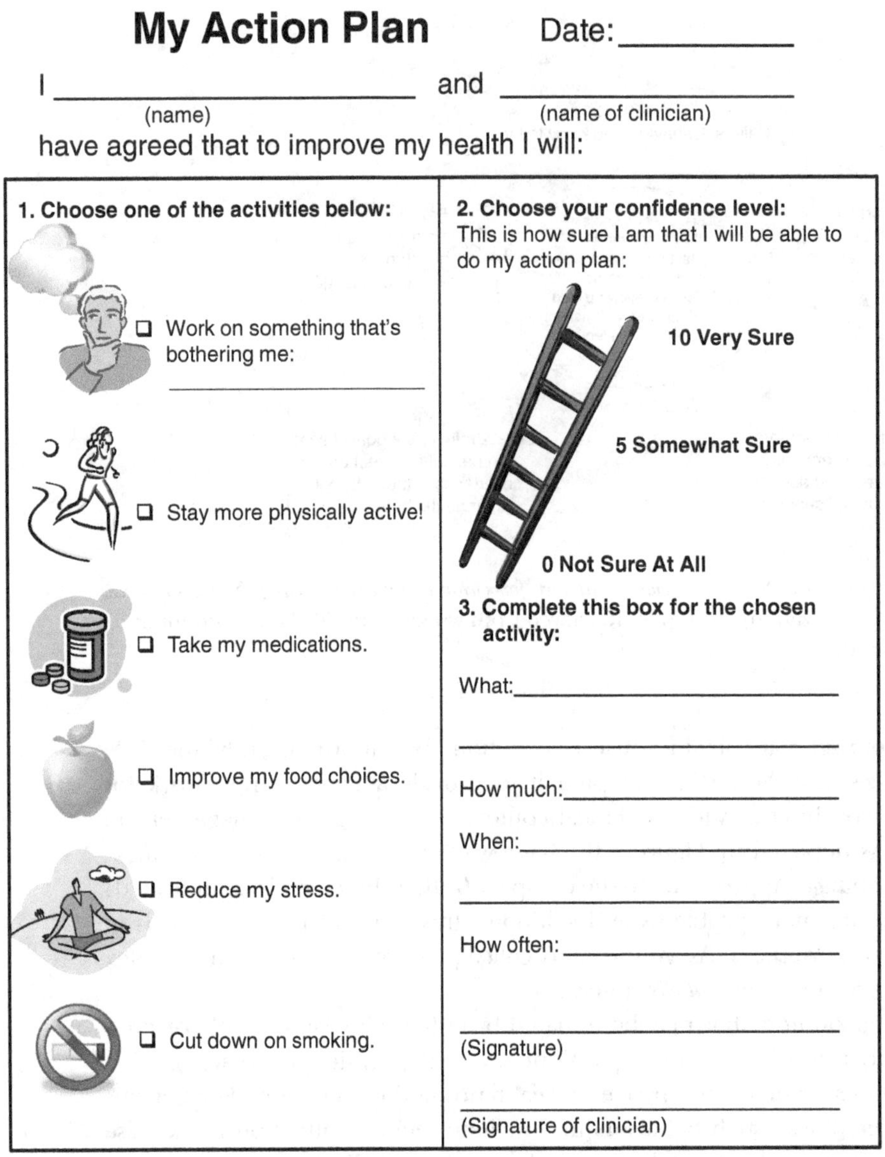

**My Action Plan**　　　Date:_____

I _____ and _____
　　　　(name)　　　　　　　　　　(name of clinician)
have agreed that to improve my health I will:

**1. Choose one of the activities below:**

☐ Work on something that's bothering me:
　_____

☐ Stay more physically active!

☐ Take my medications.

☐ Improve my food choices.

☐ Reduce my stress.

☐ Cut down on smoking.

**2. Choose your confidence level:**
This is how sure I am that I will be able to do my action plan:

10 Very Sure

5 Somewhat Sure

0 Not Sure At All

**3. Complete this box for the chosen activity:**

What:_____
_____

How much:_____

When:_____
_____

How often: _____

_____
(Signature)

_____
(Signature of clinician)

*Source:* www.familymedicine.medschool.ucsf.edu/research/research_programs/actionPlan.aspx.

barrier to health-promoting action. Again, paper or electronic action plans like the one provided in Figure 8.7 can facilitate this specific assessment. In subsequent steps of the self-management support process, clinicians or other educators advise the patient on health risks and benefits linked to behaviors the patient has identified. Based on assessment and shared information, patient and counselor then collaborate, negotiate, and eventually agree on particular behavioral goals and priorities. Members of the clinical microsystem then assist the patient in identifying personal barriers, strategies, and problem-solving techniques pertinent to the agreed-upon goals. These techniques may involve self-care, referral to other skilled providers within the same microsystem, or referral to outside support services such as community-based self-management training

**FIGURE 8.8    Implementing the 5As Model in Clinical Microsystems.**

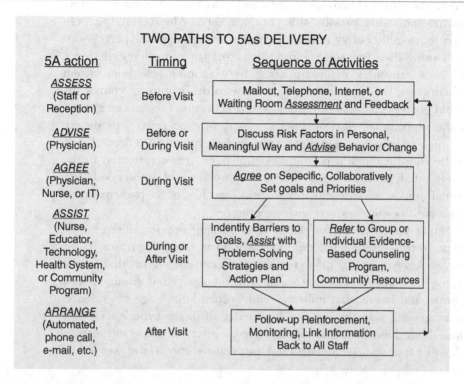

Source: World Health Organization. *Self-management support for chronic conditions using 5 As.* Geneva, Switzerland: World Health Organization, 2004, p. 12. Retrieved from www.who.int/diabetesactiononline/about/WHO%205A%20ppt.pdf.

programs. Together, the patient and interdisciplinary caregiving team arrange a specific follow-up plan that may involve repeat visits, phone check-in, and mailed reminders. Nurse follow-up calls can reinforce medication instructions discussed at the last chronic care visit or can facilitate monitoring of pain levels, exercise adherence, or home-checked blood sugar levels.

Apart from the appropriately patient-centered orientation this model hardwires into wellness-promoting interactions, the 5As are intrinsically conducive to microsystem planning and design. Figure 8.8 connects the separate interactive steps to specific inter-disciplinary members of the clinical team and frames the entire process as a sequence of interlinked activities, each of which is amenable to analysis and focused improvement. Again note there is important work for everyone in this proposed sequence. As in other care processes, success will depend upon careful defining and assigning of roles, thoughtful coordination and communication between participants, and respectful partnering at every step with the patient and family.

## CONCLUSION

This final refocusing of our attention upon role definition, communication, and partnership has implications not only for the microsystem's care of (and care with) patients, but also for its internal self-care. As Table 8.8 reminds us, one further feature of complex adaptive systems is that *precise outcomes do not always follow from precise interventions.* What is true in the care of chronically ill patients is also true in the team-building dynamics of microsystems that provide this complex care. When even the best-intentioned people join together in common cause, individual opinions and perceptions frequently differ. During their group communications, participants often experience uncertainty and also encounter many surprises. In whichever role microsystem members find themselves, the recommended response to this feature of complexity is to routinely build good principles of interpersonal process into every social interaction. Although the outcome of discrete interactions cannot be reliably predicted, overall resiliency will be strengthened in systems where these interactions occur. Long-term success in the coordinated and partnered delivery of chronic care, and in the clinical microsystem's design and improvement of that care, depends upon good communication, mutual empowerment, and the adaptive capacity of all participants to quickly learn from both positive and negative experiences.

We thus recognize the scope of complex challenges and opportunities chronic illness care presents to patients, families, and interdisciplinary caregiving teams. These participants must work together in a new, creative manner to meet goals that, in the end, they define together. They can embrace a clinical complexity that simultaneously engages head, heart, and hands: that unites the intellectual knowledge of evidence-based disease management with the emotive knowledge of illness experienced over time and that links both these knowledge domains to an interventional (and interactional) knowledge that transforms understanding into realized care in the lives of real people.

## SUMMARY

- Chronic illnesses make up the majority of patients' articulated need, occupy the majority of clinical microsystems' work time, and consume the majority of our nation's health care dollars. At the same time, the quality of chronic illness care remains suboptimal.
- The goals of chronic illness care include reduction of long term disease sequelae, minimization of impact of acute illness flare-ups, and long term optimization of function, relationships, and overall quality of life.
- Categorizing clinical problems as simple, complicated, or complex permits effective alignment of patient needs with appropriate practice interventions.
- The chronic care model links complexity principles with practical interventions to meet the needs of patients and families.
- Key components of chronic illness care include self-management support, effective decision support resources, and proactive delivery system design.

## KEY TERMS

Care over time

Chronic care model

Complex problems

Complexity science

Complicated problems

Confidence (that change is possible)

Motivation to change

Paradigm of complexity

Patient self-efficacy

Radial communications

Readiness to change

Simple problems

Three essential goals of chronic
illness care

Wetware

## REVIEW QUESTIONS

1. How is chronic care assessed in your clinical microsystem? What specific designs and processes to support chronic illness care currently exist? How might they be improved?
2. What is the impact of chronic illness care on the patients, the clinical microsystem, and families over time?
3. What are the three essential goals of chronic care?
4. How does the 5As approach advance patient self-management?

## DISCUSSION QUESTIONS

1. Identify a subpopulation of chronic illness patients in your microsystem and explore a patient's journey. (Use Carl's journey in "Case Study: The Experience of Chronic Illness" as an example.) What does your clinical microsystem do well? What might be improved? How does your clinical information system support the chronic illness care provided?
2. Discuss what the phrase "so much to take care of" means in the context of chronic illness care. Then discuss what your microsystem could do to support patients and families in their longitudinal journeys.
3. Identify the interdisciplinary roles in your clinical microsystem that are specific to chronic illness care. Then decide if these roles are matched with ideal processes that effectively meet patient and family needs. Explain your decision.
4. Identify several clinical microsystems that support chronic illness care within your clinical microsystem. Using the STAR generative tool in Chapter 8 Action Guide, discuss opportunities to enrich relationships to better meet patient and family needs.

## REFERENCES

1. Centers for Disease Control and Prevention. *Chronic disease prevention and health promotion.* Retrieved July 25, 2010, from www.cdc.gov/chronicdisease/overview/index.htm
2. U.S. Department of Health and Human Services. *The power of prevention: Steps to a healthier US.* Report issued 2003. Retrieved February 15, 2010, from www.healthierus.gov/STEPS/summit/prevportfolio/power/index.html
3. Hoffman, C., Rice, D., & Sung, H. Y. Persons with chronic conditions: Their prevalence and costs. *Journal of the American Medical Association*, 1996, *276*, 1473–1479.
4. Wagner, E. Meeting the needs of chronically ill people. *British Medical Journal*, 2001, *323*, 945–946.
5. McGlynn et al. The quality of health care delivered to adults in the United States. *New England Journal of Medicine*, 2003, *348*(26), 2635–2645.
6. Glouberman, S., & Zimmerman, B. *Complicated and complex systems: What would successful reform of Medicare look like?* Ottawa: Commission on the Future of Health Care in Canada, 2002.

7. Zimmerman, B., & Plsek, P. *Microsystems as complex adaptive systems: Ideas for improvement.* Retrieved February 10, 2010, from www.clinicalmicrosystem.org

8. Institute for Family-Centered Care. *FAQ.* Retrieved February 15, 2010, from www.familycenteredcare.org/faq.html

9. Lorig, K., Bodenheimer, T., Holman, H., & Grumbach, K. Patient self-management of chronic disease in primary care. *Journal of the American Medical Association*, 2002, *288*(19), 2469–2475.

10. Lorig, K., Sobel, D., Gonzalez, V., & Minor, M. *Living a healthy life with chronic conditions.* Boulder, CO: Bull Publishing, 2006.

11. Bodenheimer, T., Wagner, E. H., & Grumbach, K. Improving primary care for patients with chronic illness. *Journal of the American Medical Association*, 2002, *288*(14), 1775–1779.

12. Bodenheimer, T., Wagner, E. H., & Grumbach, K. Improving primary care for patients with chronic illness, Part 2. *Journal of the American Medical Association*, 2002, *288*(15), 1909–1914.

13. Improving chronic illness care. *Chronic care model.* Retrieved February 28, 2010, from www.improvingchroniccare.org/index.php?p=The_Chronic_Care_Model&s=2

14. Wagner, E., Austin, B. T., & Von Korf, F. M. Organizing care for patients with chronic illness. *Milbank Quarterly*, 1996, *74*, 511–544.

15. Centers for Disease Control and Prevention. *Deaths and mortality statistics for US.* Retrieved February 10, 2010, from http://www.cdc.gov/nchs/FASTATS.deaths.htm

16. Cherry, D., Hing E., Woodwell D. A., & Rechsteiner, E. A. *National ambulatory care survey: 2006 summary. National health statistics reports.* Retrieved July 25, 2010, from www.Cdc.Gov/nchs/fastats/docvisit.htm

17. Grant, R., Buse, J. B., & Meigs, J. B. Quality of diabetes care in U.S. academic medical centers: Low rates of medical regimen change. *Diabetes Care*, 2005, *28*, 337–342.

18. Saadine, J., Engelau, M. M., Beckles, G. L., Gregg, E. W., & Thompson, T. J. A diabetes report card for the United States: Quality of care in the 1990s. *Annals of Internal Medicine*, 2002, *136*(8), 565–574.

19. Saydah, S., Fradkin, J., & Cowie, C. C. Poor control of risk factors for vascular disease among adults with previously diagnosed diabetes. *Journal of the American Medical Association*, 2004, *291*, 335–342.

20. Parchman, M., Romero, R. L., & Pugh, J. A. Encounters by patients with type 2 diabetes—complex and demanding: An observational study. *Annals of Family Medicine*, 2006, *4*, 40–45.

21. Liu, S., Homa, K., Butterly, J. R., Kirkland, K. B., & Batalden, P. B. Improving the simple, complicated and complex realities of community-acquired pneumonia. *Quality and Safety in Health Care*, 2009, *18*, 93–98.

22. von Bertalanffy, L. *General system theory: Foundations, development, applications.* New York: George Braziller, 1968.

23. Deming, W. *The new economics for industry, government, education.* (2nd ed.) Cambridge: Massachusetts Institutes of Technology, Center for Advanced Educational Services, 1994.

24. Homans, G. *The human group.* New York: Harcourt, Brace, and World, 1950.

25. Kauffman, S. *At home in the universe. The search for the laws of self-organization and complexity.* New York: Oxford University Press, 1995.

26. Senge, P. *The fifth discipline: The art and practice of the learning organization.* New York: Doubleday/Currency, 1990.

27. Stacey, R. *Complexity and creativity in organizations.* San Francisco: Berrett-Koehler, 1996.

28. Zimmerman, B., Lindberg, C., & Plsek, P. *Edgeware: Insights from complexity science for health care leaders.* Irving, TX: VHA, 1998, p. 625.

29. Plsek, P., & Greenhalgh, T. The challenge of complexity in health care. *British Medical Journal*, 2001, *3*, 625–628.

30. Bodenheimer, T. & Grumbach, K. *Improving primary care: Strategies and tools for a better practice.* New York: McGraw-Hill, 2006.

31. Nelson, G., Batalden, P. B., & Lazar, J. S. *Practice-based learning and improvement: A clinical improvement action guide.* (2nd ed.) Oak Brook, IL: Joint Commission Resources, 2007.

32. Ostbye et al. Is there time for management of patients with chronic disease in primary care? *Annals of Family Medicine*, 2005, *3*, 209–214.

33. Batalden, P., & Davidoff, F. What is quality improvement and how can it transform health care? *Quality and Safety in Health Care*, 2007, *16*, 2–3.

34. Crosson et al. Electronic medical records and diabetes quality of care: Results from a sample of family medicine practices. *Annals of Family Medicine*, 2007, *5*, 209–215.

35. Ohno, T. *Toyota production system: Beyond large scale production.* New York: Productivity Press, 1988, p. 130.

36. Miller, W., & Rolnick, S. *Motivational interviewing: Preparing people for change.* (2nd ed.) NY: Guilford Press, 2002.

37. Glasgow et al. Self-management aspects of the improving chronic illness care breakthrough series: Implementation with diabetes and heart failure teams. *Annals of Behavioral Medicine*, 2002, *24*, 80–87.

38. Whitlock, E., Orleans, T., Pender, N., & Allan, J. Evaluating primary care behavioral counseling interventions: An evidence-based approach. *American Journal of Preventive Medicine*, 2002, *22*(4), 267–284.

39. Westley, F., Zimmerman, B., & Patton, M. *Getting to maybe: How the world is changed.* Toronto: Random House, 2007.

# Chapter Eight ACTION GUIDE

Chapter Eight Action Guide is designed to offer an additional resource in building reliable chronic care systems. The STAR Generative Relationships Tool aims to support and encourage your assessment and study of the relationships specific to chronic care delivery between your clinical microsystem and connected clinical and supporting microsystems. The intentional study and improvement or strengthening of the relationships can potentially result in more generative relationships that patients, families, and members of all clinical and supporting microsystems can benefit from.

As noted in Chapter Eight, chronic care often involves many handoffs and transitions across many settings for patients and families. It is helpful to review the External Mapping Tool in Chapter One to show the various connected microsystems where handoffs and transitions occur in the course of chronic care and to identify potential connected microsystems you wish to strengthen or improve relationships to result in more reliable chronic care systems. The complexity of chronic care that is managed over time can benefit from enhanced relationships between clinical microsystems to promote sharing of particular patient knowledge and information along with designing ideal chronic care systems where the whole system of care is enhanced through timely processes and information sharing. Better value care can be designed through seamless transfer of information and feed forward systems to help the next microsystem in the system best meet patient and family needs. The technical aspects of care can be enhanced and promoted through the human relationships between clinical microsystems, which can be developed and strengthened beginning with an assessment of the current state of relationships.

## STAR GENERATIVE RELATIONSHIPS

Once you have identified the connecting microsystems to support the course of chronic care, use the STAR Generative Relationships Tool to guide your assessment of the relationships between clinical and supporting microsystems. Look for opportunities to promote, develop, and strengthen generative relationships between microsystems. Generative relationships occur when interactions among parts of a complex system produce valuable, new, and unpredictable capabilities that are not inherent in any of the parts acting alone.[1] Generative relationships in complex systems (such as clinical microsystems and health care) offer great potential for creativity and innovation.

### Table AG8.1    STAR Acronym Defined

| S | Separateness | Differences allow for facts to be seen as interpretations. This means the microsystems or individuals in the relationship are able to offer different perspectives and considerations. |
|---|---|---|
| T | Tuning | Talking and listening provide opportunities to challenge the status quo and implicit assumptions. How often do the members of both microsystems have planned time to review and discuss processes of care in real time? Are there regular meetings to discuss the quality and safety of patient care in and between both clinical microsystems? |
| A | Action | Opportunities are identified to have the potential to result in action or to help create something new. Do the clinical microsystems engage in improvement activities together? Are new designs and models of care developed or handoff improvement PDSA cycles done regularly? |
| R | Reason to Work Together | One has a reason to collaborate to achieve mutual benefits for patients and families and staff. Do the microsystems have a shared vision for patient care and understanding that working together to provide exceptional quality of care and services will be beneficial? |

Two key components of generative relationships are as follows:

1. The relationship produces something that one member of the relationship could not have produced alone.
2. The source of value (new product or service) is created by the interaction between microsystems.

Using the STAR model, the relationships between microsystems and even individuals can be explored. The acronym STAR is outlined in Table AG8.1.

Some examples of STAR relationships shown in Figure AG8.1 illustrate how the length of each star point describes the type of generative actions that will ultimately improve the relationship.

The *STAR Generative Mapping* worksheet helps improve patient care because it identifies opportunities to improve working relationships at the boundaries based on improved tuning and intentional collaborations. Many interdisciplinary professionals can offer examples of situations when the stress of transferring a patient overshadows constructive conversations and ideal processes of transfer. Planning regular time to review the processes of handoffs and transitions could lead to improved communication (talking and listening) and system design resulting in improved patient flow. Wagner's chronic care model highlights that in order to have productive interactions with patients and families, the practice team should be prepared and proactive. Optimizing the generative relationships through the *STAR Generative Mapping* worksheet can contribute to the practice team being prepared and proactive. Figure AG8.2 is the front of the *Generative STAR Worksheet* and has instructions on creating the generative relationship assessment along with definitions of each star point. Illustrating the current relationship between another clinical microsystem through the creation of this diagram with the proper length of the star point representing the separateness, tuning, action, and reason to work together often results in thoughtful discussion within the clinical micro-

## FIGURE AG8.1   Generative STAR 1.

### Generative Relationship STAR

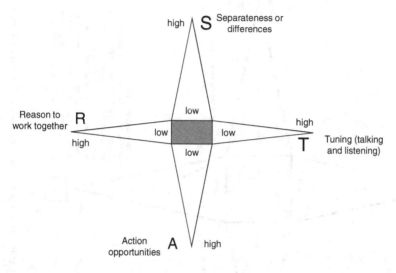

*Source:* Adapted from Zimmerman, B. J., & Hayday, B. C. A board's journey into complexity science. *Group Decision Making and Negotiation*, 1999, *8*, 281–303.

system about the etiology of current relationships and ideas about how to improve them. Examples of different types of generative relationships are illustrated in Figure AG8.3.

Engaging another clinical microsystem to consider their perspective of the relationship with your clinical microsystem can lead to a meeting of the two microsystems to discuss each other's relationship perspectives and to explore improvement possibilities including regularly planned meetings with the aim to improve patient flow across microsystems. In some instances, two clinical microsystems can meet for the first time with a goal to improve handoffs and transitions between the two, and use the *STAR Generative Mapping* worksheet to create their individual perspectives and then join together to compare and contrast with a resulting action plan for improvement activities to improve the relationship.

## REFERENCE

1. Zimmerman, B. J., & Hayday, B. C. A board's journey into complexity science. *Group Decision Making and Negotiation*, 1999, *8*, 281–303.

FIGURE AG8.2  Generative STAR Worksheet Page 1.

## STAR Mapping Worksheet for Working Across Boundaries
## Clinical Microsystem to Clinical Microsystem

**AIM**: Increase awareness of relationships between microsystems by diagnosing the current state in order to then identify possible next steps to improve relationships.

**Instructions:**

- Identify two clinical microsystems in consideration
- Complete the worksheet, and rate each point of the STAR
- Reflect on each of the "points" and what action steps you might take

Clinical Microsystem A: _____
Clinical Microsystem B: _____

**S Separateness or Differences:** There needs to be differences in the background, skill, perspectives, or training of the parties. If all of the parties are similar, they may enjoy heated debates but may leave untouched or unchallenged the assumptions upon which both sides of the argument are based. You cannot challenge an assumption which goes unnoticed. Differences allow the partners or group to see things from a different perspective. They allow "facts" to be seen as "interpretations." Value and respect for separateness.

**T Tuning (talking and listening):** There needs to be real opportunities to talk and listen to each other with permission to challenge the status quo, sacred cows or implicit assumptions of the context. The conceptual changes in a complex context can be profound. Opportunities for reflection allow the parties to grow and learn.

**A Action Opportunities:** Talk is great, but unless it is accompanied by acting on the talk, new sources of value will not be created. The parties need to be able to act together to co-create something new.

**R Reason to work together:** The parties need to have a reason to share resources, ideas or to act as allies even if only for a short period. There has to be some mutual benefit to being aligned in a project. If the parties do not see value in working together, if they see each other as adversaries only rather than as allies for this piece of work, it is highly unlikely that they will co-create something of substantial value. They may talk and learn from each other, but then do the work of creating something new alone.

**S** Separateness or Differences:
What are the manifestations of this "separateness" or these "differences"?

**T** Tuning "Talking and Listening":
What might be done to promote such "tuning"?

**A** Action Opportunities:
What might you do to start? (some have found it helpful to work on high volume, high risk interactions, some have found it helpful to begin where "work" can be removed, some have found it helpful to work to make interactions more reliable, some have found it helpful to use worksheets to structure interactions and data collection. Some have found it helpful to begin by working to monitor and manage accuracy and re-work — don't be constrained by these ideas.

**R** Reason to Work Together:
What might you use as a "frame" for working together?

*Source:* Adapted from Zimmerman, B. J., & Hayday, B. C. A board's journey into complexity science. *Group Decision Making and Negotiation*, 1999, 8, 281–303.

## System Relationship Map
## Clinical Microsystem to Clinical Microsystem

**Instructions**: Consider the relationships with ONE clinical microsystem you interact with. Map the generative star.

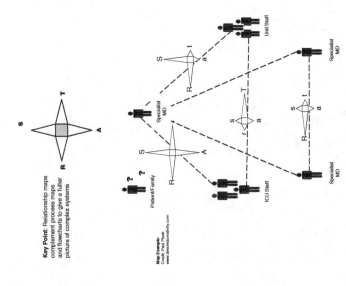

**Key Point:** Relationship maps complement process maps and flowcharts to give a fuller picture of complex systems

**Map Example:**
Credit: Paul Plsek
www.directedcreativity.com

**A few examples:**

- **STaR:** Relationship with limited action opportunities. What is blocking action opportunities? Is it bureaucratic approval process or the need for a supervisor's permission to act?
- **sTAR:** Missing separateness or differences. To enhance its capacity to generate new insights, products or services, new perspectives need to be brought into the relationship. This may require new participants or at least some structured creativity exercises to reveal hidden assumptions. Who could be added or dropped to enhance the differences in the group?
- **STar:** All talk and no action. What is preventing the relationship from moving to action? Can you change this context?
- **stAR:** Limited capacity for reflecting on the conceptual changes that are happening. It may fail to recognize shifts in patterns and thus will expend resources on experiments without capitalizing on the learning from them.

*Source:* Adapted from Zimmerman, B. J., & Hayday, B. C. A board's journey into complexity science. *Group Decision Making and Negotiation,* 1999, *8,* 281–303.

# SUPPORTING PATIENTS AND FAMILIES THROUGH PALLIATIVE CARE

Frances C. Brokaw

Joel S. Lazar

Eliza Philippa Shulman

Eugene C. Nelson

Marjorie M. Godfrey

Paul B. Batalden

---

## LEARNING OBJECTIVES

- Define palliative care from the perspective of patients, families, and health care professionals.
- Describe national variation in end-of-life care according to the Dartmouth Atlas.
- Describe how palliative care requires consideration of preventive, acute, and chronic care processes in the course of care.
- List the holistic principles that guide palliative care.
- Discuss how shared decision making informs planning and support for life-threatening illness.
- Discuss implications of palliative care for professionals in the clinical microsystem.

Palliative care addresses the needs of patients and families for comfort and dignity in the context of progressive or life-threatening illness. In the present chapter, we focus attention on the unique health needs of these patients and their families. We first consider the epidemiologic and sociodemographic shifts that have prolonged the final phase of life for most people, and that have increased the medical, emotional, and economic burden of chronic illness for individuals, their families, and society. This prolongation of the end of life has resulted in a burgeoning need for palliative care services. In the present chapter we discuss both principles and practices of such care in a variety of settings. We examine programs that focus exclusively on end-of-life-care (provided by palliative care teams and hospice), and we consider the more general integration of palliative care approaches in both outpatient and inpatient settings.

## THE NEED FOR PALLIATIVE CARE IN MODERN AMERICA

For a significant majority of Americans, the experience of life in its final months and the experience of dying that follows, are far different than they were a century ago. Thanks to successes in public health practices and in preventive medicine, and to favorable changes in the other major determinants of health, we can now expect to live thirty years longer, on average, than was the case in the year 1900. But this profound sociodemographic change has generated new health needs and challenges at the *end* of our lives, which have resulted in new care-providing systems that simply did not exist in earlier times. As Table 9.1 suggests, most of us today will live into our seventies and beyond, with chronic illnesses that entail years of potential disability (and considerable financial cost) before our death. And although those deaths once occurred most frequently (and often abruptly) at home with care from families, and perhaps a general practitioner, today we are likely to die in the hospital or nursing home often after prolonged decline in functional status, attended by numerous physicians and health professionals.[1] Physical, functional, and interpersonal losses are commonly experienced in the months and even years prior to death, and these losses demand a clinical response that is not only well-conceived and well-orchestrated, but also sufficiently flexible to meet the diverse needs of individuals and families.

In the context of inexorable disease progression, as the needs of patients and families shift from biomedical control and cure to intrapersonal and interpersonal comfort and dignity, the clinical microsystem must broaden its capacity to deliver services that are specifically palliative in nature. *Palliative care* (from the Latin *pallium*, or cloak) is

### Table 9.1   Death in 1900 and in 2000: A Comparison

|  | 1900 | 2000 |
|---|---|---|
| Life expectancy | • 47 years | • 75 years |
| Usual place of death | • Home | • Hospital |
| Expenses | • Paid by family | • Paid by third-party payers |
| Disability before death | • Not much | • Average of two years |

*Source:* Lynne, J. *Sick to death and not going to take it anymore! Reforming health care for the last years of life.* Berkeley: University of California Press, 2004.

Table 9.2    Overarching Care Needs of Patient and Family

| | |
|---|---|
| **Preventive care** | • Proactive assessment and mitigation of health risks |
| **Acute care** | • Timely attention to new or newly worsening disruption of health or function |
| **Chronic care** | • Longitudinal resiliency and support in self-management of ongoing disease |
| **Palliative care** | • Comfort and dignity in the context of underlying disease progression |

person-oriented rather than disease-oriented and directs our attention to relief of symptoms with or without treatment of underlying disease. We can properly frame palliative care as either a precise form of clinical service (many academic hospitals, for example, have developed *palliative care teams* dedicated to delivering this service) or as a more general approach to patient care that suggests numerous forms of design and implementation. We shall explore the former service-specific model later in this chapter, but our primary focus is on the more broadly conceived *approach to care* that informs multiple types of microsystem interventions. This approach is consonant with the World Health Organization's definition of palliative care as "an approach which improves the quality of life of patients and their families facing life-threatening illness, through the prevention, assessment and treatment of pain and other physical, psychosocial and spiritual problems."[2]

Table 9.2 links palliative care to the clinical continuum we have discussed in prior chapters and reminds us again that the microsystem's essential first function when planning for clinical interventions is to carefully consider the needs of patients and families. In palliative care, the overarching need is for comfort and dignity in the context of serious underlying disease. As in our prior discussions of preventive, acute, and chronic illness care, this palliative need suggests specific service design features and planning activities the clinical microsystem must incorporate into its regular work processes. In this chapter, we explore these work processes in detail. We first characterize the palliative care framework more thoroughly, with attention to key principles that can guide the design of specific services. We then explore that design itself and ask the following questions:

- What does palliative care look like at the front line of clinical service?
- What patient and family needs are most salient?
- What structures and processes must the microsystem implement to successfully meet those needs?

After examining these design features, we close with reflections on the clinical microsystem's attention to its own self-care. Because end-of-life issues touch core emotions in all participants (not only patients and families), microsystems engaged in palliative care must build their own capacity to support the well-being of team members. This support will allow caregivers to feel continually enriched rather than depleted by the intensity of their work.

## END-OF-LIFE EXPERIENCE YESTERDAY AND TODAY

For most Americans, both the trajectory of life in its final months and the experience of death have changed substantially in the modern era. Our contemporary case

FIGURE 9.1   Typical Trajectory of Health Status Preceding
Death Before the Twentieth Century.

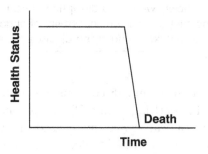

*Note:* Today there is less than a 10 percent sudden death rate (such as sudden cardiac death, trauma).

presentation, which follows, is all the more compelling if contrasted with a life and death from earlier times. Therefore, let us first consider Henry Cook, an early nineteenth-century farmer who enjoyed vigor and ongoing activity until days before his sudden death at age sixty-seven. Just half a week before dying of quinsy, an infection of the throat that restricted his breathing, Henry's physical condition remained good. Three days before his death he developed fever while chopping wood in his fields. His condition deteriorated quickly, and he died at home with family present, having been confined to his bed for just one day. Henry's life ended abruptly from an unexpected cause that would have been curable today. The trajectory of this death is portrayed in Figure 9.1. Although some individuals today also die of sudden illnesses, this was more typical in the centuries that preceded modern biomedicine.

Now consider Carl Bloom, a retired newspaper publisher whose death at age eighty-five, and whose diminishing quality of life in the two years prior to that death, are more common in our present era. After living an active and vigorous life into his early eighties, the last two years of Carl's life were marked by repeated symptom crises and illness episodes. He experienced intermittent flare-ups of both chronic obstructive pulmonary disease and congestive heart failure. Although in earlier years he had successfully managed his chronic conditions in partnership with his primary and specialist care teams (see Chapter Eight for review of chronic illness management principles and practices), with each new flare-up his recovery was slower and he returned to an increasingly poor functional baseline. On three separate occasions Carl repeated a similar (although progressively downward) cycle. This involved his traveling from his condominium (where he lived independently with his wife), to the emergency department, to the intensive care unit in the hospital, to the nursing home for 30 days of recovery and rehabilitation, and then returning to his condominium with support from home health services (whose necessity persisted, due to ongoing declines in health, functional status, and capacity for self-care).

Carl grew depressed from his losses, which were not only physical but also interpersonal and spiritual in nature. He could no longer play ball with his grandchildren, and he despaired at the loss of meaning in his own life. His wife attended heroically to his basic needs, which over time (due to his progressive weakness) grew to include assistance in walking, dressing, and bathing. She experienced occasional compassion fatigue related to Carl's continuous care requirements. In his final two weeks of life, lacking a formal advance directive to articulate his end-of-life care preferences, Carl experienced one last flare-up of respiratory distress and was admitted again to the

FIGURE 9.2   Typical Trajectory of Health Status Preceding Death for Chronic
Illnesses with Slow Decline and Periodic Crises.

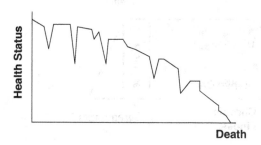

FIGURE 9.3   Typical Trajectory of Health Status Preceding Death for Chronic
Illnesses with Steady Decline and Short Pre-Terminal Phase.

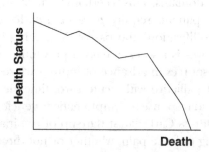

intensive care unit. For several days he was maintained on a ventilator, with two intravenous lines supplying medications and nutrients. Finally, his wife and his interdisciplinary
clinical team agreed to withdraw these high tech therapies, and he died soon after with
his wife at his side.

Carl's story is not only sad in its unfolding, but also (because it is so typical in our
times) alarming in its implications. As discussed in Chapter Eight, the great majority of
older Americans live with one (and often more than one) chronic disease, and most
will die of this disease. Because medications and other therapies can often prolong life
(without cure), the process of dying is prolonged as well. Indeed, 90 percent of
Americans will experience an end-of-life phase that follows one of two trajectories: (1)
either a slow but erratic decline (see Figure 9.2) that is punctuated by periodic exacerbations with a new, worsening baseline following each episodic flare-up (as in heart
failure and emphysema), or (2) a more predictable, steady decline (see Figure 9.3) with
a relatively brief terminal phase (as, for example, with metastatic cancer or Alzheimer's
dementia). In either case, the prolonged process of dying creates new needs in patients
and families and requires new forms of response from clinical microsystems that
endeavor to meet these needs.

## PRINCIPLES OF PALLIATIVE CARE

We have suggested in previous chapters that the parsing of microsystem care into discrete clinical domains (preventive, acute, chronic, and palliative) can facilitate powerful

**FIGURE 9.4    A Continuum of Care Model for Palliative Care.**

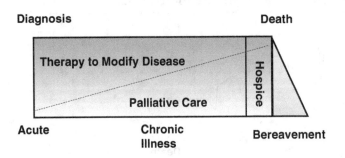

assessment and planning of discrete care components. We have also noted that the boundaries between these components are permeable, and both patient needs and system interventions may cross clinical domains. This is certainly true of high-value palliative care. Even near the end of life, patients require *preventive care*, for example, to minimize (through environmental modification) the risk of devastating falls in their home. Clarification of advance directives is also essentially a preventive activity, as it anticipates future needs and aligns resources in advance of future care requirements. Simultaneously, at the intersection of palliative with acute care, timeliness and tight coordination are manifested in the rapid response to symptomatic urgencies. How does the clinical microsystem effectively address Carl's latest flare-up of respiratory distress or a cancer patient's sudden worsening of bone pain, whether or not these symptoms require face-to-face emergency consultation?

In important respects, palliative care is also a direct and continuous extension of *chronic care*, as patient needs and priorities shift gradually over time from biomedical stabilization and control to personal comfort and dignity. Figure 9.4 depicts this continuum from chronic to palliative care, in which palliative services can both prolong life and improve the quality of that life, with a gradual shift in emphasis and therapies over time. As we suggested in Chapter Eight, optimization of function, of emotional well-being, and of personal empowerment are essential (although sometimes neglected) goals of chronic illness care, and these goals only increase in importance as care becomes progressively more palliative. Note also in Figure 9.4 that palliative interventions do not end with the patient's death, but also incorporate supports for bereavement of family and friends once the patient has succumbed to chronic illness.

As Carl's case makes clear, patients with serious illnesses are challenged by threats not merely to specific organ systems, but to their intactness as whole persons. Physician Eric Cassell states that "bodies do not suffer; persons suffer."[3] Comfort and dignity (the essential needs of palliative care identified in Table 9.1) are informed by specific symptoms such as pain or shortness of breath, but depend ultimately on the intersection of these physical symptoms with integrated experiences of personal control, knowledge, and interpersonal relationship. This whole-person orientation has special relevance to interdisciplinary teams engaged in palliative care. In his seminal work, *The Nature of Suffering and the Goals of Medicine,* Cassell writes about suffering and relationship: People can suffer from what they have lost of themselves in relation to the world of objects, events, and relationships. Such suffering occurs because our intactness as persons, our coherence and integrity, come not only from intactness of the body but also from the wholeness of the web of relationships with self and others.[3]

"The basic principle," Cassell concludes, "is that the intactness or integrity of the person must be restored."[3] Even when death is inevitable, such *restoration* is an important source of healing (as opposed to cure) in palliative care. We note here that the terms healing and wholeness share a common linguistic root, the Indo-European *kailo-*, meaning whole or intact.

In this spirit, the World Health Organization[2] has articulated the following holistic principles to guide delivery of palliative care:

- Affirm life and regard dying as a normal process.
- Neither hasten nor postpone death.
- Provide relief from pain and other physical symptoms.
- Integrate psychological and spiritual care.
- Help the patient live as actively as possible until death; maximize quality of life.
- Provide support systems to help the family cope during illness and bereavement.
- Use an interdisciplinary team to address needs of patients and families.
- Apply palliative care early in the course of illness and later in the illness trajectory.

These holistic principles can guide clinical microsystem members in the design, implementation, and improvement of palliative care processes. But principles alone do not determine care. We next examine how principles are translated into actual high-quality services.

## REDUCING VARIATION IN END-OF-LIFE CARE

It is no surprise that financial costs in the final months of life have skyrocketed in recent decades. With the aging of our population, with the substantial increase in burden of chronic illness, and with the growing availability of expensive technologies, total spending for chronically ill patients during their last two years of life between 2001 and 2005 was $289 billion dollars.[4] More surprising, and more pertinent to our current discussion, is the impressive *variation* in costs from region to region in our nation, which reflects variation in both the quantity and quality of services provided during this final year. As Dartmouth Atlas investigators have reported, and as depicted in Figure 9.5, a dramatic 2.5-fold difference in Medicare costs has been documented between high- and low-expenditure regions of the United States among comparable patients in the final six years of life.[4] This variation cannot simply reflect differences in underlying severity of disease, as populations in the Dartmouth Atlas are defined by their comparable proximity to end of life. Nor can markedly higher expenses in some regions be justified by resulting reductions in mortality in those same regions, as again, mortality across groups is identical. Rather, we have evidence here of unwarranted variation in care (and in cost) without associated improvement in outcome. We may conclude that attention to the sources of unnecessary (and often unwanted) end-of-life clinical services, and greater emphasis upon less expensive (and presumably lower technology) interventions, may improve both quality and costs associated with care.

In 2004, the National Consensus Project for Quality Palliative Care published general guidelines for the provision of high-quality palliative care services.[5] The goals of this report were to (1) provide specific suggestions to promote quality and reduce unwanted or unnecessary variation in new and existing programs; (2) develop and encourage continuity of care across settings; and (3) facilitate collaborative partnerships

FIGURE 9.5    Total Medicare Spending for Chronically Ill Patients During the Last Two Years of Life, by State (Deaths Occurring 2001–2005).

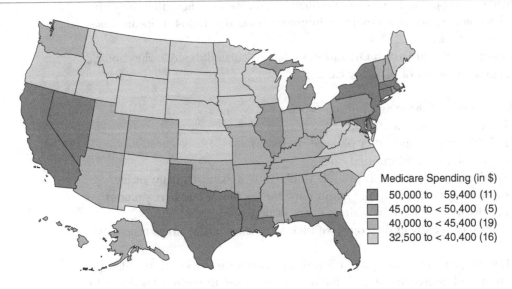

Medicare Spending (in $)

- 50,000 to   59,400 (11)
- 45,000 to < 50,400   (5)
- 40,000 to < 45,400 (19)
- 32,500 to < 40,400 (16)

*Source:* The Dartmouth Atlas of Health Care.

among palliative care programs, community hospices, and a wide range of other health care delivery settings. These guidelines address the following seven domains:

1. *Structure and processes of care.* Comprehensive assessment of patient and family needs informs a care plan based on identified and expressed values. Professional support facilitates shared decision making, alignment of care plan with identified goals, and ongoing assessment by interdisciplinary teams.
2. *Physical aspects of care.* Pain, other symptoms, and side effects are treated in a skilled and caring manner; treatment relies upon the best available evidence.
3. *Psychological aspects of care.* Psychological issues are evaluated and addressed using best available evidence by a team that includes professionals with training in counseling and communication. Bereavement risk assessment and follow-up is provided for families.
4. *Social aspects of care.* Comprehensive interdisciplinary assessment identifies the social needs of patients and families, and a care plan is developed to respond to these needs as effectively as possible. Cultural issues are assessed and addressed; regular patient or family meetings are held to address concerns, to discern goals of care, and to make referrals to appropriate support services such as psychotherapy, finance, education, employment, and transportation.
5. *Spiritual, religious, and existential aspects of care.* A spiritual assessment elicits religious, spiritual, or existential background or preferences, and related beliefs, rituals, and practices of the patient and family. Ongoing reassessments are conducted, and existential fears and concerns are addressed in a culturally sensitive manner.
6. *Cultural aspects of care.* The cultural background, concerns, and needs of the patient and family are elicited and documented, and the care plan created by the interdisciplinary team takes cultural issues into account. Communication with patient and family respects their cultural preferences regarding disclosure, truth-telling, and decision making.

7. *Care of the imminently dying patient.* Signs and symptoms of impending death are recognized and communicated, and care appropriate for this phase of illness is provided to the patient and family. Wishes regarding the preferred care setting for death are elicited and documented. Hospice referral is discussed for those who have not already accessed hospice services. The family is educated about signs and symptoms of approaching death in a developmentally and culturally appropriate manner.

The reader will note one further principle implicit in these guidelines. Palliative care is fundamentally patient- and family-centered in its orientation, even more so than preventive, acute, and chronic care. Within the general National Consensus Project categories that guide the standardization of care, specific clinical goals are entirely determined by the patient's own priorities for comfort, well-being, and dignity. What balance of pain relief versus potential medication side effects is most desirable for *this* patient? What rituals and meanings are linked with the death experience in *this* family's culture and religious system? We thus return to the key principle (discussed in Chapters Two and Eight) of *partnership* in care (between patient, family, and clinical microsystem). But here the patient is even more than partner: within the constraints of available microsystem and community resources, the entire content of palliative care (including addition and withdrawal of therapies) is guided by the patient's and family's values.

Authority, priority-setting, and distribution of activity are almost always under negotiation in clinical care. Depending on specific needs and contexts, the locus of control will appropriately shift along a continuum between clinical team members and patient and family. To some extent, this continuum is informed by the type(s) of knowledge and skill required to effect appropriate actions. In acute care settings, where patients' needs are often technical in nature, the clinical team brings resources and experiences that establish its own authority, defines priorities, and justifies its active role. As care progresses to preventive, chronic, and finally palliative concerns, where the most appropriate forms of knowledge and skill become less technical and more interpersonal and intrapersonal in nature, authority, priority setting, and caregiving activities shift naturally to patient and family. Dialogue increasingly includes not only consideration of new therapies, but also withdrawal of old ones that are no longer consonant with patients' and families' evolving needs (see also Chapter Eight discussion of complicated versus complex clinical problems).

Of course, the continuum overgeneralizes the actual dynamics of frontline care. In every clinical encounter (whether preventive, acute, chronic, or palliative), principles of *shared decision making* must inform the negotiation between clinical teams, patients, and families. As discussed in Chapter Two, all parties bring unique knowledge and skills to the clinical encounter and to the planning and design that supports such encounters. Effective collaboration is facilitated by open communication, flexibility, and mutual respect. Such qualities must be especially well-integrated into palliative care. Implementing and improving palliative care processes means inviting the patient and family to participate in decision making at every stage of the evolving work.

## CORE PROCESSES IN PALLIATIVE CARE

Palliative care may be initiated early or late in the course of a life-threatening disease, and it extends beyond the patient's death to include the period of bereavement among family and friends. As previously suggested, microsystem attention is directed to patient needs for comfort, dignity, and function. Core clinical processes include *assessment, planning, and provision* of palliative services. (These are, in fact, the very processes implied in the 2004 National Consensus Project guidelines already described.) We now discuss these three care processes in greater detail.

### Assessing the Full Health Status and Well-Being of Patient and Family

Clinical microsystems assign specific information-gathering activities to various members of the interdisciplinary team. Physicians, nurses, chaplains, social workers, and other providers may participate in coordinated assessment. Survey instruments such as pain scales, the PHQ-9 (depression screen), and the VF-12 (functional status inventory) may be incorporated into initial and follow-up care. Specific parameters of interest include the following:

- Pain and suffering
- Physical, mental, social, and spiritual well-being
- Specific disease symptoms
- Side effects of medications and treatments
- Functional abilities, including basic activities of daily living (bathing, toileting), instrumental activities (food preparation), and transportation
- Support and respite needs of family

### Planning for the Patient and Family

It is important to consider how patients' values and priorities are incorporated into present care and how future changes in health status (such as progressive decline) are anticipated. It is also important to select a setting (home, hospice, institution) where patients' needs for dignity and comfort may be most reliably served, and to know how changes in health status may affect appropriateness of that setting. Therefore, consider the following planning activities in particular: (1) advanced care planning and completion of advance directives, (2) disposition planning for home care, and (3) transition planning to nursing home or hospice.

### Providing Services to Patient and Family

Multiple domains of whole-person care (including physical, psychological, social, spiritual, and cultural domains) require anticipatory and ongoing microsystem attention. Each of these domains suggests specific interventions that, although standardized in their general features, must be tailored to the unique needs of each patient and family. A partial list of interventions is provided here:

- Pain and symptom treatment
- Clarification of goals of care and updating these as conditions change
- Assistance with decision making, aligned with values and preferences
- Withdrawal of interventions when these are no longer consistent with evolving patient needs and desires
- Crisis prevention and early crisis management
- Counseling on attaining closure in life and important relationships

- Counseling on prognosis, anticipatory guidance, and adapting to illness
- Counseling on spiritual matters
- Making available family support and counseling

The reader will note these activities are in fact further specifications of the National Consensus Project's 2004 guidelines for Quality Palliative Care.[5] Successful implementation in these domains requires that we attend to structures and processes of care and that we design our frontline clinical microsystems to address not only the physical needs of patient and family, but also the psychological, social, spiritual, and cultural needs, as these all influence comfort and dignity at the end of life. Let us next explore some specific design features of palliative care in greater detail.

## CARE COORDINATION NEAR THE END OF LIFE

As discussed in Chapter Eight, although handoffs and transitions in acute care contexts are commonly linear in nature (patient and information travel from microsystem A to B to C in a timely manner), *care coordination* of patients' chronic illness over time is complex and often displays a radial pattern. A central clinical microsystem typically coordinates care, engaging supportive microsystems for varied (and often continuous) services that address patients' wide-ranging clinical needs. This pattern of coordination is prominent in palliative care as well, and notably the patient's and family's own position at the central hub (in partnership with the clinical team) is even more essential. Clinical microsystems should not assume patients and families desire clinician coordination at the end of life. Many families have the capacity and desire to self-manage this meaningful activity in their own way.

The external resource map in Figure 9.6 (that was also discussed in Chapter One) depicts many of the coordinating relationships that may come into play in palliative care. Note that a primary microsystem (which may be a formal palliative care team, a hospice team, the patient's primary care provider, or even the family itself) aligns services to meet patients' multiple clinical needs. Note too that the breadth of these services corresponds to the previously acknowledged diversity of patient needs. When the goal is optimization of comfort, function, and dignity, consultants may include pain management specialists, pharmacists, nursing staff, psychologists, social workers, physical therapists, clergy members, alternative healers, and others. Effective central microsystems, which include the patient and family, must build resilient relationships with these varied clinical providers and community resources. The ability to coordinate care activities must be hard-wired (via physician, nurse practitioner, social worker, or other skilled staff) into the microsystem's core structure.

Figure 9.7 further underscores the intersection of multiple supportive relationships and draws specific attention to the patient's and family's centrality in the palliative care process. It is the patient and family from whom care priorities are elicited (physical, psychological, social, spiritual, cultural), and toward whom multiple clinical microsystems orient their care to honor and serve those priorities. Note as well that this entire network of relationships is embedded in an even larger network of nonclinical community supports. Although the end of life has certainly grown more medicalized in recent decades, this essential human experience transcends mere clinical domains and is deeply informed by interpersonal, cultural, and spiritual relationships that are external to traditional health care boundaries.

**FIGURE 9.6    Exploring the External Context of Coordinating Palliative Care.**

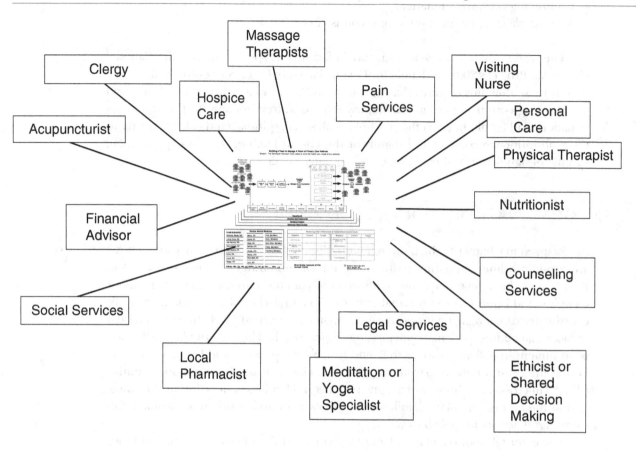

**FIGURE 9.7    The Palliative Care Team.**

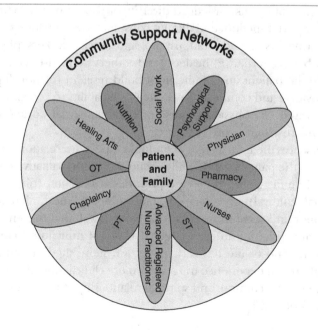

# FORMAL PALLIATIVE CARE AND HOSPICE PROGRAMS

In a growing number of settings, diverse palliative and end-of-life services are now coordinated and refined by specialty programs that incorporate whole-person and multidisciplinary care into their design. High-quality palliative care teams have emerged in many academic centers and nonacademic *hospice programs* are present in most communities as well. While these two forms of service are not identical, they share similar philosophies of care. Both place the needs of patient and family at the center of service planning, both include these recipients of care in the design and implementation of care, and both require clinicians to critically examine and potentially withdraw previously initiated interventions when they no longer serve the patient's needs and desires. In addition, palliative and hospice care programs both attend to *assessment, planning,* and *provision* of whole-person care for progressive serious illness, and both rely on interdisciplinary microsystems for full-spectrum service delivery.

While precise role definitions and boundaries vary from community to community, we note that, in general, palliative care is appropriate for any patient with *potentially life-limiting* illness, whereas hospice care is directed to people whose life is clearly drawing to a close (see Figure 9.8). As noted in Figure 9.4, the patient's overall care near the end of life is best understood as a continuum, which, over time, may include disease modifying treatment, palliative care, *and* hospice care. Alternatively, if we again consider the World Health Organization's definition of palliative care as "an approach which improves the quality of life of patients and their families facing life-threatening illness, through the prevention, assessment and treatment of pain and other physical, psychosocial and spiritual problems,"[2] we recognize hospice care as a subset of more general palliative services directed specifically to individuals who are approaching life's end.

A brief case example will illustrate the overlapping function of formal palliative care and hospice clinical microsystems (see Figure 9.9 for a flowchart of key process steps). Kathy Turner was a 54-year-old woman diagnosed (three years before her death) with pancreatic cancer. During initial oncology management, the medical center's palliative care team participated actively in management of symptoms due to cancer treatment itself. Kathy underwent concurrent radiation and chemotherapy, followed by

---

FIGURE 9.8   Disease Modifying Care, Palliative Care, and Hospice Care.

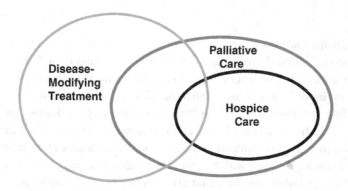

*Note:* Hospice is a subset of palliative care. Palliative care is the discipline; hospice is a way of delivering palliative care to patients who are acknowledged to be dying and to their families. In the United States, hospice care is most often delivered in the home.

FIGURE 9.9    Palliative and Hospice Care Overlap.

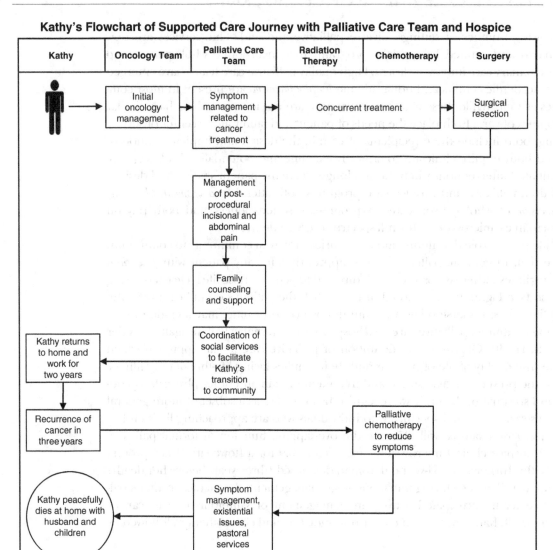

**Kathy's Flowchart of Supported Care Journey with Palliative Care Team and Hospice**

surgical resection. The palliative care team actively managed her post-procedural problems with nausea and incisional and abdominal pain. In addition, the team coordinated social service resources to smooth her transition back to her community and provided counseling to support her family's emotional transition during this difficult time. Eventually, Kathy successfully returned to work, and she remained free of disease for two years following diagnosis. In her third year, however, the disease recurred, and Kathy chose palliative chemotherapy to reduce symptom burden (but with no expectation of cure). The palliative care team assisted her with symptom management and existential issues and helped work through family conflicts that arose as her health deteriorated. Consistent with Kathy's own wishes, the family elected to care for her at home, and she received hospice care (including pain and nausea management and connection to pastoral services in her community) for three months. She died peacefully at home with her husband and children at her bedside.

## PLANNING FOR BOTH LIFE AND DEATH
## WITH ADVANCE DIRECTIVES

Of course, clinical microsystems can actively design processes to support patients' comfort and dignity even without formal palliative care and hospice teams. Many communities lack the resources to establish formal specialist programs that are solely dedicated to palliative care concerns. While specialist expertise is often beneficial, the core requirements for effective assessment, planning, and implementation of palliative care can be realized by many nonspecialist microsystems that commit themselves to reflective self-assessment (see again the 5Ps of Chapter One), interdisciplinary teamwork, and practice-based quality improvement.

One dimension of palliative care especially conducive to the microsystem's reflective engagement is the elicitation of patient *advance directives*. As we have discussed, explicit assessment of patients' present and future care preferences, and conscious planning to honor these preferences, are core clinical processes of palliative care. Unfortunately, despite the value of this work, many well-intentioned clinical microsystems have not yet defined specific roles and relationship-based protocols to query for advance directives and to document these in a manner that renders them useful to entire clinical teams. Recall Carl, the eighty-five-year-old newspaper publisher whose case opened the present chapter. Although his poor prognosis from heart failure was apparent to him and to clinical team members, no discussion was ever pursued to elicit his preferences for care in the final months of life. Nor was he queried explicitly about his desired experience of death: should this occur in the high tech environment of a medical intensive care unit or in the comfort of his own home? Absent such discussions, Carl cycled several times from home to hospital to nursing home rehabilitation, and died in an intensive care unit after one final round of endotracheal intubation, intravenous fluids, and aggressive antibiotics.

Let us contrast Carl's story with one last case study, the outcome of which was clearly more positive. Although a cure was not achieved, the engaged clinical microsystem embarked on a journey to develop new methods to assess and honor patients' care preferences not only for dignified death, but also for dignified *life* many months preceding death. Irene Belson, at the age of seventy, suffered (like Carl Bloom) from end-stage chronic obstructive pulmonary disease (COPD). In the prior year, she had been hospitalized three times for spontaneous pneumothorax (collapsed lung), and she endured several invasive surgical procedures to minimize risk of future episodes. Even so, she experienced significant anxiety when she thought about recurrent lung collapse, a very painful and frightening experience. Her COPD had progressed over time, and she now required oxygen twenty-four hours per day, although she remained short of breath even at rest.

On the morning that would change her life (even in these final years of her life), Irene arrived at her primary care doctor's office in obvious distress, short of breath, and tearful. She described how much time and energy was required to get ready for this visit and how this short but exhausting trip would impact her function for the next several days as she recovered. Her doctor felt uneasy to have compelled this frail woman to come to the office simply for a lung check and medication review. The medical team concluded, in consultation with Irene, that home-based palliative care would be a better approach for her, given her particular needs. Although an excellent hospice program existed in the community and was affiliated with the visiting nurses association (VNA), there was no local palliative care team available for formal consultation.

In response to Irene and patients like her, this primary care microsystem formed an *interdisciplinary quality improvement team* to examine processes pertinent to end-of-life care. The team's key participants included a medical resident and a geriatric attending physician, a geriatric specialty nurse, a medical assistant, and a member of the medical records department. The team met on a biweekly basis to share information and ideas and soon determined that, although many end-of-life issues required attention, advance directives needed to be tackled first. The team collected baseline data, which revealed fewer than 30 percent of frail elders in their health center had advance directives in their charts. In addition, a survey of clinicians' knowledge, attitudes, and practices confirmed wide variation in understanding advance directives, terminology, and end-of-life care. Providers expressed their desire for a common record that could be shared across care locations, and they voiced an urgent need for education on end-of-life issues such as symptom management and care planning. Finally, members of the interdisciplinary team accompanied frail elder patients during entire office visits and developed process maps to trace the actual (as opposed to the ideal) steps in care delivery.

From these varied explorations, the quality improvement group (in consultation with patient representatives) designed a dynamic electronic medical record (EMR) template with three main functions. These three components made up an enhanced advance directive that would not only capture essential information, but would also simplify *sharing* this information (most notably patients' end-of-life preferences) with all members of the care team, so actual service could be enhanced for patients' benefit. Each advance directive would be completed over time and would be updated periodically in the course of routine care. The three functional components were as follows:

1. A reliable location and standardized framework to capture legal information and goal-setting conversations with patients and families; the template provides a straightforward checklist for end-of-life planning and elicits specific preferences regarding advance directives.
2. A clinician guide to difficult conversations; specific prompts in the EMR support a values questionnaire adapted from the Vermont Ethics Network.[6]
3. Information resources that can be accessed in real time during regular office visits; these include decision support tools to guide management of symptoms in seriously ill patients.

Irene was one of the clinical microsystem's first patients to have this enhanced advance directive initiated in her chart. During the life-changing office visit we have described, she expressed her strong preference to minimize future visits to the hospital (unless absolutely necessary for symptom relief) and, instead, to spend her remaining time at home with her husband and adult children. She also voiced her desire to have symptoms of anxiety and breathlessness managed more effectively. During this office visit, her living will and durable power of attorney were reviewed and referenced within the EMR, and her doctor consulted a Web-based resource for support in treating her shortness of breath. Hospice criteria were also reviewed, and Irene and her husband agreed to meet with the local visiting nurses association as a next step in transition to home-based (rather than office-based) care.

Shortly after this important office visit, Irene experienced a symptomatic flare-up (chest pain and worsening shortness of breath) that prompted a visit to the local emergency department. The hospital team had immediate access to her enhanced advance directive, which contained details about her condition, her current symptom management plan, and her wish to stay home with her husband. Once her overall stability was achieved, she needed only a brief observational stay in the hospital to enhance her symptom management plan. She and her husband agreed the time had come for hospice enrollment. Her goals for care and comfort were clearly documented in the EMR template, and she was discharged to her home.

Now in regular dialogue with her primary care team (who visit her intermittently at home, as does the visiting nurse), Irene feels secure with self-care strategies to adjust her symptom-reducing medication as needed. She has enjoyed a full year in her home with no further hospitalizations, and recently she was even discharged from the formal hospice program because her overall condition had stabilized. She expresses appreciation for her primary care team, with whom she can now comfortably discuss difficult issues, and she is grateful that her remaining time can be spent in the intimate company of family members. She harbors no illusions regarding her clinical prognosis, but she experiences dignity in this late stage of life and anticipates similar dignity in a home-based death.

Irene's case is not unusual. The microsystem innovations in which she participated are now hardwired in this primary care practice. Within six months of the program's introduction, more than 90 percent of the health center's frail elders had established some form of advance directive in their chart, and more than half now use the enhanced directive that specifically identifies and supports patients' values and wishes at the end of life. Excellent team-based care, shared commitment to eliciting and negotiating priorities, and proactive planning to act on these priorities have together stimulated new clinical microsystem structures and processes that improve not only patients' lives, but also their dignified deaths.

## CONCLUSION

In Chapters Six through Nine, we have explored a rich variety of patient needs and experiences. We have endeavored to link these to specific microsystem resources, processes, and design principles. We saw in Chapter Six that patients' need for proactive assessment and mitigation of health risk engenders specific forms of microsystem planning for preventive care. Similarly, in Chapters Seven and Eight, we noted that patient needs for timely responsiveness (to unexpected health disruption) and resilient coaching and support (of longitudinal self-management) stimulate microsystem design and improvement of both acute and chronic care. Finally, in the present chapter, we see the progression of serious illness also mandates microsystem attention to patients' need for comfort and dignity (that is, for sensitive and respectful palliative care), as the end of life approaches.

We have also suggested in prior chapters that these compelling needs in each clinical domain are yoked to parallel learning needs of the clinical microsystem itself. As members of the care team focus (for example) on *preventive health* and risk mitigation, so too must they actively explore the safety of clinical and administrative processes. Attention to iatrogenic (health care-induced) hazards is the clinical microsystem's own form of preventive health. Similarly, as the clinical microsystem addresses new or worsening disruption of health and function in the *acute care* of patients, it must also plan for effective response to its own small or large disruptions of function (for example, unexpected staffing requirements and extended office wait times, as when a patient presents surprisingly with acute decompensation). When the microsystem refines its capacity to manage interpersonal processes in support of patients' self-efficacy in *chronic* illness, it likewise finds opportunity to improve interpersonal team processes (such as good communication, empowering of participants, and flexibility and adaptability) that make quality improvement possible.

We conclude with the observation that palliative care also impels clinical microsystems to reflect and to learn in ways that are analogous to reflection and learning in preventive, acute, and chronic illness care. Here, however, the emotional intensity of the clinical content calls for reflective response. As we suggest in this chapter's opening section, end-of-life issues touch core emotions not only in patients and families who receive care, but also in those who provide this care. Clinical microsystems engaged in palliative care must therefore build into their own work the capacity to support the team members' well-being, so caregivers feel continually enriched rather than depleted by this engaging but demanding work.

Kearney and colleagues[7] have described the risks of burnout and compassion fatigue that can undermine the effectiveness of even the most dedicated clinicians. Some microsystem members may find palliative care especially hazardous in this regard, but the challenge is real for all people who commit themselves to clinical work, to its administrative support, or to its continued redesign and improvement. Can clinical microsystems anticipate this risk and then plan for its amelioration, just as they plan for safe clinical processes in preventive care, for management of surprising disruptions in acute care, and for the demands (and rewards) of complexity in chronic care? We believe the answer is a necessary and resounding, "Yes."

The self-care recommendations in Table 9.3 were proposed by Kearney for palliative care staff and other end-of-life contexts.[7] We suggest, however, that these ideas may be

### Table 9.3    Activities That May Help Prevent Burnout

| Type of Activity | Suggested Action |
|---|---|
| Nonwork | Take time for<br>• Mindfulness meditation<br>• Reflective writing<br>• Practice of self-care activities, for example, exercise, yoga, gardening, healthy diet |
| Workplace structure | Management provides<br>• Adequate supervision and mentoring<br>• Sustainable workload<br>• Opportunities for mindfulness-based stress reduction for team<br>• Opportunities for participation in research<br>• Meaning-centered intervention for team (including alignment of personal values with organizational priorities) |
| Workplace values | Management promotes<br>• Feelings of choice and control<br>• Appropriate recognition and reward<br>• Supportive work community<br>• Fairness and justice in the workplace |
| Workplace education | Organization provides continuing education activities, including training in<br>• Communication skills<br>• Development of self-awareness skills |

*Source:* Kearney, M., Weininger, R., Vachon, M., Harrison, R., & Mount, B. Self-care of physicians caring for patients at the end of life: "Being connected . . . a key to my survival." *Journal of the American Medical Association,* 2009, *301*(11), 1155–1164.

embraced not only by palliative care providers, but by all who participate in the design, delivery, and improvement of care in any clinical domain. Interventions such as sustainable workloads, development of self-awareness skills,[8] individual and collective empowerment, and mindfulness-based stress reduction are all second order processes that can (and should) be planned by the overall microsystem, just as first order (direct patient care) processes are planned. Paying attention to the well-being of interdisciplinary team members is no luxury to be commenced when the real work of patient care is done. Rather, it is *part* of that real work, part of the true value we provide to patients and families wherever they find themselves on the health care continuum; optimal clinical care (preventive, acute, chronic, or palliative) shall always require fully engaged and high-functioning caregivers.

## SUMMARY

- Palliative care tends to be concentrated at the end of life and is part of the care continuum that also includes preventive, acute, and chronic care.
- Because people tend to live longer and the end-of-life phase is extended and burdened by chronic illness for longer periods of time, the need for palliative care is increasing dramatically.
- The primary palliative care need is for comfort and dignity in the context of underlying disease progression.
- Palliative care principles are intensively patient-centered, comprehensive, and address physical, psychological, social, spiritual, and cultural needs.
- Care coordination at the end of life is a challenging and critical dimension of palliative care.
- Advance directives help people receive the kind of care they want and need, when they are faced with life-threatening conditions.
- Both dedicated palliative care services (such as palliative care teams and hospice programs) and planned palliative care services (embedded in typical outpatient and inpatient care settings) are needed to meet patients' and families' needs for palliation and end-of-life care.

## KEY TERMS

| | |
|---|---|
| Acute care | Palliative care |
| Advance directive | Palliative care team |
| Approach to care | PHQ-9 (depression screen) |
| Care coordination | Preventive health |
| Hospice programs | Shared decision making |
| Ladder of Inference | VF-12 (functional status inventory) |
| Mental model | World Health Organization holistic |
| Pain scales |   principles |

## REVIEW QUESTIONS

1. What are the attitudes and expectations of patients, families, and health care professionals regarding palliative care in our setting?

2. What questions are raised when reviewing the Dartmouth Atlas of Health Care end-of-life variation for your specific region? Access to your regional data can be found at www.dartmouthatlas.org.
3. How are palliative care principles incorporated into the clinical domains of preventive, acute, and chronic care?
4. What are the seven National Consensus Project for Quality Palliative Care domains?
5. When would shared decision making enter into the palliative care process?
6. How does self-care apply to clinical microsystem members?

## DISCUSSION QUESTIONS

1. Explore preventive, acute, chronic, and palliative care domains in your microsystem and discuss how they are connected.
2. Assess the current palliative care processes in your clinical microsystem using the National Consensus Quality Palliative care guidelines. What are the standard processes? Is there an identified palliative care team, or is palliative care embedded within your microsystem?
3. Identity how shared decision making occurs in your current palliative care processes. Are advance directives part of your processes? What triggers palliative care processes to be activated?
4. Using the Ladder of Inference in Chapter Nine Action Guide, explore and discuss member perspectives of palliative care to gain insights into differing mental models and resultant thinking, actions, and beliefs.

## REFERENCES

1. Lynne, J. *Sick to death and not going to take it anymore! Reforming health care for the last years of life.* Berkeley: University of California Press, 2004.
2. World Health Organization. *World health organization definition of palliative care.* (p. 2) Retrieved February 16, 2010, from www.who.int/cancer/palliative/definition/en
3. Cassell, E. *The nature of suffering and the goals of medicine.* New York: Oxford University Press, 1991, p.v, p. 38, p. 287.
4. *Dartmouth atlas of health care.* Retrieved February 16, 2010, from www.dartmouthatlas.org
5. National Consensus Project for Quality Palliative Care. *Clinical practice guidelines for quality palliative care.* (2nd ed.) Retrieved February 16, 2010, from www.nationalconsensusproject.org
6. Vermont Ethics Network. Worksheets 1 and 2. Retrieved February 16, 2010, from www.vtethicsnetwork.org/PDFFiles/Worksheet12.pdf
7. Kearney, M., Weininger, R., Vachon, M., Harrison, R., & Mount, B. Self-care of physicians caring for patients at the end of life: "Being connected . . . a key to my survival." *Journal of the American Medical Association,* 2009, *301*(11), 1155–1164.
8. Byock, M., Twohi, J.S., Merriman, M., & Collins, K. A report on innovative models of palliative care. *Journal of Palliative Medicine,* 2006, *9*(1), 137–146.

Chapter Nine Action Guide explores the perspectives and conclusions that help to interpret the world we work in. The Ladder of Inference is a helpful method to explore personal experiences and resulting mental models.

## MENTAL MODELS

Mental models serve as cognitive maps that help us navigate through the complex environments we live in and work in. Mental models are images, assumptions, and stories we carry in our minds about ourselves, other people, institutions, and many other aspects of our life experiences. All of our mental maps are flawed in some way. The differences in mental models explain why two different people can observe the same event and yet describe it differently. Each person is paying attention to different details based on individual experiences. Mental models also shape our actions. For example, if we believe people are basically trustworthy, we may talk with new acquaintances more frequently than if we believe people cannot be trusted. Mental models are usually tacit and exist below the level of awareness; they are usually invisible to us until we look for them. Mental models are often untested and unexamined. To better understand how our mental models shape our thoughts, the following skills help us to increase our awareness and consider new perspectives:

1. *Reflection:* Slow down our thinking processes and examine them to become more aware of how we form our mental models.
2. *Inquiry:* Engage in conversations where we openly share our views and develop knowledge about others' assumptions.

## USING THE LADDER OF INFERENCE TO EXPLORE MENTAL MODELS

Developed by theorist Chris Argyris and popularized by Peter Senge[1] in *The Fifth Discipline*, the *Ladder of Inference* aims to explore the reasoning and attitudes that underlie human action and to create more effective learning about situations, people, and conclusions we draw (see Figure AG9.1).

**FIGURE AG9.1    Ladder of Inference.**

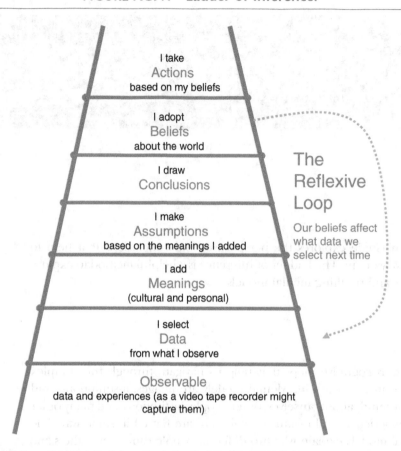

*Source:* Adapted from Scholtes, P., Joiner, B., & Streibel, B. *The TEAM® Handbook, Second Edition.* Madison, WI: Oriel, 2000.

The Ladder of Inference shows how rapidly we can leap to knee-jerk conclusions with no intermediate thought process, as if rapidly climbing up a ladder in our minds. Individuals who are undisciplined in reflective thinking have difficulty hearing what others actually say. They hear what they expect others to say, have little tolerance for multiple interpretations of events, and often believe only their own interpretation. Their mental model often offers a path of increasing abstraction, which further leads to misguided beliefs. In teams and groups, people who have not mastered a threshold level of inquiry may spend hours arguing about their ideas.

The Ladder of Inference can offer the following benefits:

- Improve your communications through thinking and reasoning (reflection)
- Help you understand how you got from the data to some abstract assumptions (reflection)
- Make your thinking and reasoning more visible to others (advocacy)
- Inquire into others' thinking and reasoning (inquiry)
- What is the observable data behind each statement

FIGURE AG9.2    Ladder of Inference for Advocacy and Inquiry.

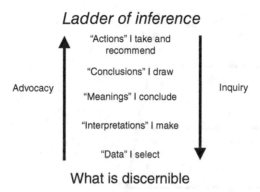

### Ladder of inference

"Actions" I take and recommend

"Conclusions" I draw

"Meanings" I conclude

"Interpretations" I make

"Data" I select

Advocacy

Inquiry

### What is discernible

*Source:* Adapted from Scholtes, P., Joiner, B., & Streibel, B. *The TEAM® Handbook, Second Edition.* Madison, WI: Oriel, 2000.

The Ladder of Inference shown in Figure AG9.2 provides a helpful tool to remind members of the clinical microsystem how to work through the process of advocacy and inquiry.

The Ladder of Inference Worksheet (see Figure AG9.3) is a helpful tool for enabling members of the clinical microsystem to practice exposing their own and others' mental models.

Consider the Ladder of Inference and one of the visits to the hospital Carl Bloom experienced. If you recall, Carl was diagnosed with both chronic obstructive pulmonary disease and congestive heart failure and was experiencing a progressive decline in overall quality of health.

In one episode, when Carl traveled from his condominium to the emergency department (ED) seeking care and support, he noticed staff to be attentive and kind in attempting to decrease his anxiety—except for one staff member. Carl noticed one nurse who kept her distance from him and overheard the nurse whispering to a colleague, "I don't understand why he comes here. We are short staffed and we need to take care of people who need emergent care . . ." and her voice trailed off.

The overheard whisper leaves Carl saddened and traveling up his own ladder as noted in Table AG9.1.

It is easy to see how quickly someone can apply their own life filters to a situation and end up with meanings, assumptions, conclusions, and beliefs that may not be accurate.

In Carl's situation, the conversation he overheard was incomplete, which left him to draw his own conclusions. The whispering nurse actually was the charge nurse for the ED who was overseeing staffing resources. Her complete statement was as follows:

*I don't understand why he comes here without his attending primary care physician calling in advance to help us understand the plan of care for him to be able to support him and his wife. We are short staffed and we need to take care of people who need emergent care and other patients like Carl and if we knew in advance what we could do to care for him or what the plan for admission to the ICU is, we could better plan resources and actions during this difficult time for Carl.*

FIGURE AG9.3    Ladder of Inference Worksheet.

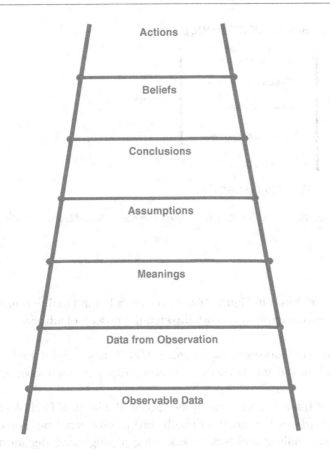

*Source:* Adapted from Scholtes, P., Joiner, B., & Streibel, B. *The TEAM® Handbook, Second Edition.* Madison, WI: Oriel, 2000.

Table AG9.1    Carl's Ladder of Inference

| Observable data | • The staff is kind and considerate except for one nurse who stands at a distance and whispers. |
|---|---|
| Selected data | • Nurse whispers "I don't understand why he comes here. We are short staffed and we need to take care of people who need emergent care . . ." Carl does not hear the end of statement. |
| Add meaning | • The nurse does not want to care for me because I am dying. |
| Assumptions | • The nurse is insensitive and uncaring. |
| Conclusions | • The insensitive and uncaring nurse doesn't want to care for dying people. |
| Beliefs | • All the ED nurses do not want to take care of me or dying patients. |
| Actions | • Carl becomes very sad, withdrawn, and tells his wife they shouldn't be in the ED. |

As noted we often can draw conclusions quickly in our own head based on data we observe. As a patient, family member, or health care professional, we should be mindful to build processes of reflection, advocacy, and inquiry into our daily work to promote deeper understanding and more effective communications.

## REFERENCE

1. Senge, P. *The fifth discipline. The art and practice of the learning organization.* New York: Doubleday/Currency, 1990.

# DESIGNING HEALTH SYSTEMS TO IMPROVE VALUE

Eugene C. Nelson

Tina C. Foster

Paul B. Batalden

Marjorie M. Godfrey

---

## LEARNING OBJECTIVES

- Define health care value and discuss value chains, value shops, and value networks.
- List four aspects of integrated high-value health systems.
- Describe accountable care organizations.
- Explore core knowledge health care leaders need to have to be effective in the twenty-first century.
- Identify ways to design and improve high-value health systems.

In this final chapter we begin with a brief discussion of the concepts of quality and value and note the clarion call for all health systems to discover ways to produce better health with greater efficiency. We then discuss complementary approaches that can be taken to improve value, promote value-based competition, relentlessly reduce all forms of waste, adopt alternative business models, start accountable care organizations, and call out domains of knowledge that health care leaders will need to produce better outcomes and lower costs. We next present the execution triangle for achieving strategic goals and discuss methods for leading change and creating change cultures. We conclude the chapter with a case study on organizational transformation in a health care system and with seven guiding principles to promote high-value health care.

## FROM PARTS TO WHOLE

In this book we have explored both challenges and opportunities in health care today. It is clear that tremendous amounts of time, energy, money, and creativity are being invested in health care and that quality and value must be dramatically improved. The data suggest the nation invests too much for health care and gets too little health for its return on investment.[1,2,3,4,5,6,7] In the first half of the book we focused on the concept of the *clinical microsystem* (the place at the sharp end where quality is made and costs are generated) and on how it serves as the basic building block of all health care systems (Chapter One). We then examined three prominent aspects of microsystems: how patients partner with providers to promote health and manage illness (Chapter Two), how safe and reliable care is delivered (Chapter Three), and how measuring and monitoring can be used to manage and improve health outcomes and system performance (Chapter Four). In the book's second half, we shifted our focus to concentrate on the experiences and needs of patients and families in varied states of illness and wellness. We explored how patients enter and are oriented to clinical microsystems (Chapter Five), how preventive care needs are addressed and health promoted (Chapter Six), how acute problems are addressed in time (Chapter Seven), how chronic conditions are managed over time (Chapter Eight), and how palliative care and services protect dignity and honor the decisions of patients and families (Chapter Nine).

But is simply understanding and improving the clinical microsystem enough? As the clinical improvement formula makes clear, scientific knowledge and an understanding of the context where that knowledge will be applied are necessary but not sufficient. The planning and execution of change that fosters ongoing improvement and innovation requires integration both within the microsystem and between microsystems and their contexts. In a sense, having dissected the clinical microsystem, we must now restore it to wholeness. At risk of oversimplifying, we might assert that quality is made by the local system at points in time, whereas value is created by the whole system over time.

To explain this idea a bit further, let us consider the Institute of Medicine (IOM) definition of quality that can be recalled using the acronym STEEEP. High-quality care

### Table 10.1  Overarching Care Needs of Patient and Family

| | |
|---|---|
| **Preventive care** | • Proactive assessment and mitigation of health risks |
| **Acute care** | • Timely attention to new or newly worsening disruption of health or function |
| **Chronic care** | • Longitudinal resiliency and support in self-management of ongoing disease |
| **Palliative care** | • Comfort and dignity in the context of underlying disease progression |

must be safe, timely, effective, efficient, equitable, and patient-centered. Although these six dimensions of quality can be realized within the clinical microsystem, to achieve high quality at the whole system level they must also be realized when handoffs occur between microsystems and within the supporting micro and mesosystems of care. The final product of the sequence of care and services can be evaluated in terms of value (that is, the goodness of health outcomes and the excellence of care experienced by patients and families in relation to costs incurred over time).

In this sense value is a rolled up or aggregate measure of outcomes in relationship to costs over the relevant time frame for a person or a population. A patient's journey through the microsystems of health care can be viewed as a *value chain*[8] with key outcomes (survival, health-related quality of life, perception of having been well-served by caring people, perception of health benefit achieved from interventions) as its output. Microsystems at their best make STEEEP quality (care that meets all six dimensions of quality) service-by-service, microsystem-by-microsystem, and patient-by-patient, but it is the cluster of microsystems that patients move through and interact with as their journey unfolds that ultimately creates value. In addition, the value chain or value network of microsystems creates an innovative, vibrant, and creative workplace for members of the microsystem. This is especially true when intentional actions enhance relationships between microsystems and move from distant or contentious relations to generative ones that focus on the patient and family.[9] This integration of microsystems with the mesosystems and the macrosystems that surround them is an essential challenge of leadership. Johan Thor, director of The Jönköping Academy for Improvement of Health and Welfare has said, "The most needed innovation in health care is on the leadership and management side. We need to find better ways to focus what we [leaders] do on a daily basis to meet the needs of the patient."[10]

In this final chapter, we present both conceptual frameworks and real-world examples of how to lead change to generate true health care value. In general, we use the term leader in its broadest sense. Most of us will not become CEOs, but, as the safety sciences and the Toyota Production System both make clear, all workers in health care can lead in large ways some of the time and in small ways most of the time. We can lead in matching what we do with what patients need, at making local improvements day in and day out, at supporting the caregivers who provide care in all the microsystems, and in using modern improvement science to help us do our daily work better. We focus the last chapter of the text, therefore, on *alignment* and *execution* for the purpose of achieving quality in the short run and maximizing value in the long run; we discuss how to reintegrate the microsystem into the mesosystem and macrosystem to attain peak performance and best value.

## NEW VISION OF INTEGRATED SYSTEMS TO PRODUCE HIGH VALUE

To meet the nation's requirement for good health status and good value health care, we must first have a new vision of integrated health systems that creatively and efficiently meet the needs of both individual patients and populations. Requirements for this new system are as follows:

- Must be responsive to the needs and desires of the informed and engaged person to help promote health, manage disease, and maximize function.

- Must strive, to paraphrase Dartmouth-Hitchcock's mission and vision, to provide each and every person the best care, in the right place, at the right time, every time . . . and thereby achieve the healthiest population possible.
- Must aspire, using IHI Triple Aim terms, to deliver (1) best health outcomes, (2) best patient experiences, and (3) lowest total costs to the patient and community.
- Must heal, using Kerr White's idea, the schism that has torn public health services away from personal health care delivery.[11]

This integrated, high-value health system will always have the patient and family at the center. It will be able to dynamically configure the essential microsystems around patients to provide just what is needed at just the right time every time. It will proactively reach out to meet the needs of the populations it serves. A diagram depicting the joining of the needed cluster of microsystems into an integrated mesosystem has been developed by Geisinger Health System and is shown in Figure 10.1.[12] The movement toward a new model of primary care medical homes is one manifestation of the mesosystem level of innovation, as is the movement to bundle payments to cover illness episodes rather than to provide siloed payments to discrete entities such as doctors, hospitals, nursing homes, and rehabilitation providers.

In addition to developing ways to align the various microsystems a patient encounters, there is a need for new *metasystems* that combine existing micro, meso, and macrosystems to address, on a population level, health and illness challenges at all stages of life. This is reflected in the development of accountable care organizations (ACOs) focused on developing integrated systems to provide high-value services to large populations. The metasystem will effectively manage the full continuum of patients' care, from preventive services to hospital-based and nursing-home care.[13] Just as the best microsystems will fail to provide optimal and innovative care if they are not able to work together, the meso and macrosystems will similarly fail to create real value if they are not able to see results and design care on a larger scale that looks at the needs of an entire population and its members.

If the new vision of an integrated health system requires both within and across system integration, then the logical next question is how the vision can be made real.

Pundits, health policy analysts, academicians, and politicians have all weighed in with answers. What follows is a brief description of some intelligent answers from thoughtful health care experts to the question, "What can be done to repair a broken health care system?"

## Create Value-Based Competition

Michael Porter, a world-renowned leader on modern business strategy, and his colleagues at the Harvard Business School have been leading a charge to reinvent health systems to focus on value creation. Porter has authored numerous articles and case studies and with Elizabeth Teisberg has published a seminal book *Redefining Health Care: Creating Value-Based Competition on Results*. The book summarizes their observations on the current health system and their thinking about future high-value systems.[8] According to Porter and Teisberg, value in health care is a function of health outcomes realized and health-related costs incurred over time for an individual. Value is not simply based on minimizing costs. It is based on maximizing outcomes and minimizing costs *over time* for people with discrete health needs. The health outcomes realized by individual people are not dichotomous (alive or dead) but multidimensional; in general, health outcomes

**FIGURE 10.1**  New Percutaneous Coronary Intervention.

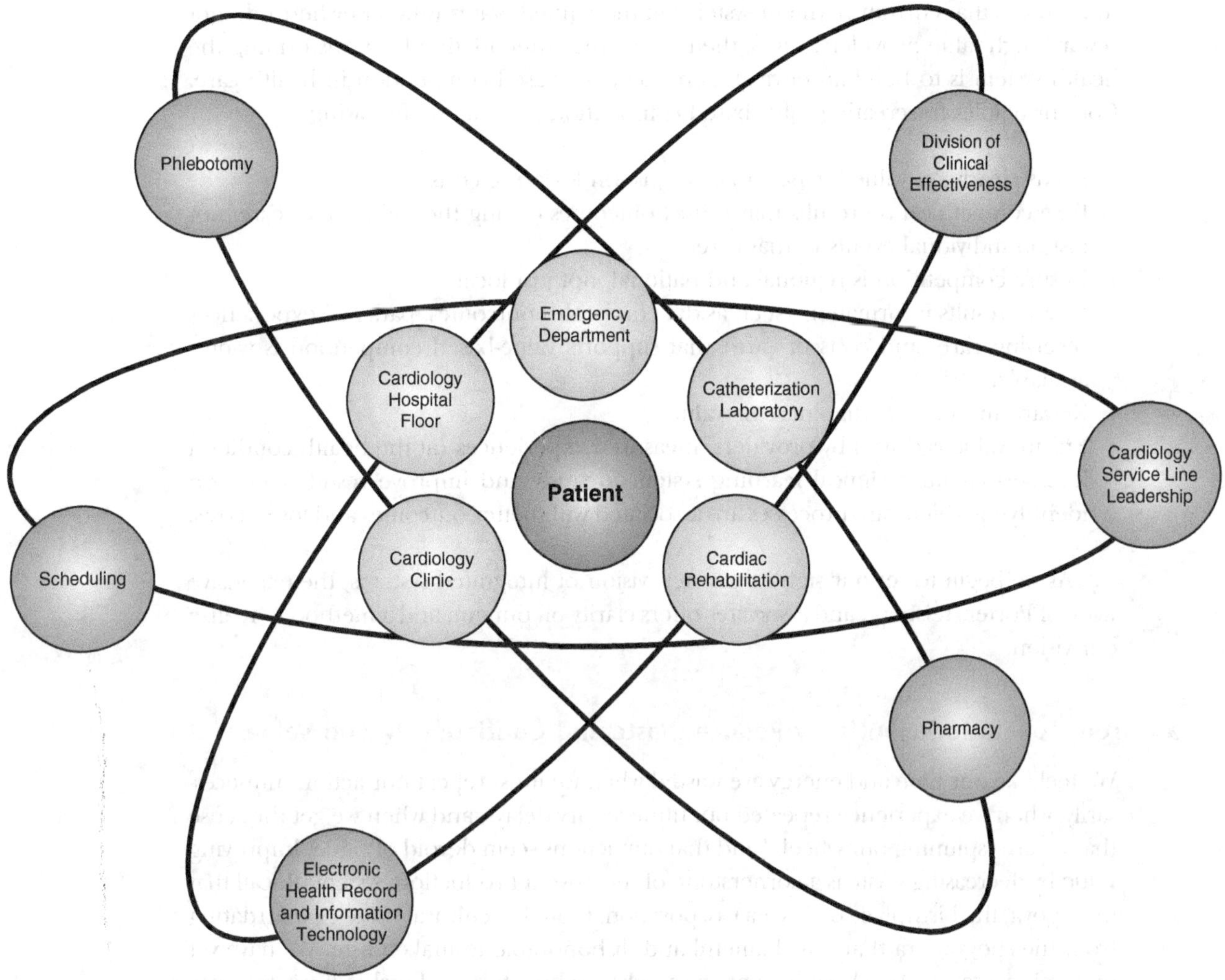

*Source:* McKinley et al. Clinical microsystem, part 4. Building innovative population-specific mesosystems. *Joint Commission Journal on Quality and Patient Safety,* 2008, *34*(11), 659.

*Note:* Professionals from many microsystems and supporting hospital services continuously revolve around the patient. Professionals from these various microsystems and services oscillate within a certain proximity of the patient during a given hospital stay. At times these are very close to or occur within the microsystem where the patient is receiving care, and at times the work done for the patient occurs without direct interaction with the patient. The sum of the interactions among the microsystems, hospital services, and professionals revolving around the patient is the newly formed mesosystem at Geisinger.

or health states fall into three major categories: (1) health risk status, (2) disease status, and (3) functional health status (physical, mental, and social domains). The dollars spent by individuals or payers are not limited to a single event, such as an operation, a hospital stay, or a clinic visit, but rather include the costs of a full set of services used during what Porter and Teisberg refer to as the full "care cycle" for a particular health problem or condition. Porter and Teisberg emphasize that value is created by frontline integrated practice units that provide care to individuals with discrete health needs (such as back problems, diabetes, breast cancer, or pregnancy) and that to measure value we must track key multidimensional outcomes of individuals and subpopulations with a given health condition during the care cycle while simultaneously tracking the dollars expended by or on behalf of those individuals. One of the contextual problems they note is that current payment systems in the United States (and elsewhere) do not reward high-value providers. Thus, their major recommendation for transforming the health system is to build an environment for value-based competition in health care. Core principles for creating value-based competition include the following:

- Focus clearly on value for patients, not just on lowering costs.
- Base competition on results that reflect outcomes during the full cycle of care, not just on individual events in that care.
- Ensure competition is regional and national, not just local.
- Ensure results information (such as data on health outcomes, patients' experiences receiving care, and costs of care) that supports value-based competition is widely available.
- Reward innovations that increase value.
- Ensure value is driven by providers' measured experiences (at the health condition level) to create a clinical learning system to study and improve results based on identifying which care processes are associated with better outcomes and lower costs.

As we begin to set our sights on a new vision of integrated systems, the expansive work of Porter, Teisberg, and associates offers clarity on our aim and a method to realize our vision.

## Learn from Toyota to Relentlessly Reduce Waste and Continuously Add Value

We feel like our time and energy are wasted when we must repeat our actions unnecessarily, when we experience repeated but unnecessary delays, and when we get the sense that we are "spinning our wheels" and that our actions seem devoid of value. Improving value by decreasing waste is a cornerstone of the Toyota Production System. Recall that in Nagoya, the birthplace of Toyota Corporation, there is a cultural value (*muda*) dating from the shogun era that it is shameful and dishonorable to make waste. We have yet to develop a sense of embarrassment about waste in health care. Taiichi Ohno, founder of the Toyota Production System, has given us seven recognizable manifestations of waste, which we can also recognize in health care:[14]

1. *Overproduction. Dartmouth Atlas of Health Care* is filled with information about the tremendous variation in volume of services, procedures, and tests across geographic areas, and the underuse or overuse of health care services. Return visits that are too soon or too frequent are another common form of this waste. We also see waste in administrative areas of health care where extra copies of documents are produced, or where both electronic and paper copies of documents are made.
2. *Time on hand (waiting).* Ambulatory care visits are legendary for the waiting involved. Patients arrive at the scheduled time and are asked to take a seat in the waiting area. No architectural design of a health care facility is complete without attention to the perceived need to wait. Another manifestation of our commitment to waiting is found in the delays in starting meetings because meeting attendees arrive later than the appointed time to begin.
3. *Transportation.* Deep in our mindset is the idea the patient should come to us. We have carried the same logic into the design of critical services such as imaging,

resulting in a situation where many hospitals have two populations: one stationary and the other in motion as they are being transported somewhere else. Lacking checklists, we often fail to complete all the actions needed at a given work or supply station, which means we then need to return to completely meet the need.

4. *Processing.* Asking patients for the same information repeatedly because the information is not readily accessible, inspecting repeatedly because the process design doesn't make it easy to do correctly the first time, and repeating lab tests to compensate for the lost results of prior tests all represent waste that is built into our work design assumptions.

5. *Stock on hand (inventory).* Rather than design the delivery systems to meet the usual demands, we often stock supplies (including medication) in the event we may one day need them. We print materials in excess of our needs and then resort to storing them in space we could use in other ways.

6. *Movement.* We design workflows that create extra motion and that necessitate trips for supplies and medications that would be unnecessary if we worked from an alternative set of design assumptions.

7. *Defective products.* We repeat imaging tests that were not properly positioned or exposed. We repeat tests when the transfer media do not allow us to use initially performed studies. We work to perform at normative rates of repeated procedures, rather than strive to reach the theoretical upper limits of performance.

Harder to see are the information gaps and behaviors based on habit rather than on scientific evidence. Often we continue to use work patterns we have become accustomed to, rather than redesign around better, scientifically supported alternatives.

## Christensen's Use of Different Business Models to Improve Health Care Value

Still harder to visualize is the waste embedded in business models we have grown to love, which have the effect of constraining our thinking and design. James Thompson identified three basic forms of work technologies: long-linked, intensive, and mediating. These technologies are involved in service and product production work.[15] More recently, Charles Stabel and Øystein Fjelstad have taken the same typology and described three distinct models for understanding, analyzing, and designing organization-level work.[16] Stabel and Fjelstad suggest it is important to explore the configuration of various attempts to create value and to carefully apply the logic of each model to the intended design of the work. The models Stabel and Fjelstad describe include (1) value chains, (2) value shops, and (3) value networks.

In a stimulating new book on the future of health care, Christensen, Grossman, and Hwang have applied the same thinking to health care reform.[17] They focus on disruptive forms of innovation that are sweeping into health care and that leverage these three business models to create disruptive innovations. *Value chains* are linked processes necessary to produce a service. They must (1) be linked in reliable ways to work well every time, (2) incorporate science and evidence directly into production processes, (3) be operated by professionals properly prepared to adhere to the processes (but not overly prepared and therefore more costly), and (4) produce the service in a timely way to meet the customer's needs. Assumptions about who does what and how are made explicit to test if a less costly, less failure-prone alternative is available. Information technology should facilitate doing what needs to be reliably done, uncovering exceptions that don't fit treatment algorithms, and assessing effectiveness so patients can benefit from this feed forward information loop. Examples of value chain models in health care include practitioner-staffed clinics in retail stores that offer limited treatments based on algorithms, and Shouldice Hospital in Toronto, Canada, that focuses exclusively on hernia repairs.

*Value (or solution) shops* are patterns of intensive application of customized knowledge to meet a particular need. Here the need must be understood to be named properly. Once named, the science needed to address it must be found, and a plan of appropriate action must be formulated. This custom work benefits from information technology that facilitates holding multiple options open while efficiently searching for relevant scientific sources. It is common for health care professionals to assume all of what is done must be designed to meet this test. Rene Amalberti refers to this error when he notes the challenge of creating equivalent actors, skilled professionals who can reliably perform with equal mastery under complex, dynamic conditions.[18]

*Value networks* are composed of linked beneficiaries who are enabled by technology to help each other. Creating and maintaining these networks has moved into a new era with the varying social linkage systems now available. The information technology to facilitate these networks must allow the linking to occur at the lowest cost (in time and resources) and facilitate protection of the members' purpose and intended social interactions. Collaborative networks in the improvement of health care (such as IHI Breakthrough Programs) or in the self-management of health needs (such as PatientsLikeMe[19] and eDiabetes[20]) are examples of this technology at work.

Christensen's analysis of the health care industry (and careful studies on other industries worldwide) suggest alternative value models might fit the work of health care better than a single model and that innovators will design new, disruptive approaches for meeting health needs with less waste and greater efficiency.

## Fisher's Work to Create Accountable Care Organizations that Provide High-Value Care

Elliott Fisher and colleagues have recognized the enormous opportunity for health system value improvement and innovation that Porter and Christensen have so clearly described. Their response has been to craft a pragmatic recommendation to create "accountable care organizations (ACOs)," that is, health systems designed to provide higher quality care and better patient outcomes at lower cost.[21,22,23] In 2009, Fisher summarized his ACO proposal as shown in the sidebar.

The hallmark of the ACO idea is that a local or regional network of physicians, hospitals, and other providers take responsibility for patients to receive services across the care continuum, across different care settings, and across time. The ACO knits together value-added care and services for patients and populations and, in return, is reimbursed for its work based on measured quality and cost performance. Shortell and Casalino have promulgated the following guidelines for starting new systems to provide accountable care:

- Patients would be encouraged but not required to be part of an ACO.

> We propose a new approach to help achieve more integrated and efficient care by fostering local organizational accountability for quality and costs through performance measurement and "shared savings" payment reform. The approach is practical and feasible: it is voluntary for providers, builds on current referral patterns, requires no change in benefits or lock-in for beneficiaries, and offers the possibility of sustained provider incomes even as total costs are constrained.[22]

- Physicians would not be required to be part of an ACO.
- Physicians, hospitals, and other health care organizations that are part of an ACO would be rewarded for improving quality and controlling costs, but would also be exposed to more potential risk.
- Tiered incentives could be created for patients to select the highest value-added ACOs based on available data.

The ACO model has been fashioned by health policy leaders to be both aspirational (has better outcomes, better patient experience, and lower costs) and pragmatic (is voluntary, feasible, mutable, and replicable). The ACO idea could accommodate Porter's ideas on how to redefine value in health care and retool the value chain through value-based competition. The ACO idea could also accommodate Christensen's prescription for disruptive innovation fueled by new business models to create a wholly new system for delivering high-value care.

## Learn What We Need to Know

Porter's, Christensen's and Fisher's proposals to transform a broken health care system explicitly focus on creating value in health care. Each proposal will require new ways of thinking about the processes, outcomes, and design of health care. Today's well-schooled leaders in improving the value of health care must be familiar with diverse bodies of foundational knowledge. We suggest the new core knowledge for leaders should include four areas: (1) lean design and production, (2) safety and reliability, (3) measurement of outcomes and performance, and (4) patient-centered design.

### Lean Theory, Principles, and Methods

The term *lean* was popularized in a paradigm-breaking book titled *The Machine That Changed the World.*[24] The book proffered a new theory for high performing organizations based in large measure on the International Motor Vehicle Program, a careful and massive comparative study of the automotive industry. The MIT-based research team found that Toyota and what many people now call the *Toyota Production System* (TPS) had proven itself superior to other competing systems for designing, manufacturing, and distributing products and services. The entire theory behind lean (and lean principles, methods, and techniques) evolved from this empirical and observational study of the automotive industry. This study showed Toyota's system for making cars, which was initially inspired by Deming and his teachings on ways to improve quality, efficiency, and productivity, was winning in the real world of the automotive industry.

The years following this book's publication have shown that TPS and lean theory principles and methods can be applied successfully to all sorts of manufacturing and services across the globe, including health care.[25] Lean thinking has come to embody today's best compendium of modern improvement knowledge as it has been applied in diverse enterprises. This body of improvement knowledge, or improvement science, is not static; it is being tested, adapted, and refined as different organizations and different people with diverse knowledge bases, skill sets, and training apply it in myriad real-world locations. Although the specific term *lean* may fade in popularity in the future, it is certain that the underlying science of improvement and innovation will continue to grow and develop as organizations of all types strive to enhance their performance.

### Safety Sciences and Human Factors Design

It has been found that high risk environments such as aircraft carrier flight decks, nuclear energy facilities, and oil rigs on the high seas can become relatively low risk environments if safety science and human factors are applied rigorously and consistently to change the way work processes are designed, executed, evaluated, and improved at all levels of the system. The movement toward safety sciences and human factors is being stimulated by a recognition of the massive amount of avoidable patient suffering that occurs while patients are receiving health care and by the low levels of reliability in providing only necessary care based on the best available medical evidence while not providing care that is unlikely to benefit that patient.[26,27]

### Performance Measurement Principles and Methods

It is difficult if not impossible to improve performance or to sustain improvements absent measurement.[28] Leading change, making change, and sustaining change all require measures that are sufficiently accurate, timely, and specific. Therefore, principles and methods for designing and implementing useful measurement systems and for displaying and communicating the results are vital underpinnings to the leader or to the health care professional who wishes to improve health care quality and value. Forces energizing the movement toward system-based and patient-centered measures include the consumer movement, the call for transparency in health care, and the reform of health care in the direction of value-based payments for care.[29] All of these forces tend to focus more attention on the patient as a beneficiary of health care and, consequently, to emphasize measuring and monitoring the patient's health outcomes, the patient's experiences in receiving health care, and the patient's health care costs in a way that makes sense to patients, families, and consumers of health care.

### Patient-Centered Design and Experience-Based Co-Design

Patient-centered design has been inculcated into mainstream health care relatively less than the three core knowledge domains of lean, safety, and measurement. It is apparent the surface has hardly been scratched. The practice of bringing the patient's and family's voices into health care by using valid patient perception surveys is becoming more widespread but is a relatively recent development.[30] Patients and family members are only rarely included in groups working on design or redesign of health care. Although organizations such as the Institute for Patient- and Family-Centered Care[31] provide excellent guidance through publications, education, and consultation, few health care organizations have integrated truly patient-centered design and improvement into their normal patterns for enhancing services. However, a deep and broad field of study about the design of goods and services has been applied outside health care and needs to be actively imported into health care. An excellent book by Bate points the way to the future; it is based on the design sciences. It features design and redesign of care based on the *experiences* of patients and families through powerful co-design principles that bring patients and families together with health professionals for the purpose of making services better.[32] The trends toward competition among providers to build loyalty and *brand recognition* and toward measuring patient perceptions as a key quality indicator are fueling the need for patient-centered design. Moreover, as stressed earlier in this text, the role of the patient should be considered as active and dynamic and includes the patient's ability to correctly self-manage illness and injury, when appropriate, and the individual's own efforts to promote personal health by adopting a healthful lifestyle.

Although we believe these four bodies of knowledge (lean, safety, measurement, and patient-centered design) could form the foundation of a new core curriculum for health care leaders who wish to improve the value of care, it is important to acknowledge the breadth and depth of this territory and to note that further exploration of the intellectual underpinnings of each core domain will be beneficial. There is much to learn from both academic disciplines (such as psychology, sociology, and economics) as well as from applied fields (such as medicine, nursing, epidemiology, biostatistics, management, engineering, and systems dynamics). What's most essential is a willingness to look across intellectual borders and to continue to explore and learn from the wide range of disciplines that explore the complexities of human work and systems.

## THE EXECUTION TRIANGLE

We have described several approaches to understanding *value* in health care and have noted some important areas of basic knowledge for those interested in creating high-value care. But knowledge alone is not enough. Fortified with a new vision of the health system, we now consider the essential problem of execution or making it so. Powerful approaches to organizational transformation include the following:

- Deming's method of organizing as a system for quality and productivity[28]
- The Baldrige process for achieving excellence[33]
- Collins's "From Good to Great" concepts and methods[34]
- Kotter's "Leading Change" and "Heart of Change"[35]
- Quinn's "Intelligent Enterprise"[36]
- Bossidy and Charan's execution framework[37]
- Toyota Production Systems[14]

These methods have been used in the real world with great success and share many common approaches. However, we have chosen here to focus on the IHI execution framework described by Nolan, which was developed specifically for transforming health care organizations.[38] Nolan's model is based on what successful businesses and health systems do to achieve extraordinary levels of performance. It recognizes the importance of effecting change at all levels of the delivery system and has been success-fully adopted by many health care organizations. Some of the common factors revealed by Nolan's research are as follows:

1. *Align goals:* set corporate-wide goals and goals in all business units.
2. *Invest and focus:* invest improvement resources in a limited number of goals.
3. *Replicate:* spread good ideas and methods around; require standardization.
4. *Provide oversight:* conduct formal reviews monthly or quarterly for guidance, adjustments, learning, and accountability.
5. *Be transparent:* make progress toward goals visible to all.
6. *Develop project portfolios:* deploy aligned projects throughout the organization.
7. *Assign full-time project leaders:* work with full-time project leaders. (Project leaders are common in industry but not in health care.)

Figure 10.2 illustrates the execution framework triangle. The apex of the triangle portrays the aim, which is to achieve strategic goals to advance mission and vision. The

FIGURE 10.2   A Framework for Execution.

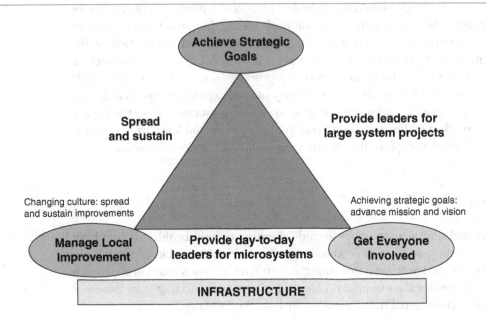

*Source:* Adapted from Nolan, T. IHI innovation series white paper. *Execution of strategic improvement initiatives to produce system-level results.* Cambridge, MA: Institute for Healthcare Improvement, 2007.

two lower corners represent key drivers: getting everyone in the organization engaged in execution and managing local improvement at the microsystem level, for example, increasing patient satisfaction, improving productivity, and increasing the use of evidence-based medicine.

The overarching theme for the right side of the triangle is leading strategic change to improve quality and value. As such, the right side of the triangle calls for senior leaders to establish an effective mechanism for setting strategic goals, deploying improvement projects aligned with strategic goals in all relevant parts of the organization, tracking progress over time, creating learning loops, and holding staff (at all levels of the system) accountable for achieving results. This is primarily top-down work that involves the following tasks:

1. Setting breakthrough performance goals and establishing a system of measures to gauge progress at different levels of the system
2. Developing a portfolio of projects to support breakthrough performance goals
3. Deploying resources to the projects that are appropriate to the aim
4. Establishing an oversight and learning system to increase the likelihood that intended results will be produced

The overarching theme for the entire left side of the execution triangle is changing culture. It focuses on real conditions at the front lines. Bottom-up improvement is anchored in local microsystem-level cultures and is crucial for making changes that are truly systemic and actually sustained. It calls for the following actions:

1. Recognizing clinical, supporting, and administrative work units as microsystems that have their own identities

2. Choosing improvement priorities that balance the needs of microsystems to generate bottom-up local improvements with the top-down strategic imperatives called for by the macrosystem

3. Promoting, testing, and implementing changes at the microsystem level

4. Getting everyone involved in improving and innovating at all levels of the organization

5. Fostering cooperation within and between microsystems by recognizing internal customer-supplier relationships and interdependencies that benefit patients while improving efficiency

6. Promoting the growth of all work units to become high performing microsystems that harmonize their work with peer microsystems up and down the value stream

Nolan describes at right the advantages of getting everyone's input and of developing improvement capacities.

The base of the execution triangle represents microsystems in the organization that do the real, hands-on, value-added work. These are the places where care is provided and where work is supported. Frontline units must find ways to improve and innovate on a day-to-day basis if they are to thrive in a changing environment. This is the place in organizations where leading change and changing culture actually meet. Leading, making changes, learning from this activity, and sustaining the changes form new patterns of thinking, acting, and believing that over time result in culture change. A case study from Cincinnati Children's Hospital Medical Center will be used to illustrate different facets of the execution framework later in this chapter.

> Organizations that have intentionally developed pervasive improvement capability in their microsystems have a strategic advantage when it comes to accelerating and sustaining system-level improvement. These organizations have an efficient and effective means of getting everyone involved to accomplish their strategic plan campaign.[38]

## LEADING CHANGE AT ALL LEVELS

As stated above, the right side of the execution triangle emphasizes leading change. To begin to master this, we must gain some knowledge about the process of leading change and being an effective leader. This subject is as important as it is vast, so our discussion will necessarily be brief and highly selective.

### The Process of Leading

The process of leading can be viewed as having three fundamental components:

1. Building knowledge
2. Taking action
3. Reviewing and reflecting

Each component flows into the next with the cycle repeating itself as a leader observes current conditions, takes action (based on prior experiences, observations, and interpretations), and then once again takes time to review and reflect on what existed, on what was done, and on what the effects were of the new actions that were taken.[39] Recall that sustained improvement in health care requires better patient and population health, better system performance, and better professional growth and development. Leaders must keep all three of these improvement domains in the foreground as they do their work, which means they must be skilled in working with both people and systems. We next explore the work of several prominent thinkers who clarify the knowledge and skills that people must have to lead successful change.

Warren Bennis,[40] whose work is cited previously in this book, suggests leading is a complex process. The effective leader takes into account the realities and demands of the current era, the complex network of individual factors, and then (within the context of organizational experience) blends the experiences and feelings people share with interpretations of these experiences and feelings so as to enable everyone in the organization to share a sense of organizational meaning that evolves over time. The competencies required to create a shared sense of organizational meaning are as follows:

- *Adaptive capacity:* hardiness, alertness, ability to learn quickly, creativity, and willingness to proactively seize opportunities as they arise
- *The ability to engage others:* creating shared meaning, encouraging dissent and dialogue, practicing empathy, engaging in ongoing effective communication
- *Voice:* purposeful, self-aware, self-confident
- *Integrity:* balancing ambition and ability with the help of a sound moral compass

Dee Hock, the founder of a new industry (personal omnibus credit cards) and a former leader of one of the major players in the credit card market (Visa), believes leaders must gain deep and extensive agreement among the organization's actors. He writes about organization members' having a fundamental need to agree on the basics of the challenge and the work at hand (see upper sidebar).

Parker Palmer, a teacher of teachers and a leader of leaders has many powerful and penetrating perceptions on leading effectively. The lower sidebar notes his provocative thinking.

Ronald Heifetz, a master teacher on modern leadership at Harvard's Kennedy School, tells his students that, as leaders, they must be able to be on both the dance floor and the balcony overlooking the dance floor.[43,44] When on the dance floor, the leader can feel the emotion, master the moves, and participate in the social interactions taking place there. From the balcony, the leader can see patterns, observe the larger context, get a sense of the whole, and learn from these panoramic views how to anticipate the future.

Karl Weick, a scholar and luminary on modern organizations, has concentrated much of his attention on complex social organizations, with a particular focus on high reliability organizations, especially those such as aviation, atomic energy, and health care that involve work with inherent danger.[45] He notes the importance of *coupling* (how activities and people are linked together). If we observe the relationships between workers on an assembly line or dancers in a chorus line, we can see that one person's actions are *tightly coupled* with the actions of the person who is next in line. On the other hand, the actions of musicians in an improvisational jazz band or members of a pal-

> Is it possible the most concise definition of organization is simply, agreement? . . . always dynamic, imperfect, and malleable . . . an ongoing process . . . not admitting of certainty or perpetuity, especially in particulars . . . revealing tolerance, trust, and mutual caring.[41]

> A leader is someone with the power to project either shadow or light onto some part of the world and onto the lives of the people who dwell there. A leader shapes the ethos in which others must live, an ethos as light-filled as heaven or as shadowy as hell. A *good* leader is intensely aware of the interplay of inner shadow and light, lest the act of leadership do more harm than good."[42]

liative care team are often *loosely coupled*. Although working for a common aim, the movements of one will not necessarily directly or predictably affect the movements of another. It is important to note, as these examples suggest, that tighter or looser coupling is not necessarily better. Rather, the nature of the underlying activity will suggest the appropriate balance of tight and loose coupling. Importantly, leaders may need to take different actions depending on whether the system is tightly or loosely coupled, as shown in Table 10.2.

**Table 10.2   Tight and Loose Coupling: Features, Characteristics of Features, and Actions for Improvement**

| Feature | Coupling Type | Characteristic of Feature | Leader Action to Promote Improvement |
|---|---|---|---|
| Autonomy | Loose | Parts are capable of semiautonomous action. | Logic, purpose, socialization |
|  | Tight | Parts are capable of contingent, dependent action. | Change parts |
| Leadership | Loose | System has many heads. | Influence, charter, data |
|  | Tight | System has one or few heads. | Change leader's mind or change leader |
| Groups | Loose | Individuals and subgroups form and leave coalitions. | Orientation, roles |
|  | Tight | Individuals and subgroups form and maintain stable coalitions. | Pick well |
| Coordination | Loose | Coordination and control are problematic. | Data, shared reviewed |
|  | Tight | Coordination and control are emblematic. | Accountability clear |
| Boundaries | Loose | System boundaries are often amorphous. | Purpose |
|  | Tight | System boundaries are pretty clear. | Next systems, different context |
| Assignments | Loose | Assignments of actors or actions to the organization or environment seems arbitrary. | Focus on effects |
|  | Tight | Assignments of actors or actions to the organization or environment fit a rationale. | Role-rationale connection |
| Focus | Loose | View shifts from structure to process. | Focus on the paths of interaction. |
|  | Tight | Focus is on perfecting the structure and using the process to understand interdependencies that contribute to overall results. | Structure or function |

# CHANGING LOCAL CULTURE

Whereas the right side of the triangle focuses on leading change *in* health systems, the left side of the execution triangle highlights the essential nature of changing the culture *of* health systems. Continuous improvement and breakthrough innovation will not take root and grow in most organizations absent a fundamental change in local frontline culture. Let us consider what the term culture means.

*Culture* can be represented by all the knowledge, beliefs, customs, and skills the individual learns by dint of being a member of a group (a society, a community, a family, an organization, or a work group). Culture is a term that is inclusive and enveloping; it is a complete design for living, working, playing, and adapting to changing circumstances for the purpose of maintaining the integrity, continuity, and survival of the group. Culture is both embodied in individuals and shared by group members. Culture has many facets that include languages, customs, traditions, norms, espoused values, philosophies, implicit rules, feelings, skills, mental models, shared meanings, stories, artifacts, tools, and physical layouts. A leading scholar of organizational culture, Schein, defines the culture of a group in the sidebar.

> A pattern of shared basic assumptions that the group learned as it solved its problems of external adaptation and internal integration that has worked well enough to be considered valid and therefore, to be taught to new members as the correct way to perceive, think, and feel in relation to those problems.[46]

Schein's definition of organizational culture highlights several important points to consider when thinking about culture change in health systems. First, culture develops and is passed on to new members because it has worked in the past and has proven to be valid in a given context. Second, culture is multilayered. It can influence individuals at the level of their naturally occurring work group (the microsystem) as well as in the collection of work groups that contribute to the care of certain types of patients (the mesosystem) and also at the macrosystem level. The most powerful culture is generally the microsystem because it is closest to the individual. Third, if one wishes to change culture, change will have to occur at the micro, meso, and macro levels of the organization, which will allow for new, correct ways to perceive, think, feel, work, act, and interact with patients, families, and colleagues. When one thinks about how fundamental and enormous this change is, one appreciates why it has been said that, under most conditions, "culture eats strategy for lunch everytime."[47] Cultural change is deep change. It is fundamental change that is easier to talk about and describe than to accomplish in the real world. Two approaches to cultural change are described next.

### Edgar Schein's View on Changing Organizational Culture

Schein, a leading scholar of cultural change in modern organizations, observes that all human groups (be they families, teams, or work groups) have one thing in common. They strive to "maintain their equilibrium and to maximize their autonomy vis-à-vis their environment."[46] This means that groups of people everywhere will try to keep doing what they have been doing in their own way despite what is happening in the world around them. This calls for dynamic action to maintain the status quo. People resist change to meet a basic need for a sense of stability, identity, and meaning.

There are times, however, when the environment compels a group to change to survive. In that case, change in culture, be it gradual and evolutionary or rapid and revolutionary, is a way for the group to attempt to preserve its "integrity and autonomy, differentiate itself from the environment and other groups, and provide itself an identity."[46] Schein describes three phases of cultural change: unfreezing, cognitive restructuring, and refreezing.

1. *Unfreezing:* takes place when something makes it impossible to maintain the old culture; this creates real motivation to change, as people perceive a threat and begin to see ways to avoid the threat that are consistent with the group's core values and ideals.
2. *Cognitive restructuring:* involves new ways of thinking and acting and of trying out and adopting new patterns of beliefs and behaviors. Although these patterns are different from the earlier repertoire, they still provide meaning and identity and increase the group's prospects for thriving in a changing environment. Trial and error and reflection and adaptation occur over time and, if deemed successful, new ways of thinking and acting replace old ways.
3. *Refreezing:* brings into play the aging of the new routines of thinking, perceiving, and acting. As time passes and as conditions improve, the new ways are no longer novel and uncomfortable but come to be seen as tried and true, until a new threat upsets the group's equilibrium and the cycle repeats itself.

When leading culture change in organizations, Schein advises leaders to avoid working directly on changing the culture or embarking on an announced cultural change campaign. He believes leaders who successfully catalyze cultural change do so by focusing people's attention on the forces that threaten the organization and its ideals, making change imperative, emphasizing what must be accomplished, and the types of behaviors and actions that will be required to thrive in the future. In this way, it becomes evident change will actually preserve the group's cherished values. The leader that has cultural savvy will recognize the stage of evolution of the organization's culture (founding and early growth, midlife and continued growth, or maturity and decline) and will use cultural change mechanisms that match the stage. For example, at a time of early growth, a focus on incremental and evolutionary change and promotion of hybrids within the organization makes sense, whereas an organization at midlife will respond better to planned change through projects and use of the organizational learning infrastructure. Mature organizations need unfreezing, which may involve bringing in outsiders or using turnarounds or truth telling to explode myths.

Leaders can choose to engage helpers to influence the cognitive restructuring. Helping roles can be present in many forms ranging from local leadership, facilitators, consultants, and coaches. Thor suggests "facilitators can help organizations manage change by assuming responsibility for demanding tasks related to improvement work . . . and transferring insights across the organization."[48] The helper role in health care can directly impact development of frontline staff and influence culture specifically during cognitive restructuring. Numerous companies and industries outside of health care routinely deploy facilitators and helpers throughout the workplace to support new ways of thinking, testing ideas, reflecting, and adapting. Health care organizations are increasingly using the helper role to move the mission, vision, and strategic plans into the workplace. Schein explores the dynamics of helping relationships and distinguishes the helping role "as consciously trying to help someone else to accomplish something."[47]

The Microsystem Academy at The Dartmouth Institute has been exploring, developing, and researching how coaching contributes to health care transformation. The Art and Science of Coaching Health Care Improvement is an educational program for people who aim to support health care improvement. Graduates of the program have formed a coaching network, and the impact of their work demonstrates increased leader ability to improve performance by working through the processes of unfreezing, cognitive restructuring, and refreezing (see www.clinicalmicrosystem.org for more information on coaching).

### Bate's Work on Organizing for Transformative Change in Health Care

Although Schein's works cover decades of study on cultural change attempts (both successes and failures) in all types of organizations, Bate and colleagues recently studied nine leading health systems in Europe and the United States that are striving to transform themselves.[32,49] Bate's work on transformational cultural change in health care is based on qualitative data (such as site visits, observations, and interviews) and publicly reported quantitative data on the performance of organizations on measures of quality and efficiency. His research question focused on gaining an understanding of the kinds "of processes that enable organizations to achieve"[49] sustained and measurable quality improvement. A hallmark of the research was that investigators studied each organization at the microsystem and the macrosystem level; researchers recognized successful cultural change is both broad and deep and that it would be necessary to understand the processes that provide the platform for successful transformation by studying the organization at both the frontline (microsystem) and front office (macrosystem) levels.

Although all nine organizations took different routes to reach the mountaintop (and therefore to sustain transformation to achieve ongoing quality improvement), they all had to put into place processes to meet six universal types of challenges: structural, political, cultural, educational, emotional, and physical and technological. Table 10.3

**Table 10.3   The Six Universal Challenges Facing Health Systems That Seek to Organize for Quality Health Care**

| Challenge | Description |
|---|---|
| Structural | Structuring, planning, and coordinating the quality and service improvement effort; embedding improvement within the organizational fabric |
| Political | Negotiating the politics of change associated with implanting and sustaining the improvement process, including securing stakeholder buy-in and engagement, dealing with conflict and opposition, building change relationships, and agreeing and committing to a common agenda for improvement |
| Cultural | Building shared understanding, commitment, and community around the improvement process |
| Educational | Embedding and nurturing a continuous learning process in relation to quality and service improvement issues, including both formal and informal mentoring, instruction, education and training, and the acquisition of relevant knowledge, skills, and expertise |
| Emotional | Energizing, mobilizing, and empowering staff and other stakeholders to want to join in the improvement effort by their own volition and sustain its momentum through individual and collective motivation, enthusiasm, and movement |
| Physical and technological | Design and use of a physical, informational, and technological infrastructure that improves service quality and experience of care |

*Source:* Adapted from Bate, P., Mendel, P., & Robert, G. *Organizing for quality: The improvement journeys of hospitals in Europe and the United States.* Abingdon, UK: Radcliffe Publishing, 2008, pp. 177–185.

provides a description of each challenge. Bate's work provides deep insight into the quality improvement journey undertaken by nine very different health systems and also offers practical guidance for assessing an organization with respect to its standing on each of the six challenges.[49]

The case study that follows reflects many of the ideas and themes that have been covered in this chapter. We will see how Cincinnati Children's Hospital Medical Center has been able to rapidly improve its performance by taking intelligent actions to "work" the execution triangle. It is undergoing organizational transformation by engaging employees at all levels of the organization to advance the health of children by applying modern improvement knowledge to advance its mission and vision.

## CASE STUDY: LEADING CHANGE IN CINCINNATI CHILDREN'S HOSPITAL MEDICAL CENTER

In 2000, Cincinnati Children's Hospital Medical Center (CCHMC) created a strategic plan to transform the organization in accord with its vision of being "the leader in improving child health."[50] In 2001, the Robert Wood Johnson Foundation funded an innovative program, Pursuing Perfection (P2), which was organized by the Institute for Healthcare Improvement (IHI), with the aim of identifying highly successful health care organizations willing to transform their patient care and management systems. CCHMC was selected as one of the thirteen P2 sites. CCHMC decided to pursue perfection rather than incremental improvement to emphasize the need for total transformation, to garner the attention of clinical leaders, and to align resources to support their vision. Physician leaders advised the CEO and chairman of the board that to gain physician commitment, the primary focus should be on key clinical outcomes, including patient satisfaction, rather than on financial efficiency.

The leadership realized the organization had limited experience with quality improvement (QI) methods. The mantra early on was "start before we're ready," as two initial strategic teams expanded their knowledge and paved the way for five more strategic teams by the end of the first year. During the next two years, additional strategic teams were added, with a goal of involving all aspects of the organization. In the start-up phase, commitment of the board of trustees to transformation was essential, and the following significant insights were learned quickly:

- *Business case for quality.* The chief financial officer engaged analysts to study the savings that could be achieved by strategic improvement teams' work in preventing nosocomial infections. Additional analyses demonstrated benefits from avoiding unnecessary hospital days as the organization experienced a significant increase in demand for tertiary and quaternary care. This analysis allowed leadership, including the board of trustees, to gain confidence that investment in quality was a good business strategy.
- *Need for transparency.* It was critical for executive leadership to support early QI efforts and to expect and accept failure as part of learning. When one of the first two strategic teams learned its clinical outcomes were average (compared to other sites), senior clinical leaders supported the frontline leaders in sharing these less-than-stellar outcomes with patients and families believing that transparency is a good thing and that being transparent would promote better results.
- *Need for improvement capability.* When the first two strategic teams began their work, only a very basic improvement infrastructure was in place and only a few leaders understood improvement science. In the next three years, twenty-four senior leaders

*(Continued)*

# CASE STUDY: LEADING CHANGE IN CINCINNATI CHILDREN'S HOSPITAL MEDICAL CENTER (Continued)

attended the Advanced Training Program sponsored by Intermountain Health Care. The CCHMC leaders realized a significant investment would be needed to build essential improvement infrastructure and that quality and data expertise from outside health care needed to be identified and recruited to support the strategic teams.

By year three (2004), it had become clear that transformation required more than strategic initiatives. It was at this point that CCHMC leaders learned about clinical microsystem thinking from the experience of the P2 team in Jönköping County, Sweden. This team was guided by a strategic plan to link strategy and improvement efforts at the micro, meso, and macrosystem levels, and had demonstrated improvements in access to care, patient-centered health care, and clinical outcomes. Guided by the conviction that high functioning microsystems are the fundamental building blocks of a transformed organization, CCHMC leaders focused on designing a strategy to support development of microsystem capability and then launched, with the assistance of Dartmouth faculty, a microsystem action-learning collaborative for six inpatient care units. During an 18-month period (December 2004–May 2006), physician and nurse co-leaders and interdisciplinary members of each microsystem-based team worked to improve specific outcomes using improvement science and teamwork skills and striving to adopt the characteristics of high performing microsystems.

Just as the microsystem leaders appreciated their roles in achieving strategic goals measured by real-time, unit-level data, strategic initiative leaders at the mesosystem and macrosystem levels began to understand the need for each clinical microsystem to be engaged in testing changes, sustaining results, and executing multiple strategic goals without overwhelming frontline staff.

Unit leaders identified the importance of building improvement expertise and developing the discipline to reach goals on schedule and negotiated a sequenced plan for achieving results. Microsystem leaders and frontline staff began to understand this was more than a series of initiatives or projects. It was instead a new way of providing care while continuously improving that care. It became common to hear frontline leaders say continuous improvement is a crucial part of their roles, and their conversations with senior leaders moved from yes or no discussions to conversations about how and when.

Strategic changes are in place at CCHMC and continue to be developed to support microsystems and their leaders through the following mechanisms:

- Ongoing improvement training in a twelve-day seminar and Intermediate Improvement Science Series (I2S2) conducted over a six-month period. The seminar includes didactic information and tools combined with between-session action and application. Over time, all micro, meso, and macrosystem leaders at CCHMC will take I2S2.
- Financial support for physicians who are serving as co-leaders of clinical microsystems.
- Increased emphasis on aligning academic pursuits with improvement work at the clinical front lines.
- Access to unit-level performance data through the organization's intranet.
- Sharing outcomes data with families, in part through outcomes data boards posted at the entrance of all units.

Annual strategic planning and prioritization is evolving. It is neither top-down nor bottom-up. Goals and plans are developed via a series of back-and-forth negotiations between micro, meso, and macrosystem leaders. This iterative process is improving each year and leads to meaningful improvement goals that are connected to the front line, where care and services are delivered, and also to the organization's strategic plan.

## Leading Change at All Levels at CCHMC

In the CCHMC example presented in this case study, we see linkages between leaders from the chair of the board of trustees all the way to the frontline microsystems, but forging this leadership chain did not happen overnight. Although the story of leading change at CCHMC has more than a single starting point, one important spark was provided by Dr. Uma Kotagal, a neonatologist who knew and understood modern improvement and worked directly with community board members on quality. Over time, the board chair, Jim Anderson, former CEO of a non-health care organization and a prominent civic leader, became the CEO of CCHMC. His vacated board seat was taken by another community leader who shared Uma Kotagal's and Jim Anderson's knowledge of and zeal for modern improvement. These three senior leaders formed a guiding coalition that came to include the chief operating officer, chief nursing officer, chief financial offer, and others. Working together, and supported by the IHI P2 Program, this lead team developed a set of whole system strategic success metrics, a coherent improvement strategy, high-priority improvement targets, and related strategic projects. They then began to identify critical mid-level leaders who could work directly with frontline clinical microsystems. One such individual was Dr. Steve Muething, a physician with a passion for quality. His first job was to deploy macrosystem strategic projects to frontline clinical microsystems in a way that would be attractive, engaging, and sustained (see Figure 10.3).

Dr. Meuthing worked with individual microsystem leaders and staff to educate them about modern improvement concepts and methods and how to apply them to their projects. Participants learned from their improvement work and were held accountable for generating desired results. Over time, existing leadership teams in frontline inpatient units became more capable at leading change. Building on this work, Dr. Michael Vossmeyer and the nursing unit director Karen Tucker created CCHMC's first high reliability unit, a model for innovation and improving outcomes, efficiency, and safety. The vision has now become a reality. A group of people led change from the Board of Trustees to the front lines of care to provide quality and value for the benefit of children and their families. In 2008 CCHMC won the prestigeous American Hospital Association's McKesson Award for being a national quality leader.

# THE PATH FORWARD FOR MAKING HIGH-VALUE HEALTH SYSTEMS

Problems facing the health system are formidable. Yet the broad outlines of a solution can be discerned. The key is to focus on value, not quality alone or cost alone, but outcomes in relationship to cost over time. In this book we have described how deep knowledge of a microsystem can be developed and used to inform the design and work of the microsystem, creating a context for ongoing improvement in which everyone participates.

## What We Need to Do

In this chapter we have made a case for ensuring microsystems are situated within functional meso and macrosystems and described how it is only with the reintegration of highly functioning microsystems into the whole that we can move from point-of-care quality to value realized over time. We have reviewed models for creating high-value care and discussed the foundational knowledge needed to make such systems real. We have explored important aspects of leading change in health care at all levels, from top-down to bottom-up (see Chapter Ten Action Guide to help guide top-down and

FIGURE 10.3 Aligning CCHMC Microsystem Improvement with Organizational Strategic Plan.

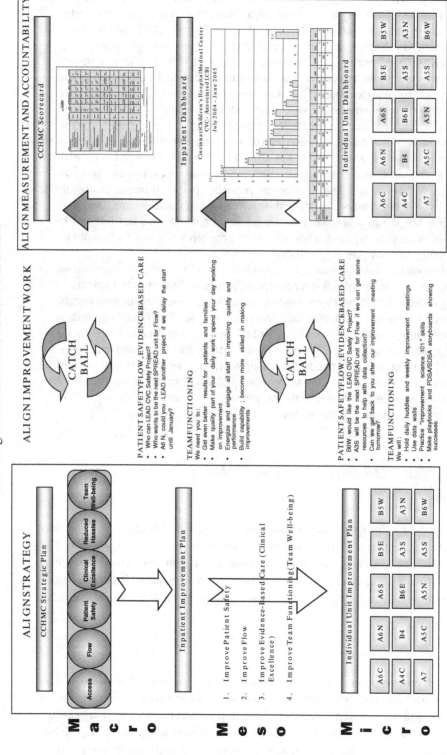

bottom-up infrastructure strategy). So where do we go from here? How do we move forward to build a system that can support this work? We propose several guiding principles.

1. *Design accountable high-performing health systems:* form high performing health systems that can deliver (and continuously innovate and improve) the value of preventive, acute, chronic, and palliative care across the life stages of populations served.
2. *Heal the schism:* align and unify public health and population health promotion with the delivery of personal health services to have a coordinated effect on the full set of health determinants.
3. *Promote personal health activation:* foster knowledge, attitudes, and practices (in individuals, families, schools, workplaces, and communities) to promote health, to prevent illness and injury, and to self-manage health problems in partnership with health professionals.
4. *Invest in infrastructure that promotes value:* direct capital toward health information and knowledge management systems and toward other infrastructures that can generate high-value, patient-centered, and population-based health services.
5. *Develop the most precious resource in the organization, the people:* intentionally develop programs and resources to support interdisciplinary health professionals' engagement with their heads, their hands, and their hearts in health care delivery and improvement. Activate the individual microsystems through the patients, families, and staff who spend their time working in them. Develop infrastructure for ongoing growth and development of each and every staff member. After all the discussion of technology, design, measurement, and technical aspects of health care improvement, it is the people who will make the difference.
6. *Make value measurements transparent:* track the health care processes (what is done) and outcomes (health outcomes and cost outcomes) of patients, subpopulations of people who share a common condition, and entire community populations. Use the measured results for payment, improvement, evaluation, and research.
7. *Change the payment system:* modify health care payments to reward high performing health systems who take responsibility for delivering and improving value and provide incentives for people who take actions to promote health, prevent illness, and intelligently self-manage illness and injury.

This book is focused on the clinical microsystem, the front line where patients and interdisciplinary health care professionals come together. We have only briefly explored the schism between population-based and individual-based approaches to care and have only touched upon how payment systems might drive change. But all these areas will be important as we look forward to a future that includes access to care for all and a meaningful focus on the creation of health. Although the problems are daunting and the potential for crisis is real, solutions are powerful and can be enacted by intelligent action by all players at all levels of the health system. To be successful, we need health professionals and health leaders at all levels of the system who have the knowledge required to take intelligent action from within the health system.

We remain committed to our belief that meaningful improvements of care will not happen without deep involvement of all those at the front lines (providers, staff, and patients and families). It is only by giving *everyone* the opportunity to create better patient outcomes, improve system performance, and continue to grow and develop professionally that we will transform our health care system and the care it provides.

## SUMMARY

- Data suggests the United States invests too much for health care and gets too little for its return on investment.
- Quality is made by the local system at points in time, whereas value is created by the whole system over time.
- Three business models for producing goods and services are the value chain, the value shop, and the value network.
- The accountable care organization approach has the potential to improve the value of care.
- Leading value improvement will require knowledge of modern improvement science, safety, measurement, and patient-centered design.
- The execution triangle for effecting change provides a cogent way for progressing strategic objectives and changing local culture mediated by building microsystem capability.
- The process of leading always involves building knowledge, taking action, and reflecting.
- Leading change and changing culture make essential contributions to transforming health care for the purpose of improving outcomes and value.
- Value improvement requires the intelligent engagement of everyone at all levels of the health system (that is, leaders, clinicians and staff, and patients and families).

## KEY TERMS

Accountable care organization

Alignment

Cognitive restructuring

Framework for execution

Lean

Loosely coupled

Metasystems

Muda

Overproduction

Processing

Refreezing

Six dimensions of quality

STEEEP

Stock on hand

Tightly coupled

Time on hand

Toyota Production System

Unfreezing

Value-based competition

Value chains

Value networks

Value shops

## REVIEW QUESTIONS

1. How is health care value defined?
2. What is a value chain? value shop? value network?
3. How would you begin to design an accountable care organization (ACO)?
4. What are the new core knowledge domains necessary for a leader in health care to be most effective and successful?

# DISCUSSION QUESTIONS

1. Consider Porter and Teisberg's core principles for creating value-based competition in health care. Describe examples of the principles.
2. Discuss waste reduction in health care. How might a microsystem take action to reduce waste?
3. Review the IHI execution framework to transform health care organizations. Select one or two of the execution framework factors and discuss how a leader might use these factors to execute a transformative plan.
4. Select one of the prominent thinkers on leading change and apply his or her thinking and recommendations to the organization you are working with.
5. Discuss how one might change local culture.
6. Identify the elements of creating high-value health systems and define the guiding principles that can help an organization achieve a higher performance.

# REFERENCES

1. Wennberg, J. E., Fisher, E. S., Goodman, D. C., et. al. *Tracking the care of patients with severe chronic illness: The Dartmouth Atlas of Health Care 2008.* Lebanon, NH: The Dartmouth Institute for Health Policy and Clinical Practice, 2008.
2. Chassin, M., & Gelvin, R. W. The urgent need to improve health care quality. Institute of Medicine National Roundtable on Health Care Quality. *Journal of the American Medical Association*, 1998, *280*(11), 1000–1005.
3. Agency for Healthcare Research and Quality (AHRQ). *National healthcare quality report.* Retrieved February 15, 2010, from www.ahrq.gov/qual/qrdr07.htm#nhqr
4. Institute of Medicine. *Unequal treatment: Confronting racial and ethnic disparities in health care.* Washington, DC: National Academies Press, 2002.
5. The Commonwealth Fund Commission on a High Performance Health System. *Why not the best? Results from the national scorecard on U.S. health system performance, 2008.* New York: The Commonwealth Fund.
6. Centers for Disease Control. *National Center for Chronic Disease Prevention and Health Promotion.* Retrieved February 23, 2010, from www.cdc.gov/chronicdisease/index.htm
7. Cunningham, P. *Trade-offs getting tougher: Problems paying medical bills increase for U.S. Families, 2003–2007.* Retrieved January 15, 2010, from www.hschange.com/content .1017/#ib5
8. Porter, M., & Teisberg, E. O. *Redefining health care: Creating value-based competition on results.* Boston: Harvard Business School Press, 2006.
9. Zimmerman, B., Lindberg, C., & Plsek, P. *Edgeware: Insights from complexity science for health care leaders.* Irving, TX: VHA, 1998.
10. Producer, Anders Lennberg and Max Rangner, and Director, Helena Hvitfeldt. Medical Management Center, Karolinska Institute. *Medical moves.* [video]. Unit for Bioentrepreneurship, Stockholm, Sweden, 2009.
11. White, K. *Healing the schism: Epidemiology, medicine, and the public's health.* New York: Springer-Verlag, 1991.
12. McKinley et al. Clinical microsystem, part 4. Building innovative population-specific mesosystems. *Joint Commission Journal on Quality and Patient Safety*, 2008, *34*(11).
13. Reforming provider payment: Moving toward accountability for quality and value. Issue brief. *Accountable care organizations.* Washington, DC: Englebert Center for Health Care Reform at Brookings and The Dartmouth Institute for Health Policy and Clinical

Practice, March 2009. Retrieved July 25, 2010, from www.brookings.edu/events/2009/0311_aco.aspx

14. Ohno, T. *Toyota production system: Beyond large production.* Tokyo: Diamond, 1988.

15. Thompson, J. *Organizations in action: Social sciences bases of administrative theory.* New Brunswick, NJ: Transaction Publishers, 1967.

16. Stabell, C., & Fjeldstad, Ø. D. Configuring value for competitive advantage: On chains, shops, and networks. *Strategic Management Journal*, 1998, *19*, 413–437.

17. Christensen, C., Grossman, J. H., & Hwang, J. *The innovator's prescription: A disruptive solution for health care.* New York: McGraw-Hill Books, 2009.

18. Amalberti, R., Auroy, Y., Berwick, D., & Barach, P. Five system barriers to achieving ultrasafe health care. *Annals of Internal Medicine*, 2005, *142*(9), 756–764.

19. PatientsLikeMe. *Find patients just like you.* Retrieved February 24, 2010, from www.patientslikeme.com

20. Wikipedia. *Ediabetes.* Retrieved February 24, 2010, from http://en.androidwiki.com/wiki/EDiabetes

21. Fisher, E., Staiger, D. O., Bynum, J. P., & Gottlieb, D. J. Creating accountable care organizations. *Health Affairs*, 2006, *26*(1), w44–w45.

22. Fisher et al. *Fostering accountable health care: Moving forward in Medicare.* Retrieved July 25, 2010, from http://content.healthaffairs.org/cgi/content/abstract/hlthaff.28.2.w219v1

23. Shortell, S., & Casalino, L. P. Health care reform requires accountable care systems. *Journal of the American Medical Association*, 2008, *300*(1), 95–97.

24. Womack, J., Jones, D., & Roos, D. *The machine that changed the world: The story of lean production.* New York: Harper Perennial, 1991.

25. Womack, J., & Jones, D. *Lean thinking: Banish waste and create wealth in your corporation.* New York: Simon and Schuster, 1996.

26. Leape, L., & Berwick, D. M. Five years after to err is human. What have we learned? *Journal of the American Medical Association*, 2005, *293*, 2384–2390.

27. Orszag, P., & Ellis, P. The challenge of rising health care costs—a view from the Congressional Budget Office. *New England Journal of Medicine*, 2007, *357*(18), 1793–1795.

28. Deming, W. E. *Out of crisis.* Cambridge: Massachusetts Institute of Technology, Center for Advanced Engineering Study, 1989.

29. Institute of Medicine. *Performance measurement: Accelerating improvement.* Washington, DC: National Academies Press, 2006.

30. Sitzia, J., & Wood, N. Patient satisfaction: A review of issues and concepts. *Social Science & Medicine*, 1997, *45*(12), 1829–1843.

31. Institute for Family-Centered Care. Retrieved February 24, 2010, from http://www.familycenteredcare.org

32. Bate, P., & Robert, G. *Bringing user experience to healthcare improvement: The concepts, methods and practices of experience-based design.* Oxon, UK: Radcliffe Publishing, 2007.

33. Baldrige Program. *Criteria for performance excellence.* Retrieved July 25, 2010, from www.nist.gov/baldrige/publications/criteria.cfm

34. Collins, J. *Good to great. Why some companies make the leap and others don't.* New York: Harper Business, 2001.

35. Kotter, J., Dan, S., & Cohen, D. S. *The heart of change: Real-life stories of how people change their organizations.* Boston: Harvard Business School Press, 2002.

36. Quinn, J. B. *Intelligent enterprise: A knowledge and service based paradigm for enterprise.* New York: Free Press, 1992.

37. Bossidy, L., & Charan, R. *Execution: The discipline of getting things done.* New York: Crown Business, 2002.

38. Nolan, T. IHI innovation series white paper. *Execution of strategic improvement initiatives to produce system-level results.* Cambridge, MA: Institute for Healthcare Improvement, 2007.

39. Nelson, E., Batalden, P., & Godfrey, M. *Quality by design.* San Francisco: Jossey-Bass, 2007.
40. Bennis, W. *On becoming a leader.* Cambridge, MA: Perseus Books, 2003.
41. Hock, D. *One from many.* San Francisco: Berrett-Koehler, 2005.
42. Palmer, P. *Let your life speak.* San Francisco: Jossey-Bass, 2000.
43. Heifetz, R. *Leadership without easy answers.* Cambridge, MA: Harvard College, 1994.
44. Parks, S. *Leadership can be taught: A bold approach for a complex world.* Boston: Harvard Business School Press, 2005.
45. Weick, K. Management of organizational change among loosely coupled elements. *Making sense of the organization.* (chapter 17) Oxford: Blackwell, 2001.
46. Schein, E. *Organizational culture and leadership.* (2nd ed.) San Francisco: Jossey-Bass, 1992.
47. Schein, E. *Helping: How to offer, give and receive help.* San Francisco: Berrett-Koehler, 2009.
48. Thor, J. et al. Learning helpers: How they facilitated improvement and improved facilitation—lessons from a hospital-wide quality improvement initiative. *Quality Management in Health Care,* 2004, *1*(13), 60–74.
49. Bate, P., Mendel, P., & Robert, G. *Organizing for quality: The improvement journeys of hospitals in Europe and the United States.* Abingdon, UK: Radcliffe Publishing, 2008.
50. Godfrey, M. M., Melin, C. N., Muething, S. E., Batalden, P. B., et al. Clinical microsystems, Part 3. Transformation of two hospitals using microsystem, mesosystem and macrosystem strategies. *Joint Commission Journal on Quality and Patient Safety,* 2008, *34*(10).

Chapter Ten Action Guide provides a helpful tool to guide organizations in transformation activities and planning: the M3 matrix, or the micro, meso, and macrosystem framework.

## MICRO-, MESO-, AND MACROSYSTEM MATRIX

The micro-, meso-, and macrosystem (M3) matrix identifies specific actions leaders can take at the three main levels of the health system to foster whole system transformation. Macrosystem actions are taken by the senior leaders, for example, the chief executive officer (CEO), chief nursing officer (CNO), chief informatics officer (CIO), and chief operating officer (COO), who are responsible for enterprise-wide performance. Mesosystem actions are taken by the midlevel leaders who are responsible for large clinical programs, service lines, and clinical and administrative services, for example, the vice president of inpatient surgical services, vice president of perioperative services, and vice president of ambulatory services. Microsystem actions are taken by leaders of frontline clinical systems who engage in direct patient care, provide ancillary services that interact with patient care, or provide administrative services that support patient care, for example, the director of Post Anesthesia Care Unit, director of Neuroscience Unit, director of Intensive Care Unit, and director of Dermatology and Allergy Clinic.

The M3 Matrix displays actions to lead organizational transformation not only according to the three system levels but also according to time frame, suggesting actions to consider taking immediately (within months one to six), in the short term (during months seven to twelve), and in the next phase (during months thirteen to eighteen).

Leaders of health care systems can use the M3 Matrix for developing a specific action plan to begin the journey toward organizational transformation. The timeline reinforces the fact that deep cultural change usually takes years.

Organizations cannot transform themselves without positive engagement of the workforce. Improvement is everyone's responsibility and needs to be communicated and expected by all leaders at all levels of the organization. The leaders of health care systems can adapt the M3 Matrix to develop an intentional and specific eighteen- to twenty-four-month action plan that affects all levels of the organization.

Beginning with transformational activities at the clinical microsystem level, the development continues to the meso and macrosystem levels, bringing the smaller systems together and promoting in whole organization transformation.

## FIGURE AG10.1   Micro-Meso-Macro Framework: M3 Matrix.

**Microsystems Developmental and Organization Transformation Journey: The Stages**
**Microsystems Developmental and Organization Transformation Journey: The Stages**

1. Create awareness of flow of work and the clinical unit as an interdependent group of people with capacity to make change.
2. Test some changes to address some of the "embarrassing stuff."
3. See ourselves as a system of care.
4. Respond to strategic challenges and invitations.
5. Measure performance.
6. Learn to integrate multiple improvement cycles while taking care of patients.
7. Unending curiosity about and pursuit of "best known" world class processes and outcomes.

| Microsystem Level<br>"Inside Out" | Mesosytem Level<br>"Creating the Conditions" | Macrosystem Level<br>"Outside In" |
|---|---|---|
| **0-6 Months** *Pre-work: Visit www.clinicalmicrosystem.org Rea<br>Part 1, 8, and 9 of series/watch Batalden streaming video | | |
| • Form Interdisciplinary Lead Team including patients/families | • Link strategy, operations, and people: "Make it Happen" | • Develop clear vision for meso/microsystems |
| • Dartmouth Microsystem Improvement Curriculum | • Support and facilitate meso/micro system protected time to reflect and learn | • Set goals for improvement |
| • Learning to work together using effective meeting skills | • Identify resources to support meso/microsystem development including information technology and performance measure resources | • Make clear distinctions between what the system will do and what it will not do. |
| • Rehearsing within studio course format | | • Design meso/microsystem manager and leadership professional development strategy |
| • Practicing in clinical practice | | • Engage board of trustees with improvement strategies |
| • Daily huddles, weekly Lead Team meetings, monthly all-staff meetings | • Develop measures of microsystem performance | • Expect all senior leaders to be familiar and involved with meso/microsystem improvement |
| • Learning sessions (monthly) | • Address roadblocks and barriers to micro/mesosystem improvement and progress | • Expect all staff to engage in learning and improvement |
| • Conference calls (between sessions) | • Set goals/expectations | • Provide regular feedback and encouragement to meso/microsystem level staff |
| | • Link improvement with "evidence" | • Articulate the contributions of the clinical microsystems and how they advance the organization's worthy aim and enhance the well-being of the whole enterprise |
| | • Advocate for the microsystem and the macrosystem | • Create an appreciation for the regulatory environment of health care and the reimbursement mechanisms and how these external forces influence all levels of the health care system: micro, meso, and macro |
| **6-12 Months** | | |
| • Staff reinforcement by leadership | • Convene meso/microsystems to work on linkages and handoffs | • Expect improvement science & measured results from meso/microsystems |
| • Colleague reinforcement | • Focus on the patient journey within and between microsystems | • Develop whole system measures & targets/goals |
| • New habit development through repetition | • Focus on the "flow" of care, information, and patient and staff needs | • Attract cooperation across health professional discrepancy traditions |
| • Improvement science in action | • Facilitate system coordination | • Design Review and Accountability quarterly meetings for Senior Leaders |
| • Add more improvement cycles | • Link with electronic medical records | • Track and tell stories about improvement results and lessons learned at meso/microsystem levels |
| • Build measurement into practice | • Link business initiatives/strategic plan to microsystem level | • Develop budgets to support and develop strategic improvement |
| • Measures/dashboards/data walls | • Attract cooperation across health professional discrepancy traditions | • Ensure resources to support meso/micro system (e.g., IT) |
| • Playbooks and storyboards | | • Plan time in schedule (develop the habit) to round at meso/microsystem levels to observe where learning, improvement, and change must happen |
| • Relationships between microsystems (linkages) | • Track and tell stories about improvement results and lessons learned at meso/microsystem levels | |
| • PDSA-SDSA Improvement | • Include improvement as regular agenda item | |
| • Best practice using Value Stream Mapping/LEAN design principles | | |
| **12-18 Months** | | |
| • Continue "new way of providing care, continuously improving and working together" | • Link performance management to daily work and results | • Develop professional development strategies across all professionals |
| • Actively engage more staff involvement | • Support and coach microsystem leadership development | • Design HR selection and orientation process linked to identified needs of macro/microsystems |
| • Multiple improvements occurring | • Provide resources to support microsystem development | • Link performance management to daily work and results |
| • Network with other microsystems to support efforts | • Provide feedback and encouragement to microsystem | • Align recognition, incentives, and rewards for individuals and groups to foster accountability for improving and maintaining quality, efficiency, and flexibility |
| • Coach network and development | • Encourage and support search of "best practice" | • Create system to link measurement and accountability at micro/meso/macro levels |
| • Leadership development | | • Develop "Quality College" for ongoing support and capability building throughout organization |
| • Annual review, reflect, and plan retreats | | |
| • Quarterly system review and accountability meetings to meso-macro leadership | | |

Leaders at all levels of the organization can create the conditions for improvement to flourish and for excellence to emerge. The M3 Matrix offers ideas of what leaders might do to engage all staff and bring forth energy and creativity to result in a culture of high-quality, high-value care and services.

The macrosystem level senior leaders need to clearly set expectations with a compelling vision, mission, and measured goals. The M3 Matrix refers to the macrosystem as "outside in," which represents senior leadership providing the guiding vision and expectations.

The mesosystem leaders "create the conditions." Notice in the first six months, the mesosystem leaders focus on linking strategy, operations, and people to "make it happen." "It" is the vision and measured goals determined by the senior leaders. The leaders actively support members of the micro- and mesosystems to meet regularly to reflect and learn about current performance and improvement. Mesosystem leaders collaborate with the microsystems to find ways to create the protected time and space for learning. Additionally in the first six months, the mesosystem leaders identify resources within the organization to support frontline staff development. Organizational resources from information technology, performance measures, and organizational development are important to identify and articulate the important support they can offer to the microsystem improvement activities. Mesosystem leaders actively address roadblocks and barriers to create the conditions for microsystems success. Creating the conditions also includes reminding microsystem members of the expectations and goals of improvement over time and expecting improvement to be linked with evidence and best practices.

The macrosystem leaders support and encourage staff development from the "inside out." The mesosystem leaders set expectations from the organization perspective that is the "outside in" while the microsystems take actions from the "inside out." In the first six months, the microsystem can form a lead improvement group including patients and families to begin to assess, diagnose, and treat their clinical microsystem. The Dartmouth Microsystem Improvement Curriculum provides a tested path to guide the members of the microsystem through reflection and improvement sessions and cycles. The clinical microsystem interdisciplinary lead team meets weekly to develop skills and new habits to be able to provide exceptional care and continuously improve the care and services. Daily huddles provide time to advance the developmental journey of the microsystem and keep conversation and actions alive in the daily work of providing care and services to patients and families.

The levels of the organization begin to transform as all staff acquire knowledge, skills, and abilities to provide care and services and improve. The developing workforce identifies new needs and resources over time as represented in the different time periods in the M3 Matrix.

The micro-, meso-, and macrosystem leaders and staff work simultaneously to move closer to the vision and goals to become a high-performing transformed organization. The transformed organization consists of many small interconnected systems with engaged interdisciplinary staff who understand their work is to provide care and services and to find ways to improve every day. The timeline and activities listed on the M3 Matrix can help provide a potential path of action for all levels of the organizations.

human factors design, high-value health systems,
312–313

## I

I PASS the BATON, 172, 175
iatrogenic hazards, mitigating risk of, 208
ICN (Intensive Care Nursery), at Dartmouth
  background, 89
  case study, 88, 90
  discussion, 92–93
  implementing patient safety, 89–90
  near misses, errors, and adverse events, 89
  prevention of nosocomial infections, 91–92
if-then formulations of algorithm-based care, 227
IHC (Intermountain Health Care), 137, 141
improvement, measuring within levels of health system,
132–133
improvement equation, 22–23
Improvement Triangle, 140–141
Improving Patient Access to Care workbook, VHA, 191
*in situ* simulation, learning from errors, 104
indirect assessment, of downstream outcomes, 177
infants, preventive care activities, 199
informants, patients as, 65–66
information
  in chronic care model, 259–260
  diagnostic errors from failure to synthesize, 100
  for full health status assessment in palliative care, 286
  patient safety and, 130
  scoring with MAT, 41–44
  sharing in patient-centered care, 51
information environment
  fostering rich, 138–139
  measuring what matters, 132–133
  in top performing microsystems, 14
information flow for high-value care
  balanced scorecards, 143–145
  balanced scorecards vs. compass, 145–146
  cascades metrics for, 148–149
  dashboard metaphor, 146–147
  designing, 140
  feed forward and feedback, 140–141
  Measure What Matters worksheet, 149–150
  Patient Value Compass, 141–143
  summary review, 150–152
information prescriptions, 63–65
information technology
  guidelines for scoring with MAT, 41–44
  patient safety, 130
informed decision making, 58, 63
initial assessment, in plan of care, 178–180
Inpatient Unit Profile, Greenbook, 34
inpatients, evaluating access to care, 167–168
inquiry
  how mental models shape, 297
  using Ladder of Inference to explore, 297–301
Institute for Clinical Systems Improvement, 227
Institute for Healthcare Improvement, 148
Institute for Patient and Family-Centered Care, 51, 82–83
institutionalized adults, preventive care activities, 199
integrated systems, high-value, 306–307
integrity
  leadership, 316
  restoring in palliative care, 282
*Intelligent Enterprise* (Quinn), 2
Intensive Care Nursery. See ICN (Intensive Care
  Nursery), at Dartmouth
interdependence
  guidelines for scoring with MAT, 43–44
  patient safety, 129

interdisciplinary
  effective care plans as, 181
  preventive care as, 211
  quality improvement team, 291
Intermountain Health Care (IHC), 137, 141
Intermountain Health Care, Utah, 16
International Motor Vehicle Program, 311
interventions, practices for patient safety, 90
interviews, for patient knowledge, 65–66
inventory (stock on hand), decreasing waste, 309
IOM (Institute of Medicine)
  chain of effect, 7–9
  definition of quality, 304–305
  on fundamental aim of health care, 48
  patient safety goal, 88
  Ten New Rules for health care, 49–51

## J

Josie King story, 106
just culture school of thought, patient safety, 99

## K

Kano model of satisfaction, 53–54
knowledge, creating value, 311–313

## L

laboratory, as supporting microsystem 5P, 38
Ladder of Inference, 297–301
latent conditions, causing medical errors, 97
latent failures, HRO sensitivity to, 123–124
leadership
  executing organizational change, 314, 323–324
  as most needed innovation in health care, 305
  patient safety within microsystems, 105, 124–126, 129
  process of, 315–317
  scoring with MAT, 41–44
  in top performing microsystems, 13
  transitions and handoff processes, 172
  using M3 Matrix for transformation activities,
332–333
lean theory, 311
levels of organizations, 6–7
life expectancy
  burden of chronic illness, 246
  and palliative care, 278–279
line-of-sight measures, cascading metrics, 148
little dot microsystem levels, 148
live actors, rehearsal through, 120
local culture
  case study, 321–323
  changing, 318–321
  executing organizational change, 314
loopholes, HRO sensitivity, 123–124
loose coupling, 316–317
lost productivity, in chronic disease, 247

## M

M3 (micro-, meso-, and macrosystem) Matrix, 331–333
macrosystem
  cascading metrics for, 148–149
  chain of effect and, 9
  chronic care model and, 257–258
  horizontal/vertical care levels, 9–11
  M3 Matrix for transformation activities, 331–333
  nesting of clinical relationships in, 7
  research on microsystem in, 15–16
  role of mesosystem in, 19–20
mammography, preventive activity of, 217–218
management, of institutional imperatives, 132–133
many-to-one relationship, health care today, 2